S0-CQT-538

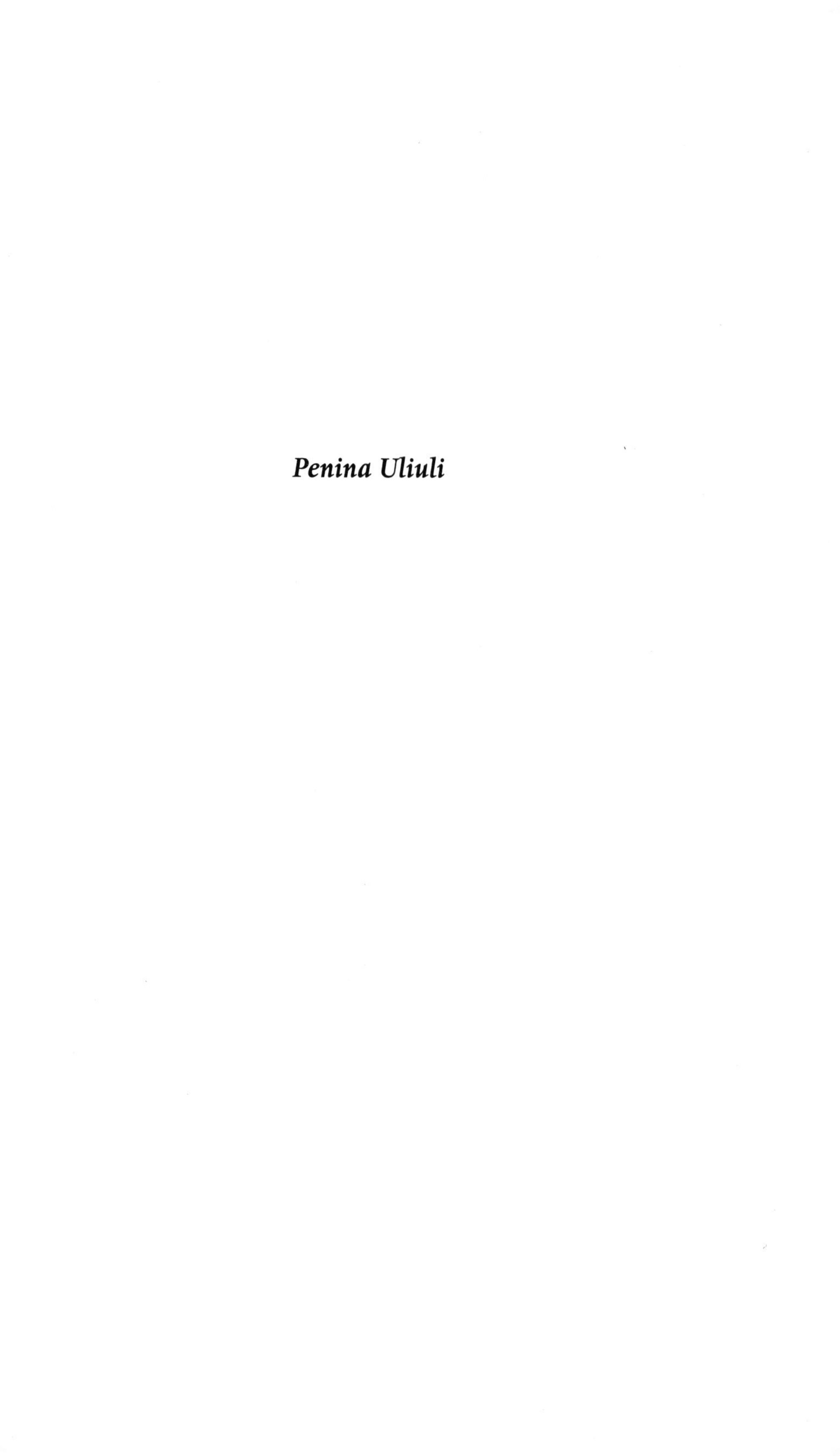

Penina Uliuli

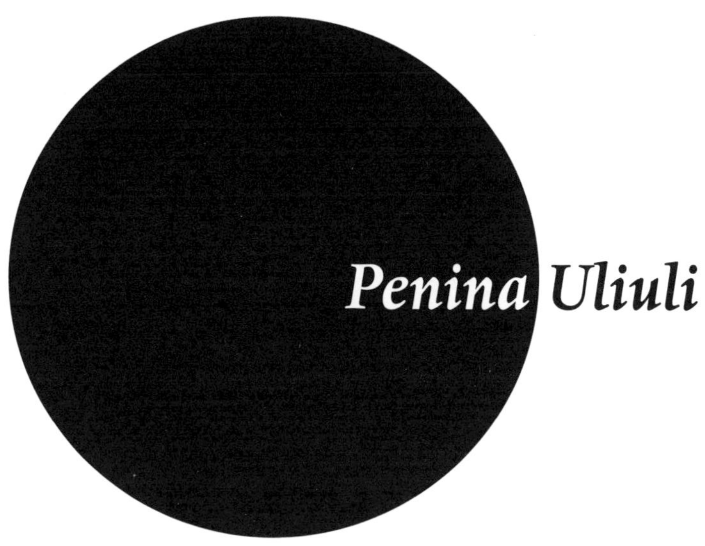

Penina Uliuli

Contemporary Challenges in Mental Health for Pacific Peoples

PHILIP CULBERTSON *and*
MARGARET NELSON AGEE, *Editors*
with CABRINI ʻOFA MAKASIALE

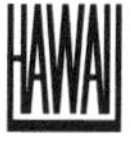

University of Hawaiʻi Press
Honolulu

Printed in the United States of America
12 11 10 09 08 07 6 5 4 3 2 1

Library of Congress Cataloging-in-Publication Data
Penina uliuli : contemporary challenges in mental health for Pacific peoples / Philip Culbertson and Margaret Nelson Agee, editors ; with Cabrini Ofa Makasiale.
p. ; cm.
Includes bibliographical references and index.
ISBN 978-0-8248-3194-3 (hardcover : alk. paper) —
ISBN 978-0-8248-3224-7 (pbk. : alk. paper)
1. Pacific Islanders—Mental health.
2. Pacific Islanders—Mental health services.
I. Culbertson, Philip. II. Agee, Margaret Nelson.
III. Makasiale, Cabrini Ofa.
[DNLM: 1. Mental Health. 2. Oceanic Ancestry Group. 3. Mental Disorders—ethnology. 4. Mental Health Services. 5. Spirituality—Islands of the Pacific.
WA 305 P411 2007]
RA790.7.P25P46 2007
616.890099—dc22 2007020603

University of Hawai'i Press books are printed on acid-free paper and meet the guidelines for permanence and durability of the Council on Library Resources.

Designed by Chris Crochetière,
BW&A Books, Inc.
Printed by The Maple-Vail Book
Manufacturing Group

Contents

Editors' Note

Every day in the depths of the Pacific Ocean, among the coral, fish, and seaweed on the ocean floor, nestles the *tifa* (oyster). Its shell sometimes opens, and it feeds by filtering plankton and nutrients from the warm currents as they pass through its flesh.

●

Occasionally a parasitic organism, a biological intruder, will drill through the oyster's shell, and in defense the oyster will form a protective barrier, or mantle, around it. Over the course of years, a mantle of nacre forms, layer by layer, around the irritating intruder. The end product radiates an array of various colors—from shades of blue and purple to tints of platinum and green. This is the rare and precious gem, the "pearl of great price," the Pacific black pearl, or *penina uliuli*.

●

This book is named after that pearl. It started with an idea, a need to produce a resource by Pasifika for Pasifika, about treatments, conditions, issues, protocols, and processes faced by Pacific peoples. From that nucleus, this resource grew, layer by layer, as more mental health professionals, researchers, practitioners, counselors, psychotherapists, and community workers joined in. The end result is a precious, rare, and colorful resource, radiating the unique and indigenous shades of the Pacific.

Introduction
On Building a Fale

On a sunny Auckland spring day in October 2003, Margaret Agee and Philip Culbertson, faculty members at the University of Auckland, were enjoying a collegial cup of coffee. Philip had just received notice that his 1997 book, *Counselling Issues and South Pacific Communities*, was going out of print, and the two were sharing their frustration at how difficult it is to locate the formally and informally published work of Pasifika colleagues in the field of counseling. This lack serves as the primary impediment to the dissemination and advancement of multicultural theories and creative developments in practice in the mental health field throughout the Pacific and internationally.

Eventually they began to dream of facilitating a new edited collection, designed to serve both the training and ongoing professional development needs of mental health professionals, to increase their skills in addressing mental health issues particular to indigenous Pasifika peoples. Philip and Margaret realized that they needed a Pasifika person on the editorial team, and so invited Cabrini Makasiale, a Fijian-born Tongan psychotherapist, to serve as the advisory co-editor. In March 2004, the three co-editors began to approach mental health professionals in Auckland about contributing to such a book. The response was immediate and enthusiastic.

The Birth of a New Community

A letter of invitation was sent to a list of Pasifika mental health workers, inviting them to a breakfast to learn about the project. The co-editors' dream was a book in which mental health workers indigenous to the Pacific would take creative ownership of the contents, while the co-editors would provide the tools and machinery to get this collection into print. In this way, the co-editors hoped that a purer Pasifika voice could emerge, without the taint of further colonization by the pālagi West. We believe that in this collection, the voices of indigenous writers can be heard speaking for themselves, in their own way.

The initial breakfast meeting in late June was attended by eight Samoan and Tongan women, in addition to the co-editors. The group was welcomed and the food blessed by the Rev. Dr. Winston Halapua, a Tongan minister who is also a faculty member at Auckland University. The ensuing discussion yielded a number of points, which by the end of the book remained in the forefront of the minds of many of the writers:

- Language is a key tool for healing, underlining the importance of discipline in the way we use words with one another in therapeutic processes.
- Challenging language used by experts in the field—both with reference to mistaken diagnoses, as well as in terms of assumed meanings, for example, "connectedness"—highlights the need to create new expressions to communicate greater depth of conceptual meaning.
- The importance of creating new models for assessment relates to the above point with regard to critiquing the language and concepts currently used.
- In working with families, cultural concepts, for example, relating Tongan constructs to issues that families are encountering in the pālagi world, are valuable tools for fostering resiliency and creating points of connection.
- Models of community development and management that best suit Pasifika need to be identified and built upon. A lot of cultural "recipes" have been attempted that have not successfully met the needs of their target groups in the twenty-first century. Instead, it is necessary to return to the roots of these models—in terms of both intention and process—deconstruct them, then replace them with new models that better equip Pacific peoples to thrive in a multicultural and global world.
- It is exciting and challenging to be part of creating something new that reflects our lives in the present, evolving out of our valuing of history and tradition. The theme of moving forward emerged very strongly, expressed in terms of our recognizing that we live in a new era, as a new generation, needing to develop new models and to look ahead two to three generations. In reflecting on the responsibilities this presents, the following were noted:
    - The need for a balance between cultural respect and challenge.
    - The *what* remains the same; the *how* changes.
    - The need to address the issue of what happens when traditions no longer serve their original purpose but become destructive —to address the roles that traditions play.
    - The challenge of redefining the *'āiga/kāinga/'ohana* (extended family) in the urban environment, and examples of adaptation.
    - The need to flatten hierarchical structures so that young people have a voice.

Feeling the Way through the Process

Auckland-based members of the group met approximately once every two months throughout 2004 and most of 2005 (the Honolulu-based members were kept in touch via frequent emails). As the project developed, others heard of our work and asked to join the group. Some who wished to write found that they weren't ready, or were overwhelmed by prior commitments, or didn't yet have the writing skills to contribute, so they withdrew. A variety of styles emerged as the manuscripts developed, each chosen in order to fit the content of what needed to be said. Some articles were produced via interview; others were produced by audiotaped group discussion; most were through-written by their designated authors.

In group meetings, several important topics were raised. Philip and Margaret remained the primary drivers of the group process, though alert to the complex effect of their whiteness. The shadow of colonization hangs heavily over the Pacific. As well, postcolonialism, particularly in relationship to the early work of anthropologist Margaret Mead in Samoa, raises serious questions about how much white academics can ever understand the voice of indigenous people, unless they are allowed to speak for themselves.

A second important topic was the evident tension between the island-born Pasifika writers and the New Zealand–born Pasifika writers. This difference highlights the complexity of the South Pacific. The Hawaiian writers in this book, like the Māori of New Zealand, still live in their own land, which has been colonized by Europeans. Samoan, Tongan, and Niuean writers here, while deeply attached to their island heritages, do not live in the homelands of their ethnicity, but have chosen to immigrate to complex societies in which they are often viewed as outsiders. Pasifika is therefore a diverse community in transition. While many issues addressed in this book immediately stem from the process of immigration and communities in transition, in other respects they also have their roots in traditional structures and hierarchies of island life.

Third, the group spoke often of what wasn't being written about and what wasn't being said. Certain topics are obviously missing or underdeveloped in this book—the role of traditional healing in the mental health process; the fact that so much training methodology in mental health is inappropriate in that it recolonizes the very people it professes to serve; the difficulty of surviving in mainstream mental health agencies; the way that Christianity has distorted the wisdom of indigenous Pacific cultures; the silencing of so many voices within the Pasifika community by the Pacific elders themselves—to name but a few. These and other topics await the continuing development of Pasifika voices within the mental health community, who can contribute even more writing about the richness and problems of the proud and beautiful cultures that originate in the Southern Ocean.

On Building a Fale

In November 2004, the group met to talk about what might hold this book together, given that it is written by people from several Pacific cultures with a wide variety of educational and professional backgrounds. On reflection, the range of author backgrounds relates to the question of how the term *Pasifika* is used in this book. Both *Oceania* and *the Pacific* are contested terms, in that they are applied to an area that covers one-quarter of the globe. Oceania and the Pacific may apply to Polynesians, Melanesians, and even to the relative handful of Caucasians who have disappeared into the indigenous cultures since the early 1800s. Our authors in this book identify themselves primarily as Samoan, Tongan, Niuean, and Hawaiian, but as a group they carry other identities as well, including Tokelauan, Māori, Chinese, English, German, Irish, and Swedish. For the time being, rather than entering into the territory of contested terminology, we have used the term *Pasifika* to describe the cultural identities and issues of people who identify as Polynesian, with roots in the Southern Pacific. Even among these groups, there are important cultural differences, but they elected the term *Pasifika* as their preferred self-descriptor.

Our group discussion began with two questions: What does it mean to write a book together? How can we find our own voices and yet disagree with each other? The cultural metaphor that emerged was of the *fale*, the distinctive architectural structure traditional to Samoan and Tongan cultures—a structure used for various purposes, including as a family's primary dwelling and for village meetings. In Tongan culture, a traditional fale is generally oval-shaped, with a domed roof and flimsy walls of woven mats, or more recently, something more substantial. In Samoan culture, a traditional fale is generally round, with a domed roof and woven mats that roll up and down to create the effect of external walls. In both cases, the emphasis is minimally on a foundation, some supporting poles, and a roof. Between the foundation and the roof, a complex open space is constructed.

The foundation of the fale. A fale is only as strong as its foundation. In unpacking the metaphor, group members offered various interpretations. One option was that "the foundation is the blood that is in us. Historians say that we Polynesians came from one source, and before the fale was, we were." A respondent observed that the image of blood suggested "our collective hearts" as the foundation. Another observed that "we survive in non-Pacific environments because, whether we are Tongan, Samoan, Niuean, or whatever, we pull together as Pacific people." Another observed that the foundation of the fale is "the past we cherish, the present we live in, and the future we anticipate."

The bones or pillars of the fale. Each writer in this book has a unique identity, sometimes referred to as one's social location. Each has a unique genealogy, life experience, belief system, and connection with an indigenous culture or combination of cultures. These interact with a person's class, age, gender, philosophy, economic position, and political affiliation, to form a particular way of seeing and understanding the world that is individual and irreplaceable—or, as one participant put it, "you see the elephant from where you are." Another member of the group began to articulate her social location with the words, "I am a Tongan woman marginalized commoner feminist migrant. Another Tongan woman can speak from the same social location, and that will highlight both our similarities and our differences. We each come from multiple realities." The writers of this book come from multiple realities and multiple points-of-view, just as the pillars of a fale come from many different trees, carved and polished in many different ways, holding both difference and sameness. To the fale, the writers bring their individual diversity, and together they draw strength from each other to hold up the roof so that others can shelter beneath it. To accentuate the diverse social locations represented in this book, and in keeping with Pacific protocol, each essay begins with the writer's self-introduction.

The space in the fale. The essayists in the discussion were attracted to the fiction that they were sitting together in a fale, having a *talanoa* (conversation) about family matters. Talanoa always includes agreement and disagreement. But what norms would govern this family? One participant observed, "It is *our* space, so we can create our own norms, and don't have to borrow anyone else's." Another added, "The prime purpose of the fale is shelter. The good, the bad, and the ugly of any family can find rest there." A fale, then, is where a family can come together with its own way of doing things, and do that in a mutually owned, shared space. Yet how complex this space is: even in a family, and certainly in this group, the members bring many different perspectives—a colonized perspective and a noncolonized perspective; a Western analytical way of thinking and a very metaphorical way of talking that is also philosophical. The complex space is never empty, yet not everything is visible.

The roof of the fale. Interpretations of the cultural metaphor of the fale ranged widely at this point. One participant offered: "our Pan-Pacificness." At the opposite end of the scale, another answered: "Whatever else holds us together, we are also held together by marginalization. One might say that what holds us together is blood; another might say it is Hawaiki, but what also binds us is that we are all colonized." It seems that in this time of transition, Pacific peoples are struggling to articulate what point of unity they can shelter under, as if the past were clearer than the future.

A village of fales. Some of the essayists spoke, with gales of laughter, of visiting the Polynesian Village in Hawai'i. But in a sense, this community is, at least, a village of professional fales, for the essays are, variously, by educators, counselors, community social workers and developers, clinical psychologists, and psychotherapists. Unanimously, the participants hoped that, with their work, new voices could be heard among the talanoa in the fale—voices that could speak even more about the future than about the past or the present. All hoped that the future would be different because of what they were doing in the present.

Ultimately, the essayists included here understand this book as a contribution to an ongoing talanoa. As Pacific peoples, cultural restrictions (*tapu*) have been observed in the writing. The essayists have tried to tell the truth as they experience it personally and professionally, and yet some things are in riddles (*heliaki*), left to the reader to unpack. This is the Pacific way: to speak in symbol, metaphor, and poetry, so that sometimes the heart understands long before the head does. But this book is intended to be as open as a fale, where there are many entrances and exits and almost limitless opportunities to engage the complex spaces.

Conclusion

This "pearl of a book," then, is the essayists' *mea-alofa*, or gift, to the future. We offer it to counselors and psychotherapists; social workers and practitioners; teachers and teacher aides; mental health workers and community workers; educational psychologists; faculty and trainers in educational institutions; university students, including professionals in training; anthropologists, sociologists, and cultural theorists; policy developers, administrators, and researchers; ministers and church workers; members of Pacific communities in their diversity; and all others in a variety of fields wherein the "multiple worlds of other" are relevant.

This project was supported in part by a grant from the University of Auckland Staff Research Fund, and by grants from St. Johns Theological College and the Faculty of Education and the School of Teaching, Learning, and Development with the Faculty of Education of the University of Auckland. Thanks go also to the editor of *Forum: The Journal of the New Zealand Association of Psychotherapists* for permission to reprint a shortened version of "The Use of Symbol and Metaphor in Pacific Counselling" by Cabrini 'Ofa Makasiale, from volume 6, 2000, pp. 17–31; to Fuimaono Karl Pulotu-Endemann for the use of his Fonofale drawing; to Dr. Melenaite Taumoefolau of the University of Auckland and Ms. Fia Turner-Tupou for help with the correct diacritical markings in Tongan and Samoan. Thanks go also to the Rt. Rev. Dr. Winston Halapua of the College of the Diocese of Polynesia for praying this project into existence, and to William Hamilton, director of the University of Hawai'i Press, for his courteous and always-punctual encouragement.

Margaret would like to thank her husband Tom Agee for his unfailing support as well as his technical assistance, her Pasifika clients and students over the years who have been her teachers and her inspiration, and every member of the team that contributed to the building of this fale, which held us and sustained us in the process of creating this book. Philip would like to thank the deans and staff of St. Johns Theological College, Auckland, particularly Helen Edwards, who was always ready to rescue us in emergencies, and Rekha Bahsin and Belinda Dolan-Roberts for their timely production assistance. Cabrini would like to thank the community with whom she lives, and all those who turned out for our meetings over the course of developing this book. Each, whether their names are visible here or not, has made a significant contribution to the successful completion of this project.

Philip Culbertson
Margaret Nelson Agee
Cabrini 'Ofa Makasiale
January 2007

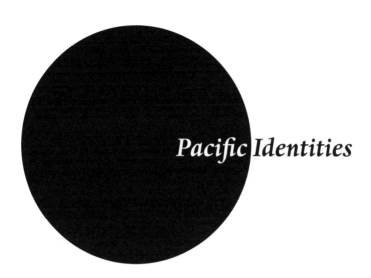

Pacific Identities

Editors' Introduction

The first five essays provide insights into aspects of Pacific identities. As a professional working with young people, Siautu Alefaio introduces some of the challenges faced by Pacific youth—including both New Zealand–born and immigrants—growing up within a contemporary urban environment. For a young person whose identity is formed within the collective contexts of family and church, the associated values, roles, and expectations are in many ways at odds with the other formative contexts in which they live their lives. These include the culture and values of Western society, the expectations of schools and tertiary educational institutions, as well as contemporary urban youth culture and global society. Positive role models and mentoring are identified as important in helping them navigate their way successfully through the conflicts and challenges they encounter.

These are the focus of Emeline Afeaki-Mafile'o's discussion of her holistic approach to developing community-based mentoring programs for Pacific young people. Her initiative in creating these programs, which reflect collective Pacific values, was inspired by her personal and professional awareness of the complexity of young people's worlds, identities, and developmental processes. Particular challenges can be encountered by those who have multiple cultural heritages and are *'afakasi* (half-caste).

Knowing oneself through knowing one's body is the theme of the next two essays in which the authors address a range of issues through the medium of reading the male body as text. From a Samoan perspective, Tavita Maliko's reading of his body reveals the personal shame engendered by colonial practices and the need to reclaim the body from gender-based messages and the colonial gaze. In Maika Lutui's essay, the influences of Tongan cultural values, traditional myths, and the overlay of Christian myth are implicated in creating confusion and negativity toward the body. From a therapeutic perspective, the result can be dissociation, or an internalized split, between one's sense of identity and the awareness of one's body, impairing personal integration and wholeness. These two essays provide interesting points of comparison between Samoan and Tongan constructs of masculinity. They also indicate the subtle and extensive ways in which particular influences, including cultural structures, social control, and political hierarchies, affect the individual.

Challenges and benefits associated with being 'afakasi—integrating one's identity out of multiple cultural heritages—have not been widely acknowledged or addressed in the context of mental health and wellbeing among the Pasifika community. In the final essay in this section, an exploration of these issues is based on a facilitated discussion among four Samoan women professionals of their own personal experiences of being 'afakasi. The implications for their own sense of identity and belonging, their parenting of their children, and their work as professionals are complex, pain-laden, enriching, and intriguing, inspiring a commitment to further research on the part of this group.

1

Supporting the Wellbeing of Pasifika Youth

SIAUTU ALEFAIO

Twenty-nine years ago a man from the villages of Manunu (Upolu) and Fagamalo (Savai'i) and a woman from the inner-city village of Mātautu tai-Apia (Upolu) gave birth to me, their middle child and only daughter, Siautu Tiomai Alefaio. The man left a prominent position in the police department's Criminal Investigation Branch in Samoa to become a factory worker in Hellaby Meats of Mt. Wellington, New Zealand. The woman, a beautiful dancer in Aggie Grey's dance troupe and also an upcoming photographer at the age of 12, left all her aspirations of education to attain a job in order to make enough money for the prospective dream of making it big in the "land free-flowing with milk and honey"—Aotearoa/New Zealand. For some years Aotearoa was exactly that, with money enough to bring over all their other siblings and eventually their mothers.

My father (now a parish minister of a Presbyterian church) and mother (an early-childhood educator) both self-sacrificially gave up their own hopes and dreams to pursue a bigger one—of prosperity for future generations. As a registered educational psychologist I have seen many journey stories similar to mine, and it is my own hope and dream that our contribution as Pacific people here in Aotearoa/New Zealand will inevitably pave the way for future generations to embrace all that they are and become all that they have been called to be.

Having reached the shores of the Promised Land—Aotearoa/New Zealand—the process of working the land has taken its toll. Telling the truth about acculturation for Pasifika youth in New Zealand will hopefully contribute to the understanding of Pasifika youth identity and how we can begin to welcome the journey ahead.

Our story is different . . . our story is about family, about church and that's why it's gonna change . . . I can see a Pacific—yeah a New Zealand Pacific culture coming up—and that's the way we'll express ourselves—a New Zealand Pacific identity. (cited in Alefaio, 1999, p. 51)

Growing up in South Auckland, the heart of Polynesia in Aotearoa/New Zealand, was never an easy feat. The stories of young people describing their journeys as they experienced living in two worlds, the Pasifika world and the pālagi world, became significant to me as a young adult finding my way through life in a tertiary institution. These stories prompted me to undertake a thesis investigating young people's perceptions of their identity in the context of their families and communities and the process of adjustment that occurs when the unfamiliar norms and values of the host culture are encountered. The experience of walking in two cultural worlds has been investigated in many countries, including our own, mostly where the host culture is the dominant Western culture, governed by Eurocentric ideals and cultural norms (see Anae, 1997; Crosbie, 1993; Rodriquez, 2003). Certain issues and challenges are commonly experienced by ethnic minority youth in transition within mainstream cultural environments. In order to understand the worldview of Pasifika youth in Aotearoa/New Zealand, and to provide them with effective practical support on their journey as they navigate their way through their cultural worlds, it is vital that their unique perspectives are sought and their voices heard.

Le Malaga—*Our Journey*

Pasifika people currently comprise 6.5 percent of Aotearoa/New Zealand's total population, and are one of the most youthful and fastest-growing minority groups. The wave of migration from the Pacific, which occurred during the 1950s to 1970s due to the demand for labor in New Zealand, created the largest Pacific ethnic minority group in Aotearoa/New Zealand, next to the indigenous Māori, or *tāngata whenua* (people of the land). The term *Pacific* is itself a homogeneous term used to describe a group of island nations from the region of the Pacific, including Samoa, Cook Islands, Tonga, Niue, Tokelau, and Fiji. Meleisea and Schoeffel (1998) have described the New Zealand–Pacific relationship through the migratory period as "a kind of extension of the country's colonial relationship with the Pacific" (p. 166).

The majority of the Pasifika population in New Zealand is located in the urban Auckland region, which is also projected to have the largest increase of Pacific people residing within its boundaries (Statistics New Zealand, 2002). Associated with this "Pasifika-browning phenomenon" is an increasing contribution of Pacific cultures over the past six decades to Aotearoa/New Zealand as a nation. The significant impact of these can be experienced in many arenas, including the rugby field, where the sporting prowess of taro-fed "Pacific-Black"' (Pasifika members of the All-Black rugby team) such as Jonah Lomu and Michael Jones has been celebrated, in the African American/Pasifika-hip-hop inspired music and arts scene, in live theater, and in the visual arts. Pasifika youth are emerging as an influential force in youth culture in New Zealand today. However, these highly visible pockets of Pasifika talent mask the reality of overcrowded housing, poor health, low incomes, and tail-end educational achievement.

The journey of Pasifika youth is born out of a historical, migratory past filled with hopes and dreams of a new utopia—a new way of living, a better life with a hope-filled, expectant future. Today, however, we encounter, on a daily basis, issues such as abuse, teenage pregnancy, suicide, drug and alcohol use, violence and crime, and Pacific peoples are disproportionately represented in these areas of concern. In order to address the issues facing Pasifika youth, we need to understand the context that has arguably the greatest influence over their developmental process. The role of families and family relationships in the identity development of our young people needs to be understood if we are to provide effective support and intervention to reduce the harm that is occurring in young people's lives.

Family: Collectivism and Cohesion

When we look back historically, research highlights the importance of the family as the primary social context in which identity develops. McAdoo (1993) has described the experience of growing up in the confines of the family as being the place where we first begin to get a sense of who we are, what we are, and what direction our lives will take:

> When we examine ourselves, we find that who we are and who we can become depend in great part upon who we started to be. This is found within our families. Our ethnicity cannot be separated from our families. Within the security and insecurity of our families, as they face all of the developmental changes that families must, by definition, go through, we become firmly established in our time and place. (p. 3)

Describing the influence of family on the development of ethnic identity more specifically, Phinney and Rosenthal (1992) noted:

> the family is the source of children's first experiences related to ethnicity, and it is generally with the parents and other family members that children make their first identifications as part of a group. Family and significant others are the principal sources of information and influence providing a cultural context . . . families that participate with pleasure in their cultural traditions and express positive feelings about their group are likely to lay a basis for a positive ethnic identity. (p. 152)

The importance of a family's own positive cultural identification in healthy ethnic identity development is highlighted here.

Two key aspects of Pacific families found to have a significant impact on young people are family structure with regards to collectivism and the environment of the family in terms of cohesion. Understanding the strength of these two elements is necessary in order to understand the need of Pasifika youth for connectedness in their current environment as a minority group within mainstream society.

Collectivism

International studies have investigated the relevance of structural collectivism in ethnic family groups. Taule'ale'ausumai (1997) vividly illustrates the importance of collectivism through a description of the Samoan family structure:

> Unlike the nuclear family of western society, Samoa's social existence is collective and corporate. Family life extends out beyond the nuclear family, incorporating uncles, aunties, both sets of grandparents and many cousins. Therefore children are thought of as belonging not only to their parents but also to the wider kin group and, in the case of Samoans, to the village community, inclusive of the church. (p. 166)

As a result, for youth of Pasifika heritage, who we are and how we see our ourselves are generally inextricably linked to our *'āiga/kāinga* (family). Identity development occurs within the heart of the family for Pasifika youth; the context of each young person's family defines who he or she is, in character and deed. In the words of Hunt-Ioane (2005), the socialization of Samoan children "always begins in their home and then permeates every area of activity and interpersonal relationship that they engage in and experience as individuals" (p. 95). Pasifika youth must therefore be embraced as a product of the "we," since the majority do not consider themselves as individuals but rather as part of the family. Their roles within their families, although at times very difficult, are powerfully influential in the development of their identities and worldviews.

Understanding family values and roles is therefore fundamental to understanding the worldview of Pasifika youth. As Pilato, Su'a, and Crichton-Hill (1994) have explained:

> The preservation of family unity, integrity and credibility is of paramount importance . . . The prevailing belief of Pacific Island people is that individual achievements are directly related to the nurturing and support of the family. In almost every case the individual edifies and attributes the source of their success to their family. (p. 5)

An individual's whole identity is interconnected with the extended family, not isolated or alone. In this environment, conformity and family allegiance are emphasized over individuation. In the words of one young person:

> I'm not really an individual, just the fact that I perceive Islanders as a very communal people, like I think you can hardly ever see Islanders by themselves . . . they've always got somebody with them. When they eat—they eat big, you don't just have a small feed, you invite everybody to come . . . I see it as collective . . . it's hard to be an individual within the family, you actually have to probably physically remove yourself to be an individual, because there's always conformity within the family, you have to conform, you have to do what your parents want you to do, what your family wants you to do. (cited in Alefaio, 1999, p. 42)

In this collective context, Pasifika youth are taught to share resources and place the needs of family and community ahead of their own, as one young person has described:

> Even with money, you can't be an individual, like as soon as you get money, a portion of it goes to Mum and Dad, and then after that when it's just me, a portion of it goes to the church, and then when there's money just by myself and I'm out with friends a portion of it goes there . . . it goes down to—eating food—the littlest thing, if you go out with your friends even if you have only one pie—you know five bites each—it's expected, you have to share. (cited in Alefaio, 1999, p. 43)

For Pasifika youth growing up within New Zealand society, the collective nature of the family means they simultaneously have to process the competing value systems of the individual versus the collective. Collective living and being is challenged every day for them when they enter the school, socialize with peers, and are exposed, in the competing global media market, to a barrage of images that promote success-driven, individualistic principles. Our customary way of sharing a pie among five people—meaning we might only get a bite each—gives way to competing self-interests. We are taught at school to work hard and do our own homework so that we will succeed to our own benefit. However, at Sunday School, when preparing for Scripture Union exams, we work together with our friends, we all share the stories we learn, we encourage one another, and, yes, laugh at each other, nurturing each other's strengths. We might not ever win the ultimate prize of sitting at the front table at the big Sunday celebration feast at the end of exams, but we know that together we've enjoyed each other's company, and that together we study, we learn, we eat, and we do well.

Cohesion

Within a strongly collective family structure, the more cohesive the family environment is in terms of the strength of family relationships, the more likely it is that a young person, wherever he or she lives, will develop a strong Samoan ethnic identity (Alefaio, 1999). Cohesion in the family is associated with the degree of commitment, help, and support family members provide for one another. Cohesive families provide youth with emotional support and security as they develop autonomy and establish age-appropriate, close relationships with peers. Moreover, by reducing psychosocial stress, family cohesion also appears to decrease levels of delinquent and acting-out behavior (Wentzel & Feldman, 1996).

Cohesion within Pacific families means principles of mutual respect, service, and reciprocity. These principles, while naturally *lived* in the island context, are more often *grown* in the Western context, where the differences in lifestyle and the pressures of contemporary urban life make the application of those principles more challenging. In New Zealand, the application of these principles within each young Pacific person's life is associated with the developmental process; cognitive maturity enables a young person to grow in her or his understanding of these values. This process of attitudinal change has been reflected upon by one youth, who has also described the Pacific principle of reciprocity, where one's responsibility as one grows older becomes more entrenched in the family:

> My perception of family has changed since I was younger, now that I have a real job, you really start to honor your family, and you see the influence of your family . . . with our culture it's not weird to still be at home and working. A lot of my peers within the work place they always ask me—why haven't you ever left home and that, but you know it's my duty and obligation . . . I've been through my vacation, I've been through that *ta'a* (muck around/goof off) stage, and now it's time to work back for the family . . . I remember Mum and Dad always said to us, when we were younger, "you've got to come back and *galue* (work) within the *'āiga* (family)." (cited in Alefaio, 1999, p. 39)

In a Hawaiian study (Joe & Chesney-Lind, 1995), where Pacific Islanders included immigrants from the respective island groups, family was described as the core of the Pacific Island community. In Samoa and other Pacific Islands, where families live in open *fales*, behavior is clearly visible and, hence, children's behavior is directly controlled. When a child is unruly, he or she can be sent to stay with relatives, given the understanding and availability of extended family there. The Hawaiian study also found, however, that the arrangement where the traditional social and economic activities took place in the family was severely disrupted in the Western economic context.

Challenges to Family Cohesion

With the changes associated with migration, new patterns of living and working have called for multiple levels of adaptation and new modes of thinking. New trades have had to be learned and new skills acquired, shifting from the plantation to the factory floor. When support was no longer necessarily accessible from the extended family, Pasifika migrants have had to turn to friends and peers. Given the limited availability of extended family to help with child care in particular, parents have had to decide how best to manage shift-work hours and child-rearing responsibilities.

Coping with these competing demands without the support of the wider social structures that were in place traditionally within the village context has meant that some families have had adaptation experiences of "village isolation." This means the quality of relationships that help create a cohesive unit within the family/'āiga have been jeopardized. In a five-year longitudinal study conducted by Arrendondo (1984) with young adult migrants, values based on family modeling and teaching were described as an important part of life for all participants. In the context of village isolation, when parents are absent, the village role modeling of these values is lost, thereby creating a generation of youth who substitute the values of a culture that is unfamiliar to their parents for the values that have been lost, in turn creating a cultural divide within the family.

This is clearly visible through the growing youth gang culture and the aspiring affiliation of some young Pasifika people with the African American hip-hop culture (Zemke-White, 2004). Crosbie (1993) has argued that the influence of American pop culture on Pasifika identity is because of its relevance to their cultural colors. It is perceived not as a copycat syndrome, but as an affiliation of identity. It has become apparent, however, that this value-shift affiliated to identity is associated with the developmental journey of Pasifika youth. As one late adolescent has observed, a lack of family connectedness or cohesion with family, and limited achievement and/or motivation within the education system, are influential factors from his perspective:

> I've grown up with a lot of guys that have turned to hip-hop, a lot of them they're really strong in their *fa'a-Samoa* [the Samoan way], but it's their education —they're lacking heaps in learning and education. So because they're lacking in that they just go with the flow . . . they're hardly there with the family, so they have to look for another group where they can be somebody. (cited in Alefaio, 1999, p. 50)

In the process of developing a mature understanding of Pacific principles of cohesion within a family, struggle is inevitable as Pasifika youth contend with competing values and interests. Many times Pasifika youth journey a full circle; as the young person quoted earlier explained, the ta'a (muck around) stage is a period of exploration. Nurturing this time and allowing youth to explore will help Pacific families foster cohesion. This is not easy, however, for families that are themselves already under considerable pressure, including the stresses of poverty, disadvantage, and the associated social problems.

In a study conducted by Strier (1996), the coping strategies of immigrant parents were investigated. The results revealed that the social cognitions, child-rearing ideologies, expectations, norms, rules, and beliefs adhered to by parents tend to preserve meaningful elements of the original culture. Family distress was viewed as being more pronounced in families with adolescents in which developmental stress and intergenerational differences interact with cultural conflicts.

Such stressors were identified by Hunt-Ioane (2005) in discussing the complexities of expectations in the contemporary environment. The competing cultural practices that influence the migrant Pacific child in different environmental contexts, such as school, peers/friends, and family, convey conflicting messages that must be negotiated. Parental expectations of Samoan migrants can be difficult to sustain in face of their children's exposure to a variety of types of behavior, lifestyles, and other influences that represent values and principles that differ from those of their collective cultural upbringing.

Every day, counselors in schools support Pasifika young people in coping with the conflict that this inevitably creates within them, especially if their parents do not "have an awareness or minimal understanding of how life is very different for a child raised in New Zealand as opposed to their upbringing in Samoa" (Hunt-Ioane, 2005, p. 37). Many youngsters struggle to cope without support beyond that of their peers, and as a result become caught in a destructive cycle of harmful behavior associated with confusion and dislocation.

Our Wider Family/'Aiga: *The Church*

The church, as an extension of family at the heart of Pacific communities, can play a vital role in supporting young people. Pasifika peoples are often described as being rooted in biblical principles, an assumption proceeding from their high level of affiliation with churches. *Fa'avae Samoa i le Atua*, the national motto, means "Samoa is founded on God." Most Pacific nations have strong affiliations to Christianity and a belief in God through the influence of the early missionaries to the Pacific region. The values and beliefs of the Pacific are underpinned by the concept of Christian love. When migration to New Zealand occurred, churches became the epicenter of community life.

Taking the role of the church into account is imperative in any practical response for nurturing the generations to come. For many Pasifika youth, their religious faith is a strong source of support and sustenance. This is described in the voice of one Pasifika young person, who, when elaborating on her developmental journey, referred to the impact of Christianity:

> Yeah, family's important but it's not the central thing that holds us together, it's mostly our Christian relationship with God and just the fellowship we have with our Christian brothers and sisters . . . the church within my life is really important, I really enjoy it, helping me out in my fa'a-Samoa. (cited in Alefaio, 1999, pp. 39–40)

The challenge that lies ahead for those who are nurturing this generation of Pasifika youth is to assist the church to accommodate the changes and needs affecting these young people and their families.

Because of the importance of family, church, and wider community to them, many young people embrace the added demands upon them as integral to their lives as Samoan youth:

> I think that's the challenge . . . growing up in New Zealand, for me it's unique. I think it's easier for pālagis to succeed because there aren't as many things in their lives. Whereas Polynesians are church oriented plus your school and work and you're supposed to make everything fit together. So I enjoy it, and I see it as a challenge. I don't see being a Samoan as a disability, it's just that God has chosen me to be a Samoan child, and so I do my best to be the best Samoan. (cited in Alefaio, 1999, p. 47)

Many, however, struggle to meet these different, and often conflicting, expectations, and require more effective support and understanding from within both their Pacific and pālagi communities.

This struggle is about issues of the heart, of identity and belonging for youth trying to discover who they are, in the context of a dominant culture most dissimilar to their own heritage. Their identity development is inevitably influenced by the values and beliefs of the host culture, which challenge and compete with their Pacific cultural worldview.

The Last Word: Supporting the Wellbeing of Pacific Youth

As the voices of Pasifika youth are increasingly heard, and their experiences and needs are better understood, their strengths and resilience can be celebrated and more effective ways of supporting them in their developmental journey can be devised. This includes the concept of mirror imaging, associated with mentoring and represented in the diagram below, which illustrates the elements that are proposed as central to understanding Pasifika youth identity development.

Mirror imaging refers to knowing who you are through familial mentoring and role models: not the *I* but the *we*. The mirror image one sees is a communal one, utilizing Pasifika mentors and role models that can be found within our wider network of connections, including family, church, and community. A sense of belonging is therefore nurtured through familial connections and cultural practices. This, in turn, encourages what is a

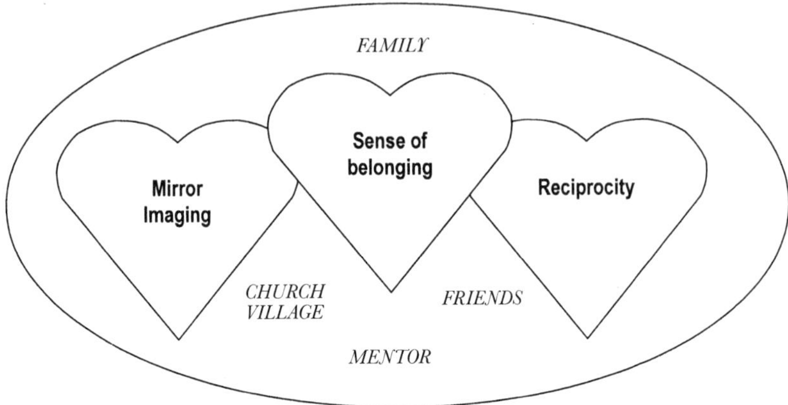

traditional practice of our heritage: reciprocity, giving, and growing in our families, churches, schools, communities, cities, and nations.

In shaping the destiny of our youth, it is therefore the resources associated with these elements in young people's lives that can provide appropriate support for them within their cultural contexts. In particular, relationally based mentoring of Pasifika youth by Pasifika mentors/role models themselves is developing strongly within our community. We are building our own confidence in our capacity to find creative and culturally based strategies for supporting Pasifika youth in their developmental journeys, and growing within them the vision, not only to cope with their daily circumstances, but also to see beyond them, to the possibilities of what they are capable of becoming.

References

Alefaio, S. (1999). Impact of family structure and family environment on the ethnic identity of Samoan young people in New Zealand. Unpublished master's thesis, University of Auckland.

Anae, M. (1997). Towards a New Zealand-born Samoan identity: Some reflections on "labels." *Pacific Health Dialog, 4*(2), 128–137.

Arredondo, P. M. (1984). Identity themes for immigrant young adults. *Adolescence, 14*, 977–993.

Crosbie, S. (1993). Americanisation: American popular culture's influence on Maori and Pacific Island identity. *Midwest, 3*, 22–29.

Hunt-Ioane, F. (2005). Physical discipline in Samoan families. Unpublished master's thesis, Massey University, New Zealand.

Joe, K. A., & Chesney-Lind, M. (1995). Just every mother's angel: An analysis of gender and ethnic variations in youth gang membership. *Gender and Society, 9*, 408–431.

Kroger, J. (1996). *Identity in adolescence: The balance between self and other.* London: Routledge.

McAdoo, H. P. (Ed.). (1993). *Family ethnicity: Strength in diversity.* Newbury Park: Sage.

Meleisea, M., & Schoeffel, P. (1998). Samoan families in New Zealand: The cultural context of change. In V. Adair & R. Dixon (Eds.), *The family in Aotearoa New Zealand* (pp. 158–178). Auckland: Longman.

Phinney, J., & Rosenthal, D. (1992). Ethnic identity in adolescence: Process, context, and outcome. In G. R. Adams, T. P. Gullotta, & R. Montemayer (Eds.), *Adolescent identity formation* (pp. 145–172). New York: Sage.

Pilato, T., Su'a, T., & Crichton-Hill, Y. (1994). A Pacific Island perspective. *Social Work Now, 11,* 25–29.

Rodriquez, R. (2003). "Blaxicans" and other reinvented Americans. *Chronicle of Higher Education, 50*(3), B10.

Statistics New Zealand. (2002). *Pacific progress report: A report on the economic status of Pacific peoples in New Zealand.* Wellington: Ministry of Pacific Island Affairs and Statistics, New Zealand.

Strier, D. R. (1996). Coping strategies of immigrant parents: Directions for family therapy. *Family Process, 35,* 363–376.

Taule'ale'ausumai, F. (1997). Pastoral care: A Samoan perspective. In P. Culbertson (Ed.), *Counselling issues and South Pacific communities* (pp. 215–237). Auckland: Snedden & Cervin.

Wentzel, K. R., & Feldman, S. S. (1996). Relations of cohesion and power in family dyads to social and emotional adjustment during early adolescence. *Journal of Research on Adolescence, 6,* 225–244.

Zemke-White, K. (2004). Keeping it real (indigenous): Hip hop in Aotearoa as community, culture, and consciousness. In C. Bell & S. Matthewman (Eds.), *Cultural studies in Aotearoa New Zealand: Identity, space, and place* (pp. 205–228). Oxford: Oxford University Press.

2

Affirming Works
A Collective Model of Pasifika Mentoring

EMELINE AFEAKI-MAFILEʻO

From an early age I have been driven by my passion for youth, especially youth of Pacific Island descent. I am a New Zealand–born Tongan (Kolofoʻou and Haʻapai), Samoan (Falefa and Savelalo), and Māori (Ngāti Awa). The heritages of my multicultural migrant parents have allowed me to receive an abundant world of knowledge. I have benefited from my parents' sacrifices by reaping opportunities in education, by gaining a bachelor of social work (honors), a postgraduate diploma in social sciences, and a master's in philosophy in social policy.

As a result of my qualifications, I have been able to contribute to the wider Pacific Island community in New Zealand. I am the founder of Affirming Women (AW) Ltd, a social service agency based in South Auckland that employs a group of vibrant young men and women to deliver a Pacific worldview of mentoring and education to children and young people. I have had the privilege of representing Pacific youth issues in many areas, such as the Pacific Youth Court Community Liaison Panel in Manukau, and regional and national Pacific mentoring roles.

Pacific peoples from many islands have made the journey of migration to New Zealand. Despite the differing traditional social structures among diverse Pasifika cultures, these provide a common basis for Pasifika people's sense of collective identity. In Auckland, sometimes called the largest Polynesian city in the world, the Pacific population comprises many different ethnicities. The five major ethnic groups that are scattered among the population of Auckland are Samoans, Cook Islanders, Tongans, Niueans, and Tokelauans. Smaller Pasifika groups include Fijians, Tuvaluans, Tahitians, and Kiribatis. Within this large Pasifika population, almost 60 percent are New Zealand–born (Statistics New Zealand, 2002).

In an effort to assist their development and self-determination, the New Zealand government has resourced the settlement of Pasifika families since they began to migrate to the country fifty years ago. Today, the Pasifika population in this nation is particularly young. The median age for Pasifika peoples is 21 years, compared to 35 years for the national population. Almost one-quarter of all Pasifika peoples in New Zealand are between 12 and 24 years old, with an even larger percentage in the 0- to 11-year-old age range.

Statistics concerning Pasifika people also clearly identify slow but steady progress in addressing the inequalities of educational background that immigrants experience. Due to the high birth rate, the number of Pasifika children entering the compulsory school system continues to rise, and as well, Pasifika young people are staying longer in secondary education. The number of Pasifika students in tertiary education is also increasing. However, the proportion of Pasifika graduates with a university degree is still considerably lower than the national figure. In general, such statistical information highlights that Pasifika people are no longer just visitors in this land, but a significant and established part of the population of New Zealand.

The effects of migration have infiltrated all aspects of the life of Pasifika young people, even as they seek wellbeing and holistic development (mind, spirit, body, and family relationships) in their growth toward adulthood. Inherent in Pacific thinking is the belief that an individual is born to become useful for his or her family, community, and country. It is imperative, therefore, for Pasifika young people to undertake a process of acquiring a constructive self- and communal identity in order to achieve adulthood. This quest indicates the importance of mentoring for Pasifika youth, and more specifically, of Pasifika people's mentoring their own young toward a secure and prosperous future.

Searching for the Pacific Self

Reflecting on my own development through adolescence, as both a New Zealand–born and ethnically mixed woman, I have realized that as I have become more mature, I increasingly cringe at the many external influences that attempt to define me as a "this" or a "that." I now believe I have the right to determine, and to live out, what I believe to be my true self.

Self-truth, self-choice, and self-development are the foundations of a person's self-identity. Even though I come from a communally defined culture, I deliberately and consciously use the word *self.* Each of us, whether Pasifika or pālagi, searches for a self within the context of our nation, community, and family. As a Pasifika woman living in New Zealand, I have learned to journey through a global world, using the strengths that come from my culture as protective factors that allow me to live resiliently.

My self-identity began as a young girl growing up in the Auckland suburb of Mangere and attending an English-speaking, predominantly Pacific Island church. The dominant cultures within the congregation included my own Tongan culture. As a child, the pride of my Tongan identity was reinforced in my relationship with my parents and among those like them. They taught me to unashamedly identify myself as a product of Tongan communality and as a descendant of the Pacific's oldest kingdom. My Tongan pride, undergirded by parental support, inspired me to represent Tonga in sport and cultural performances, and to remain involved in youth groups and Tongan festivals. My identity as a Tongan in these social contexts has grounded me. Being accepted within these groups has given me a sense of belonging—first to my immediate family, in particular to my parents, and then to those with whom I celebrate life.

In a multicultural society, each person tends to identify with one of the particular ethnicities within that cultural mix; this is sometimes termed *aspired identity* (Bovens, 1995). I have spent my life so far trying to contribute to my own aspired identity by working in education, counseling, lecturing in Tonga, completing a book on Tongan history, mastering my native language, and investing myself in Tongan youth groups. These involvements neither increase nor decrease my biological Tonganness, nor do they wipe out the importance of the less obvious ethnicities that I carry biologically—my Māori, Samoan, and pālagi inheritance. The richness of my personal journey and my infectious passion for community development serve as an acknowledgment and response to the various cultures I carry in my body and my heart.

Not until I was in high school did it come to my attention that my grandmother, whom I love deeply and for whom I am named, was of another culture. My grandmother is a wonderful woman and it was through my relationship with her that I learned to love the members of my Samoan family. Then later, I became aware that my paternal and maternal lineages included Māori and pālagi ethnicities, in addition to my grandmother's Samoanness. My heart has extended its love to the cultures that I aspired to know, in addition to my Tongan ancestry. My inheritance is an eclectic cultural wealth that is also part of my identity. The personal expressions of love from family members extended the territory in which I found my sense of belonging.

That territory was further expanded through my university studies, as I learned more about appreciating the cultural diversity I embody. As a social work practitioner, I applied the theories I had learned in my training to the communities that I felt connected with through my own diverse lineage. However, my inherent Tongan environment and upbringing meant that my cultural Tonganness overrode the uniqueness of the smaller ethnic influences in my life, at the same time complementing them. And of course, I am a young resident of New Zealand's major urban center, so part of my identity is shaped by twenty-first-century technology, including cell phones, text-, photo-, and video-messaging, mini-discs, and DVDs. As I followed my own journey through this exciting, but sometimes confusing, mix, I became increasingly aware of how much I and others like me could be helped by some sort of mentoring system.

Mentoring Pasifika Migrants

Pasifika people, motivated by concern for the next generation, migrate to Western countries with the desire to achieve a higher living standard. But first-generation New Zealanders need assistance in understanding what it means to live as an ethnic minority, and their parents, who may see their cultural identity and traditions jeopardized, need New Zealand–born mentors who can provide culturally appropriate support. A developing Pasifika generation needs to know how to navigate two worlds and two sets of expectations—the pālagi one and the Pasifika one. We need to know when and how to function well in Western systems, and when and how to submit to the timeless cultural standards that our parents personify.

I believe that appropriate mentoring for Pasifika young adults must be structured around four values: lifestyle-led, family-oriented, community-contributed, and culturally encouraged. I identified these four values by examining my own cultural journey toward self and holism. In a *lifestyle-led* program, mentors must believe in the practice delivered—walking the talk—because they themselves are initially setting examples by role modeling their expectations for mentees. *Family-oriented* highlights the importance of a sense of belonging to the collective, including the wider extended family, while *community-contributed* gives the young adult or mentee the opportunity to grow responsibly within, and in relationship to, her or his own community and nation. *Culturally encouraged* means that appropriate Pasifika mentoring assumes that, in the absence of a mentor, the mentee's culture will continue to provide protection that encourages sustained development and a sense of resiliency.

In addition to the values of a structured program, mentoring within the Pasifika context involves the willingness to learn through the observation of cultural values. It is the universally shared Pasifika principles of support, love, humility, and respect that motivate Pasifika families. Our parents teach us these principles, which develop in us as attributes as we grow into adulthood. Traditionally, it is within this large family and community collectiveness that we as Pasifika people are mentored. I understand this effect from the experiences of my own life and the various choices I have made. My choices are never a reflection of myself alone, and neither are the consequences. My parents and family are never isolated from what I do, as they have always been the backbone of every decision I have made.

Maintaining a cultural and communal identity as an ethnic minority among a pālagi majority is an ongoing challenge. Pālagi culture seems to expect a great deal from us, at the same time that it misunderstands us. As

Pasifika people, we share commonalities that set us apart, such as our religious and family beliefs, our identification with culture, our inherently collective response, and our shared history of migration. We have also attempted to import the values and principles found in our home cultures to New Zealand, in order to keep our families healthy. The pālagi majority seems to expect that we should have left part of ourselves and our culture back in the islands, making sacrifices so that our children could fit in. Despite the impact of migration and colonization, however, it is clear that we have established systems within our communities that support and maintain our development and culture in the midst of our inherited status as migrants.

A significant support for Pasifika people as migrants in a new land has been the church, acting as a safe place for people to be uniquely Pacific. As the hub of the Pasifika community, the church is often referred to as the mirror reflection of village life back in the islands. The church is a place that breeds Pacific ownership, both through financial growth in buildings and assets, as well as models of organizational capacity and decision making. The church is a place where our language is taught, our people accepted and acknowledged, and our indigenous styles of leadership validated.

Mentoring through Affirming Works

In order to support young Pasifika adults as they move forward toward resilience and holistic wellbeing, Affirming Works was developed as a vehicle to transport Pasifika principles, through the process of mentoring, into mainstream organizations. Affirming Works is a registered company that I began four years ago as a result of my own exploration of my self-cultural-communal identity. It is a social service company that specializes in the provision of mentoring and education by delivering wellbeing programs from a Pasifika perspective, but designed for all cultures. We have successfully created, developed, and implemented a variety of unique educational mentoring programs in many schools in the Auckland area.

Affirming Works is characterized by the shared enthusiasm of young, vibrant Pasifika people who seek to contribute to their community. Although the team is newly created, the members bring with them solid qualifications and experience as youth service providers and community workers within the Auckland region, as well as sound knowledge of other existing networks.

Positive role models who are representative of diverse Pasifika groups show others how it is possible to succeed, thus counteracting pervasive negative stereotypes created by the media or pālagi racism. By matching younger people with successful adult members of the same group, role models will have a specific impact on the mentees' cultural identity and aspiration levels (Evans & Ave, 2000). When built on trust and mutual esteem, mentoring involves more than just dialogue; mentors teach actively, through role modeling and demonstration. The aim of mentoring is holistic personal development. As benefits are transferred from the mentor, the mentee becomes empowered.

While mentoring in Western cultures is often conceived as an individual, one-to-one relationship, we do not deem such a model to be appropriate or effective in dealing with young Pasifika adults. Cultural empowerment is an important goal in mentoring these young adults, as is family trust. Pasifika people may be suspicious of individual mentoring outside the family, especially if the mentor does not reflect the same values and beliefs as the mentee's family. A conflict of values and beliefs between mentor and mentee has also proven to be quite confusing for the young adults involved.

To address the need for culturally matched and culturally appropriate mentoring, Affirming Works has developed a model known as the Collective Model of Mentoring. This model has been structured to embrace a young person's collective way of life, which is an integral part of fostering the holistic development of any young person, irrespective of ethnicity. Through the Collective Model of Mentoring, mentors have the potential to influence and engage young people in their own environments.

This model is collective, in that mentees are held in a secure package of support as they grow. Above the mentee stand the upward mentors, that is, the Affirming Works staff, who assess the needs of the mentee and organize encouragements and activities designed to bring into fullness the talents and skills inherent, but underdeveloped, in the mentee. The Affirming Works mentor provides the scaffolding for peer mentoring to be established through peer activities, that is, how peers in the program can

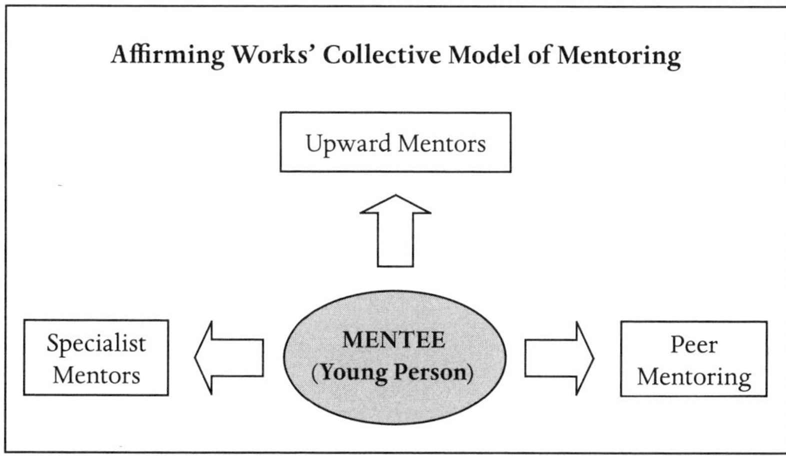

learn to exercise specific leadership skills. On the other side stand various specialist mentors, that is, support people called in to meet some specific need of the mentee, such as a psychologist or a social worker, or perhaps a rugby or public speaking coach. The following case study illustrates the way in which the program works.

A CASE ILLUSTRATION

Sala is a young woman of joint Samoan and pālagi heritage, who has found a way forward for herself through Affirming Works. Sala was identified by her school as being at risk, due to noncompliant behavior displayed both in and outside the classroom. Too quick to share her own opinions, Sala found it difficult to interact with others in the program. However, with the support of her mentors and close friends, Sala completed two more years of high school.

When Sala was initially assessed by her mentors at Affirming Works, these were some of the identified challenges she faced:

- Sala spoke to mentors about her disengaged relationship with her mother. Frequent heated arguments between them often resulted in her staying at other people's homes.
- Sala tended to argue with teachers or other school staff. What frustrated her most were those school staff who encouraged her to leave school, and indeed, eventually she was suspended.
- Sala showed signs of depression and suicidal ideation. The Affirming Works social worker supported her as a specialist mentor.
- Sala was associated with gangs (because of the involvement of some of her cousins), and on occasion had displayed volatile behavior by fighting. Sala was assaulted two or three times by members of other gangs, both male and female.
- Sala exhibited signs of substance abuse, and had easy access to drugs and alcohol.
- Sala was half-caste and beautiful (she worked part-time as a fashion model). She was sometimes the brunt of ridicule and had been accused by female peers of trying to steal someone's boyfriend. At parties or school events, Sala was approached by girls she did not know, wanting to fight her.
- Sala crashed her parents' car and was made to complete hours of community service as part of her sentencing.
- Sala had an acrimonious disagreement with her best friend, after which they did not speak to each other for almost a year.

In her first two years of mentoring, Sala was in Affirming Works' Tupu'anga (Origins) program. Tupu'anga is our three-tier model for mentoring students in their last three years of high school. The overall program is constructed to ensure that it aligns with the specific focus and objectives of each year level, as follows:

Year 11 (Sophomore): Vision and Engagement—Holistic personal development, learning tools to effectively engage in their academic environment, and the setting of personal goals.

Year 12 (Junior): Careers and Leadership—Development of leadership skills through initiating, organizing, and implementing activities in their community. Students formulate and develop their post-school transition plans.

Year 13 (Senior): Ambassadors—Students continue to develop and follow through with their post-school transition plans. Students exercise leadership in their school, family, and community, and also have the opportunity to act as ambassadors for their cultures and nations.

Given the multiple and complex issues with which Sala struggled, it clearly would be difficult for her to remain in a mainstream school. Yet even after she was suspended from school, she continued to access support from Affirming Works, and decided to attend our incubator-mentoring transition program, called Bounce Higher.

Bounce Higher is a thirteen-week pre-mentoring program founded on the principle of resiliency, and seeks to teach students how to use their own strengths. A transitional plan forms the pathway into further education or employment. Its sister program, Bounce High, is designed to assist youth ages 16–18 with low qualifications, who have left school and are in need of support to further their transition into employment or higher educational opportunities. Each student is encouraged to set personal goals toward further education or employment. Identifying potential barriers to personal success and creating plans of action to deal with such barriers emphasize an integral resiliency skill. Students are actively monitored by their Affirming Works mentors to implement their individual plan, focusing on their short- and long-term goals.

There are many other ways in which Affirming Work promotes the well-being of youth. We believe that all our programs are reflected accurately in our agency's mission statement: "to empower young people to reach their full potential in life."

The culturally appropriate mentoring that Sala received from Affirming Work eventually supported Sala in achieving the following results:

- Sala earned high academic marks.
- She reached the final year in her high school education. Unfortunately, early in the year, Sala dropped out of school, unable to cope with the many conflicts that were affecting her, including falling

out with her best friend. However, drawing on her newfound sense of resilience, Sala decided to give school one more try, and so re-enrolled. Sala's successful acceptance was supported by a staff member who believed in her potential. Despite her attempts, Sala was unable to complete the year.

- Upon leaving high school, Sala enrolled in Bounce Higher to assist her transition into either further study or employment. When she did not receive high enough marks in the national educational achievement exams, Sala revised her options and decided to apply to the New Zealand army. While awaiting a response to her application, Sala showed growth and personal development by undertaking a fitness program, including running in the mornings and cutting down on smoking. Unfortunately, her application was declined for health reasons.
- She reduced her consumption of alcohol and use of drugs.
- She stopped self-harming.
- Sala's self-worth and self-esteem increased, and she became more confident in her abilities and skills, not wanting to stay idle. Bounce Higher helped Sala explore other possible career pathways. Eventually, Sala was able to put a resume together and begin the search for employment. After a successful interview, Sala was offered a job as a retail assistant at a local mall. Soon after, Sala was offered a promotion to the role of assistant manager. Obtaining employment meant that she could begin paying back her parents, which was one of her personal goals.
- Sala's court-ordered hours of community work were completed at Affirming Works, including cleaning, administrative duties, and opportunities to share her own personal journey with students currently in school.

Through the many challenges she has faced, Sala's self-esteem and confidence has developed. She is a very resilient young lady, who continues to remain employed at the retail store. Sala has begun to consider traveling abroad to Europe, and has decided not to settle for anything less than her best. Traveling to unfamiliar surroundings and meeting new people would demonstrate Sala's confidence as she continues to pursue her personal goals. Sala's most recent milestones were the purchase of a new car, a trip to Tonga, and the consolidation of her debt to her parents.

Conclusion

Affirming Works promotes an environment that is culturally safe and appropriate, interactive, enjoyable, and professional. This collective approach to learning is responsive to client needs. The youthfulness of the Affirming Works staff allows for natural relationships to form; as well, the knowledge of culture-specific protocols facilitates parental involvement in the program. Affirming Works encourages family meetings, and since most of the staff members speak a Pasifika language, Affirming Works is able to overcome language barriers that students' parents might otherwise encounter.

Furthermore, working cooperatively with the major tertiary providers in Auckland allows students in the Bounce Higher and Tupu'anga programs to be exposed to higher academic organizations and networking opportunities. During our program's camps, various tertiary providers, career services, and training organizations have the opportunity to meet with us and provide workshops or expos to further engage students in positive transitioning pathways, community responsibility, and business shadowing.

Positive pathways and transitions encourage Pasifika young people to remain in school so as to further their education, and subsequently strive for better employment, in turn resulting in less dependency on state benefits. Successful transitions for Pasifika youth will shape the changing face of New Zealand's future for our people. By mentoring individuals who are claiming a cultural identity, a self-identity, and a true identity, we can contribute to an effective and resilient communal identity for young people who desire to find and improve themselves. Successful individuals contagiously affect their peers, and that in turn promises a better future for us all.

References

Bovens, L. (1995). The intentional acquisition of mental states. *Philosophy and Phenomenological Research, 55*(4), 821–840.

Evans, I., & Ave, K. (2000). Mentoring children and youth: Principles, issues, and policy implications for community programmes in New Zealand. *New Zealand Journal of Psychology, 29*(1), 41–49.

Ministry of Pacific Island Affairs. (2003). *Ala fou, new pathways: Strategic directions for Pacific youth in New Zealand.* Wellington: Author.

Statistics New Zealand. (2002). *Pacific progress report: Report on the economic status of Pacific Peoples in New Zealand.* Wellington: Ministry of Pacific Island Affairs and Statistics New Zealand.

3

Canoe Noses and Coconut Feet

Reading the Samoan Male Body

TAVITA T. MALIKO

My mother gave birth to ten children. The first three died within a month of their births. The firstborn was a girl, who died at one month; the second a twin boy, born on Sunday, and a girl, born on Wednesday, both of whom passed away at age one-and-a-half weeks. Mom hadn't even known there was another twin coming until the second one arrived. She went into labor seven more times, and all survived. The second to last was another set of twins, both girls. Of these ten, I am number five, but the second-born of the surviving kids.

I commented to Mom the other day, "You must have been doing too much work in the latter days of your first pregnancy." Her reply was devastating. I saw a tired, heavily pregnant woman with a big load on her back, walking the whole three miles from the plantation in the rain. She went into labor for the first time the next day. My heart was broken; it still is.

My parents. I see their joy and their pain, their laughter and their tears. I hear their pain in their voices, and I see it in their eyes. It is written on the wrinkles of their aging bodies. I see it every day.

I am a Samoan-born male who completed the four-year training at Malua Theological College in Samoa, to be a minister in the Samoan Congregational Church. I moved to New Zealand, where I completed my bachelor's of theology and master's of theology (first-class honors) at the University of Auckland. I am now preparing to do my PhD, after spending four years in the workforce.

> Using a new machete / he follows the old tracks / to a not so distant past / meeting his ancestors along the way / capturing them on canvas / mapping out their stories / so they will never be lost / and his own children / will be able to find them. (Mila, 2005, p. 16)

Niko Besnier (1994) comments upon the fusion of Christianity and cultural traditions in Pasifika:

> For many contemporary Pacific peoples, Christianity and "tradition" are so embroiled with one another that they have become the same in certain areas

> . . . As a result, many social formations and cultural processes in the Pacific cannot be successfully understood without reference to the Christian context in which they are embedded, and, in turn, Christianity in the region can only be studied in tandem with society and culture. (p. 339)

Though Besnier is writing about Nukulaelae atoll in Tuvalu, his observation is true of most Pacific nations today. It is therefore essential to begin this essay by revisiting the social constructs, attitudes, and values imposed upon Samoans by the missionaries who first brought Christianity to the Pacific. Contemporary Samoan understandings of the male (and female) body are a result of their colonized and racialized bodies, or what Albert Wendt (1999) calls the postcolonial body. Deconstruction of the Samoan male body therefore also means uncovering the beholder whose gaze and values helped fashion and reshape our bodies into their present traditional and religious ideal form.

The White Man's Gaze

When European missionaries arrived in Samoa, they were shocked to discover the sensual nature and practices of the Samoans, including their natural state of undress. Turner (1884), a Wesleyan missionary who began working in Samoa in 1841, wrote in his diary:

> During the day a covering of ti leaves (*Draccena terminalis*) was all that either sex thought necessary. They sewed ti leaves together, and made themselves an apron. The men had small ones about a foot square, the women had theirs made of longer ti leaves, reaching from the waist down below the knee, and made wide so as to make a girdle covering all round. They had no regular covering for any other part of the body. (p. 118)

Missionary John Stair was even more frank: "Both sexes, but frequently the males, appeared in little better than a state of nudity, whilst all children went entirely unclothed until ten or twelve years of age" (1897, p. 113).

The early missionaries were scandalized by what they judged to be the evil heathen immodesty of the Samoans. The missionaries undertook to change the way of life of the islands' local people. The near-nakedness of the Samoans was a major concern to the missionaries, and they saw clothing the Islanders' nakedness as a starting point of their mission. Yet contemporary Samoan author Albert Wendt (1999) correctly points out that the Samoan concept of "being clothed (*lavalava*) had little to do with clothes or *laei*. In pre-pālagi times, to wear nothing above the navel was not considered 'nakedness.' To 'clothe' one's arse and genitals were enough" (p. 400).

The Racialized Body

As early as the fifteenth century, Portuguese historian Gomes Eannes de Azurara provided theological justification for the enslavement of Africans by Europeans (Raboteau, 1996). The biblical figure of Ham, Noah's son who discovered his father drunk and naked, was punished with the curse that his descendants would have dark skin. Gunson (1978) notes that these racist arguments also found a welcome in the Pacific. Particularly strong comment was directed against the Fijians who, as Melanesians, have quite dark skin; Samoans, as lighter-skinned Polynesians, were spared the most intense condemnation, but their bodies were racialized nonetheless. As Gunson (1978) writes:

> Despite the fact that the Evangelical Missionary Societies were foremost in the ranks of those who sought to end the slave trade, a view persisted that the darker races were of inferior stock and somewhat less than brothers . . . Certain traits and popular racial prejudices were kept alive by the missionaries themselves, some simply due to color consciousness, but others due to the various arguments which asserted the superiority of the white races. (p. 200)

Their social doctrine of the cross was to transform people to live like Europeans. As missionary John Williams wrote, when planning a spacious house for himself and his family in Samoa, "The missionary does not go to barbarize himself, but to elevate the heathen; not to sink himself to their standard, but to raise them to his" (Gutch, 1974, p. 19).

The Body, Colonized and Resistant

The missionaries' attempt to annihilate traditional Samoan custom was successful in many ways. Gilson (1970) describes the missionaries' objective as

> to Christianize the law of the land—to ban the activities and relationships, social and personal, that by mission standards were immoral or tainted with "heathenism" associations, and to prescribe the ethics and conventions of puritanism . . . the prohibition of obscenity in word and action; the imposition of new standards of dress, including "full coverage" for women and, when at worship, shorts or coats for men, but not shoes for either; the adoption of hair styles "appropriate" to the individual's sex, meaning long for women and short for men, the reverse of traditional styles. (p. 96)

Unquestioningly, most Samoans believe that we have always lived that way.

In Samoa's hot climate, it is customary to see men with their naked upper bodies at work, at play, fishing, and the like, except at church or during family devotional services. Every village in Samoa has some kind of curfew after sunset that lasts from twenty to thirty minutes for evening household devotions. During the brief curfew, every male person dons a shirt or singlet—just for the duration of the devotion. If a man does not have a shirt at hand, he will ask for a *lavalava*, a towel, a sheet, or anything he can use to cover his upper body or his back. Men who have been roaming outside the house will rush in to do the same. After the service they peel off these coverings so as to feel the evening breeze once again.

A Samoan *matai* (chief) who takes the floor to speak on behalf of others in the open *malae* is obliged to remove his shirt before he speaks; it is most disrespectful not to do so. This traditional speech is called the *lāuga*. Ironically, the pastor's Sunday sermon is also called the lāuga, but for the performance of this pastoral duty, the minister's body must be covered, usually in white clothing. The implied message is that God does not want to see the human body, though it was created "in His image" (see Eilberg-Schwartz, 1997).

Today in Samoa, as in most Pacific Island countries, a suit that covers most of the body is considered the only appropriate way of dressing for men during church services, despite the heat being unbearable in a closed-in church in a tropical climate. This is a clothing standard imported by the Victorian missionaries, but now deeply engraved upon Samoan church protocol. Church services can be miserably hot for ministers and worshippers alike.

Despite the missionaries' efforts, pockets of Samoan culture still resist the covering of the body with clothing. For example, during traditional entertainment, men expose their upper bodies and most parts of their legs. Missionaries were also unable to stop traditional tattooing for both men and women, yet today, both the Congregational and the Methodist churches in Samoa still exclude tattooed congregants from partaking in holy communion as punishment for "having spilled blood."

I remember an incident from my village in the early 1970s. More than a hundred people were in church that day and one matai had worn a new blue long-sleeve shirt with a tie. The minister condemned him from the pulpit for wearing blue when everybody was expected to wear white. I now interpret the minister as saying that one was not acceptable before God if one did not cover up one's black skin with white clothing. This is what we learned from the missionaries.

The Mythological Body

According to Samoan mythology, Nāfanua, born as a clot of blood, grew up to become a woman warrior of extraordinary prowess. She was sent by her parents to avenge the suffering of her people in the village of Faleālupo.

She slaughtered everyone in her path, pursuing the enemy fifteen miles to the west of the island. When the battle reached a certain place called *o le pā i Fualaga*, the wind blew up her top, exposing her breasts. The retreating men realized that she was a woman, after all, and felt greatly shamed. At that very moment, the battle ended, apparently because no man wanted to fight anymore. Today that place is called *o le malae o le ma* (the field of shame), for there a woman shamed men. Today, the field of shame is a warning to any man defeated or subordinated by a woman, in whatever sphere of life, and this theme of the shame of men echoes time and again whenever the myth is retold.

Between my own village of Asau and another, Aopo, sit two huge rocks, said to be the bodies of Si-Āsau and Si-Āʻopo (a man from Āsau and another from Āʻopo). These two men were to decide the boundary between their respective villages, situated next to each other. They agreed that each was to sleep in his own village and in the morning they would walk toward each other; their meeting point was to be the boundary between the two villages. When they met the following morning they fought, each pushing the boundary farther from his homeland. Eventually, they murdered each other, and turned into the two rocks that lie side by side. This landmark is still the boundary of the two villages today.

Si-Āsau and Si-Āʻopo literally put their bodies on the line for the sake of their heirs for many generations in the future. Their stone bodies marked their own respective piece of the earth, which will belong to their children and their future generations.

Traditional Samoans believed in body theism. A god could, therefore, be found in any form or shape, be it a fish, tree, rock, bird, or whatever. These were not abstract gods; each had a body and was found within the realm and life cycle of human existence and understanding. The traditional gods were embodied and celebrated in Samoan arts and life rituals, as gods whose biological sex or gender made no difference, and in the totality of whose bodies, in all shapes, forms, and colors, Samoans found comfort. This stands in great contrast to the invisible Christian God, who was portrayed to Samoans as having a male body.

The Gendered Body

Discussions of the body in any culture cannot escape the necessity of defining sexual assignment and gender identity via ideals of masculinity and femininity. One basic definition is presented in Suaʻaliʻi (2001):

> Sex refers to the biological or physiological make-up of a person, determinable at birth through recognition of male or female genitals. The sex of a newborn child is established by locating, either before or at birth, the child's genitals. The child is then "labeled" male or female. (p. 161)

Old Samoan traditions reflected sexual assignment symbolically:

> If the little stranger was a boy, the umbilical cord was cut on a club that he might grow up to be brave in war. If of the other sex, it was done on the board on which they beat out the bark of which they make their native cloth. Cloth-making is the work of women; and their wish was that the little girl should grow up and prove useful to the family in her proper occupation. (Turner, 1884, p. 79)

Gender identity in Samoan culture, based on social role, must be carefully distinguished from sexual assignment, which is based solely on biology. Sua'ali'i (2001) continues: "Gender, on the other hand, is established by non-biological factors: those psychological, social and cultural factors imposed by society on the male or female person/personality" (p. 161). Samoan culture has at least three genders: masculine, feminine, and *fa'afāfine*. In general, only two genders are assigned, corresponding with genital configuration, but a third gender—fa'afāfine—may emerge in the course of child or adolescent development. Research also indicates that once gender is assigned at birth, it is defined and reinforced primarily by culturally sanctioned roles, as well as by status, rank, and what are understood to be traditional cultural values (the *fa'a-Samoa*, the Samoan way of life). For example, the titles given to wives of matais dictate their respective roles in the community: *faletua* and *tausi*. A faletua is the wife of the sacred high chief (*ali'i*), while a tausi is the wife of the more secular talking chief (*tulāfale*). Faletua means "house at the back." It is said that no matai can function well without a *tautua* (servant) and, likewise, no front house exists without a house at the back. Two meanings are encompassed in the title faletua: one is that the wife serves the male ali'i (who resides at the house at the front) from the back, and second, the ali'i depends entirely upon his wife for his well-being and to make sure that he carries out his duties properly. Tausi, on the other hand, literally means "to nurture." The tausi's task is to nurture her husband (tulafāle).

According to Mirsky (1996):

> All masculinities share two central components: the negatively defining characteristics of being not feminine, or like woman; and the positively defining characteristics of having more power (social, physical, cosmic and so forth) than that which is feminine, or women. (Femininity and women are conflated in this understanding, because that is exactly how the patriarchal structuring of gender functions). (p. 31)

Any binary gender construction traps both men and women in rigid roles, so that neither has adequate opportunity to freely explore the boundaries of their assigned gender role without social discrimination.

These scripted behaviors and gendered relationships are embodied within much of the Samoan culture, including the matai (chiefly) system. The majority of matais are men; in my own village, there are over three hundred matais, and not a single female matai. The village of 'Iva on the island of Savai'i prohibits the conferring of chiefly titles upon women. In such a setting, it is easy to tell a woman to shut up when men talk, especially in village and church political affairs and in the decision-making processes. Hence women's voices are filtered through the tight funnel of their husbands and fathers, who make the rules.

The Tattooed Body

The tattoo is one of the most obvious sites of resistance to colonization. Despite attempts by missionaries to stop traditional tattooing, it has survived as an important part of Samoan culture. The origin of the Samoan tattoo is told in the traditional myth of the twin sisters Taemā and Tilafaigā (Tilafaigā is Nāfanua's mother), who swam all the way from Fiji, bringing with them the *'ato au* (bag of instruments for making the tattoo). As they swam, they sang their song: *E tatā o fafine ae le tatā o tane* (the women will be tattooed but the men will not). As they neared the reef of the village of Faleālupo, they spotted a huge *faisua* (clam) on the sea bed, so they dived down to get it. When they reemerged, the men and women had switched gender in the song, thus reversing who was to be tattooed. Their new song became: *E tatā o tane ae le tatā o fafine* (the men will be tattooed but the women will not).

Tattooing is an extremely painful experience, and pain is often associated with manliness. It is commonly said that a Samoan man is not really a man without a tattoo. But it must be remembered that the tattoo was brought to Samoa by women, and given by women to men. On the other hand, the word *faisua* (clam) is often a slang synonym for the word *vagina*. In the myth, the faisua is the very object that generated the reversal of the lyrics from tattooing women to tattooing men. Samoa, known by European merchants as the Navigator Islands, is home to many myths about skilled men navigating the Pacific. In this myth, the twin sisters were even better navigators—they surpassed the men by swimming to Fiji and back, a feat never before achieved by a man. But all this came to nothing because of the faisua. Their diving down to the faisua symbolizes their fatal weakness: because they possessed the faisua (vagina), they were not good enough to possess the tattoo, and it became attached to masculine socially constructed ideals.

People look at the tattoo with pride and admiration. It is a mark of endurance and manly beauty. As a public symbol, it must be exhibited for others to see; it serves no private purpose. All these associations with the tattoo are also characteristic of masculinity and patriarchal cultures.

Samoan young men are supposed to have a traditional tattoo that runs from the upper part of the stomach and lower back, down to below their knees. To display their tattoos, men wear their lavalava dropped below the waist and gathered above the knees. It is often said that a man is no man without a tattoo. Turner (1884) explains:

> Until a young man was tattooed, he was considered in his minority. He could not think of marriage, and he was constantly exposed to taunts and ridicule . . . as having no right to speak in the society of men. But as soon as he was tattooed he passed into his majority, and considered himself entitled to the respect and privileges of mature years. (p. 88)

Reading My Own Body

Turner (1884) gives a glimpse into the beautifying of newly born Samoan children in the early nineteenth century:

> During the first two or three days the nurse bestowed great attention to the head of the child, that it might be modified and shaped after notions of propriety and beauty. The child was laid on its back, and the head surrounded with three flat stones. One was placed close to the crown of the head, and one on either side. The forehead was then pressed with the hand, that it might be flattened. Our [European] "canoe noses," as they call them, are blemishes in their estimation. (pp. 79–80)

A newly built canoe is sharp in the nose area as opposed to an old canoe, whose nose is flattened, worn out, and hammered from years of work and service to the family and community. Instead of plastic surgery, newborns receive a gentle massage, a little push, and some guidance in the right direction, so that from an early age, they conform to the Samoan construction of beauty. They do not remain newborns for long: whether male or female, they are already being fashioned to perform specific tasks in the life of the community.

In my younger years I played flanker, a position that requires speed, in two schools' leading rugby teams. But I was not a speedster; I have wide feet, and short legs that resemble those of Alfy Langer, the Australian Rugby League player, or of Taufusi Salesa, perhaps the most locally famous Samoan rugby player. Mine are the kind of legs that seem twisted inwards from the knees down, each eye-balling the other as if in constant confrontation. But for both Langer and Salesa, this particular leg formation has generated the magic that has won matches, and team mates and whole countries have come to rely on such unattractive legs for victory. Their legs and feet have not only left marks on the playing field, but on the whole sports world. Their legs and bodies have been their passport to success and to seeing the world. Such feet have established for them a particularly superior personal identity.

My feet have not had the same success on the sports field, yet they bear the history of my own life. I look at Samoan women and town boys; they do not have wide feet as I do. I guess my feet adapted themselves to my way of life. I grew up in a country village far away from town, hardly ever wearing shoes. At least three times a week, I would walk or run five miles up the mountain to the plantation, do some eight hours' work there, then walk another five miles back to the village with a huge load of foodstuffs on my shoulders that at times more than doubled my body weight. I had to develop wide feet to anchor my frame while walking long distances.

I had mastered the art of coconut climbing by age 10. I would climb two hundred-foot coconut trees, with bare hands and feet as if I were running on the beach, even on windy days when the tall thin trees would sway at least six feet from side to side. It felt like swinging on a kindergarten swing. I had no fear at all, because I had reliable wide feet, coconut feet, which had centimeter-thick calluses from years of walking barefoot, and a good strong pair of hands. I could smell the strength of the wind, which informed me when I was in danger; hence I knew when to hold on tight. My chest used to bear the scratch marks of such climbing, for at times I would slip, and then grasp the coconut trunk tight for dear life's sake. My body had become accustomed to these tasks, so much so that my body's reflexes were faster than my mind's.

When I was a kid, one of our major activities was to swim in the many pools in our village. We boys would hang out with each other, and when we went for a swim, we would race to the pool, slowly undoing our lavalavas as we ran, throwing them to the side of the pool as we jumped in. We would swim or run around naked at the side of the pool, without a care in the world. Each boy would put a two-meter-long log in the water, then lie horizontally on top of the log, facing downwards, paddling about with both hands and feet. If someone followed behind one of these logs, one could clearly see the male testicles squashed against the log underneath the body weight. I even saw teenage boys riding logs in such a manner.

After one such swimming session, my older cousin deliberately took my lavalava from the side of the pool and left it two hundred meters from the pool—a childish way of shaming me, because I then had to walk naked all that way under the gaze of so many eyes. I chased him all the way home and hit him so hard with a rock that he never did it again. Why was I that angry? I remember well that I was not only angry; I was also ashamed to be seen naked outside the comfort zone of the pool area. I was over 10 years old then, and my older cousin, who apparently already knew the shame of nakedness, had a cruel way of teaching me this social taboo. At that age, it was all right to be seen naked around the pool, but not between the pool and home.

Before our village had access to tap water, everyone had to go to the pools for washing (there was another specific pool for drinking only). There was a pool for men only, another for women; the two pools were on either side of the main road, and people bathed mainly in the evening. Children were not allowed in the pool during the adults' evening time. Children had their turn during the day, bathing only in the women's pool. A shack was erected by the side of the pool, occupied by women who took turns not only watching over the children, but also enforcing the pool regulations, such as the specific bathing time for children. So the children's nakedness in the pool was made possible not only because they were by themselves most of the time, but also because the adults tolerated it. As soon as children left the pool, holding their lavalavas in their hands, the first adult they would meet would order them to cover up. Adults were teaching children to be ashamed of their naked bodies.

Early in life I got the message about what was expected of me as a person born with a penis. If I wasn't physically strong enough to do a particular task that was asked of me, my mother would say, "What a waste of that hanging thing [referring to my penis]! Had it been given to [my sister] it would have been more useful." I heard many other mothers say that to their young boys, and I must admit that I hated it then as much as I do now.

Children call each other names, and I was called a *fa'afāfine* (like a woman)—thankfully not by other children, but regrettably by my own immediate family. These are the wounds I still carry around within me that have shaped my relationship to women, and especially to gay men. Because I hated being labeled a fa'afāfine, I learned to keep as far away from that gender as possible, depriving myself of intimate friendships with men in general.

At age 20, I remember being in the back seat of a car with two other guys. We couldn't possibly sit comfortably, as our shoulders would push against each other's, so the guy in the middle (my very good friend) rested his extended arms on the two sets of shoulders on either side of him. It was the longest ride of my life because I was not enjoying this body contact with another man. I didn't say anything because I knew my friend to be a genuinely friendly guy, and I didn't want to hurt his feelings. I had played in the position of prop in rugby, where the hooker would extend his arms on my shoulders in exactly the same way. But that was rugby, where men have to bind together to form a stronger, purely physical oneness, and to tough it out, smashing against the opposite set of eight skulls. In any other setting, even shoulder rubbing is just not allowed.

I've learned within my own social, cultural, and religious context that men are not supposed to form any kind of bond with each other, physically or emotionally. This was part of a defensive stance, because to behave otherwise might entail humiliating consequences, such as confirmation that I was indeed a fa'afāfine. The overall result was that I was never in control of my own self or body; it was controlled by the hyper-masculinity of family, culture, society, and religion.

My mother and I went to see her family in another village. While we were there my cousin took me to the village pool where another kid my age was playing with those small crawling creatures that live within shells. This kid had short hair, just like mine, and as I talked to him, my cousin recoiled and waved at me to come. He whispered, "Didn't you know that that's a girl? She's not a boy; she's a girl!" and he laughed. I suppose my cousin was taking the same journey as I was: to be as far away from women as possible, in case we became feminized. A penis possessor was to be an almighty warrior, fearless, powerful, unyielding to pain, and certainly not anything like a woman. At this young age we already had tons of presumptions and prejudice about the opposite sex—the other—without knowing anything else about them. Yet, that other is the very body that embodied us for nine months and nurtured us all, whether male or female (Moltmann-Wendel, 1994, p. 103).

Final Words

These are some of the many theological, social, and cultural ideals that have isolated my own Samoan male body, as if it were something foreign to myself. This essay began with the missionaries' efforts to stamp out traditional forms of clothing, which celebrated the body in a more revealing and natural way. As in an Auckland nightclub, the body is the visual and concrete part of the Samoan dancer that makes the connection between the performer and the audience, or with other performers. The body is the site of communication, entertainment, and effective healing. At cultural gatherings and celebrations today, Samoan men take off their shirts; at worship they cover up their bodies, usually without questioning the reason. Such missionary-dominated cultural views of the body are deeply tattooed upon our real culture and traditions through the multigenerational process. Unfortunately, we now claim Victorian Christianity as our own, as the way Christianity should be, and as the way Samoan culture and traditions have always been. This confusion is not easy to untangle. Traditions have authority, cemented by religion, sanctioned by God—and who dares battle against such a combination?

These kinds of belief and the accepted devaluing of our bodies, as well as their multiple implications and consequences, have been taught and passed on throughout the history of humanity, and from one culture to another, so that today we are thickly clothed with multigenerational layers of disembodied bodies. We all bear the scars of our history; whether we like it or not, our bodies are shaped by, respond to, perform, and in one way or another, sustain the beliefs and actions deeply embedded within ourselves by family, culture, and religion.

This theological, social, and cultural heritage has inflicted deep wounds within our psychological, spiritual, and physical selves—multigenerational injustices that need to be corrected in order to heal our wounded beings. As a Samoan man, I have missed out on the richness of intimate relationships with many men and women—just because I am a man. Alienation of the body from our selves may be a foreign and transplanted concept, but it is now up to us to begin the healing, to reclaim our identity and values that celebrate our bodies as part of our selves. We must reclaim and celebrate our bodies in their unity and all their diversity of color and sexuality. We can only appreciate the other if we accept and appreciate our selves first, in our totality. As Elizabeth Moltmann-Wendel (1994) says:

> A theology of embodiment . . . seeks to give people once again the courage to use their senses, which atrophy in a rational culture, to stand by themselves and their experiences and accept themselves with their bodies, to love them, to trust them and their understanding, and to see themselves as children of this earth, indissolubly bound up with it. (p. 104)

We also must acknowledge that this is a long, bumpy road to travel. I know that whatever I am made of—body, soul, self, spirit, conscious and unconscious mind—the only reality I know about myself is my body. I can only express my emotions through my body; hence I can only relate and be in relation to other bodies and beings through my body and their bodies. I am satisfied that whatever shape or color that my body has, it can be faithful to my cultural and personal values. This body has served my family, village, church, and personal ambitions. Whatever is embodied in my body—visible or invisible—I know that I have a unique place in this world.

My body has matured now. It has lost the macho physique it once had, but it still bears the marks of my own history as a personal, cultural, and religious being. All that is embodied within my body is my self. I do not *have* a body; I *am* my body, created in the divine image of God, whom I glorify for my uniqueness.

References

Besnier, N. (1994). Christianity, authority, and personhood: Sermonic discourse on Nukulaelae Atoll. *The Journal of the Polynesian Society, 103*(4), 339–378.

Eilberg-Schwartz, H. (1997). The problem of the body for the people of the Book. In T. K. Beal & D. M. Gunn (Eds.), *Reading Bibles, writing bodies: Identity and the Book* (pp. 35–55). New York: Routledge.

Gilson, R. P. (1970). Samoa *1830 to 1900: The politics of a multi-cultural community*. London: Oxford University Press.
Gunson, N. (1978). *Messengers of grace*. Oxford: Oxford University Press.
Gutch, J. (1974). *Beyond the reefs: The life of John Williams, missionary*. London: Macdonald.
Mila, K. (2005). *Dream fish floating*. Wellington: Huia Publishers.
Mirsky, S. (1996). Three arguments for the elimination of masculinity. In Bjōrn Krondorfer (Ed.), *Men's bodies, men's gods* (pp. 27–39). New York: New York University Press.
Moltmann-Wendel, E. (1994). I *am my body: A theology of embodiment*. London: SCM Press.
Raboteau, A. J. (1996). *Slave religion: The invisible institution in the antebellum South*. Oxford: Oxford University Press.
Stair, J. B. (1897). *Old Samoa*. London: Religious Tract Society.
Sua'ali'i, T. M. (2001). Samoans and gender: Some reflections on male, female and fa'afafine gender identities. In C. Macpherson, P. Spoonley, & M. Anae (Eds.), *Tangata o te moana nui: The evolving identities of Pacific peoples in Aotearoa/New Zealand* (pp. 160–180). Palmerston North: Dunmore Press.
Turner, G. (1884). *Samoa: A hundred years ago and long before*. [London] Auckland: Southland Reprints.
Wendt, A. (1999). Afterword: Tatauing the post-colonial body. In V. Hereniko & R. Wilson (Eds.), *Inside out: Literature, cultural politics, and identity in the New Pacific* (pp. 399–412). Lanham: Rowman & Littlefield.

4
Jonah, Arnold, and Me
Reading the Tongan Male Body

MAIKA LUTUI

Mālō e lelei! *My name is Maika Lutui. I am 26 years old. I was brought up in the Kingdom of Tonga, on the island of Tongatapu in the village of Tofoa. I am the third of six children who belong to the family of Hainiala Lutui and Viliami Niulala Lutui of Tofoa. I have two older brothers (Kilisimasi and Aleki Uilisoni Lutui) and three little sisters (Mele Atilili, Emeline, and Fakavamoeatu he hakau Lutui).*

All my life I was raised in Tofoa on a little farm that my grandparents, Uluaki Tuai and Mele Atilili Tuai, had planted for our family needs. I did all my early studies in Tonga. I attended the Havelu Tofoa primary school; from there I went to Tonga College, and finished my secondary education at Tonga High School. In 2000 I entered Sia'atoutai Theological College, graduating in 2002 with a bachelor of divinity.

In 2003 I moved to New Zealand to further my studies. In 2004 I gained a graduate diploma in theology from Auckland University's School of Theology. Currently I am working on my master's of theology there. I wrote this essay for one of my master's courses, with the help of Philip Culbertson, and I am honored to contribute it to this book.

Exploring the social construction of the physical body is, for a Tongan, like being born into a whole new unknown world. I am a 26-year-old Tongan male, born and raised in Tonga all my life, until two years ago, when I moved to Auckland. In my whole life thus far, I have never been encouraged to think about my own body, even for a moment. I don't understand why; perhaps it is because the society I have grown up in did not allow me to think about my body. My mind and my soul, yes, but not my body. As I begin, I still do not understand why I am writing this essay. I still do not understand the meaning of this phrase: "I do not have a body, I AM my body" (Moltmann-Wendel, 1994).

How can I understand my male body within my Tongan culture? Reading my own body is a good starting point because I am a Tongan man. It should be able to tell me how I as a Tongan understand my body. But I do not know how to talk about any male body because I cannot read my own body, much less explain the phrase "I am my body." What does "I am" mean as a person growing up in a communal culture? How can I talk about men's bodies without women's bodies? I have been taught that, as a communal person, addressing both male and female bodies is the only way that will give me a clear picture of my physical, sexual, cultural, and spiritual identity.

I have faith, however, that Tongans need to see their bodies as they are, in order to help them in their journey in this world. In saying that—although this will challenge me—I know that I will have to go against the grain in order to articulate Tongan understandings of the physical body, and give voice to my own body.

Reading My Own Body

Trying to read my own body has been one of the hardest challenges I have undertaken in my life. To gain some insight, I asked my Tongan friend what he thought about his body. He did not give me an answer straight away. Instead, he answered me with another question: "What do you mean?" I asked my girlfriend (she is a Tongan) what she thought about her body and the same thing happened. She just smiled and laughed and said, "What do you mean?" I don't know why she smiled and laughed, but I am sure she was signaling me that she had no clue how to answer. Maybe no one does; in my research, I have found no Tongans in the past who have tried to read their own bodies. Perhaps they do not think about it. Perhaps I am the first Tongan ever who tried to see his own body.

My body includes two short big legs, two small ears, one nose, and a mouth. My upper body is full of muscle balance, while my lower body and my arms are big and full of muscles. This already tells a story about where I grew up. I grew up on a farm, where I left very early every morning to work on the family's plantation. This seems to confirm Morton's (1996) observation that "as soon as [Tongan] children can understand a request made of them they begin to 'work' and that before they are six" (p. 137). I helped my grandfather out while my father worked at the Tongan government post office. I was not supposed to stay in the house to help my mum because I have a male body. As I understand now, being born with a penis mandated my being at the plantation where the real man's work exists, in the eyes of Tongan culture.

In primary school I was one of the strongest-looking boys my age. This was because, as a rugby player, I was one of the hardest boys to put down during the game. Yet I don't remember ever being told, during that time, that I had a strong body. More often the praise I heard was that I was "a boy with a big heart." I do indeed have an inner self that contains no fear, as is expected from Tongan males. But this contrast indicates how we Tongans deny our bodies. In our society, everything concerns the mind and soul, not the physical body.

When I was a younger man in Tonga, I loved to watch videos. The body builder I most loved watching was Arnold Schwarzenegger. He had a huge body, full of muscles because of his hard work at the gym. I remember thinking that one day I would like to have his body. I did not understand why I wished to have someone else's body. Now I understand that all bodies are socially constructed—they are only the product of the limited way we can see ourselves and what we desire.

One day in my village in Tonga, my friends and I went for a swim at the village beach. Other children were already there enjoying themselves in the sea when we arrived. Suddenly I saw the boys swimming back to shore, trying to get out of the water as fast as they could. I wanted to know why. I thought there was a shark or something, so I called to my cousin, one of those in the sea, to ask what had happened. He just said, "Because girls are in the water, too!" I realized at that moment that these boys had grown up in the same environment as me. We were told to stay away from women. This indicates a culturally constructed sense of differentiation. I am a man; I was not going to be with women because I am more valuable than they. This is because I am not like women; I have a penis. At this young age I had already taken advantage of the opposite sex without knowing anything else about them. Yet the opposite sex is the body that embodied us for nine months, whether one is male or female.

How Other Tongans Read My Body

Fifteen years ago in Tonga I could run around naked in my house. At that time our family consisted of my parents, my two older brothers, and me. I never heard my parents comment on my nakedness as a little 5-year-old in our home. Five years later my twin sisters were born and, although they were still babies, their birth changed the way I behaved at home. I was not allowed to run around naked in the house; even half-naked was not acceptable. This is often referred to as *tapu* (forbidden) in Tonga. After that time, whenever I ran around naked, both my parents would shout at me to go put on some clothes. I did not understand why but the way they usually said it was: "Hurry up and put on some clothes. Can't you see that your sisters are here?" I silently questioned why I wasn't allowed to be naked, or half-naked, when my twin sisters were only 3 months old. Did I have a body too ugly for the twins to see, or was there another reason? I never did really understand, but the message was, "That is our Tongan way." Still today I am left with the unanswered question: Is the Tongan body sinful, or is it holy because it is a gift from a Holy God?

When I was still a small boy, my relatives and older people liked to hold me. This went on for many years. I never understood why until now: it was because of my body. This past year I was at a kava ceremony held at a friend's house. I arrived and saw a man sitting and talking to my uncle, but I did not know who he was. As I tried to figure out who he was, I noticed him looking at me. Soon, he stood up and came to sit beside me. He asked, "Do you remember me?" I said, "Sort of, but not really." When he introduced himself, I suddenly remembered. He was one of the senior boys in our village while I was still young. This was the first time we'd met after fourteen years. The first thing he told me was how he and the other senior boys loved to hold me when I was young because I was so strong and handsome. I smiled because I never knew that, but I was happy to hear his story about my body.

Now, as an adult, I wonder what they expected from a little boy's body? What did they see in my body? Why did they like to hold a little boy's body like that? What does handsome mean when they looked at me? Does this mean that all the other boys my age in our village were all ugly? If so, how did they judge that? Who told them that? What does ugly mean anyway from the perspective of a Tongan?

I played rugby when I was younger. Playing rugby at certain achievement levels reveals something about the changes in young men's bodies. When I was still at high school, a new rugby coach arrived to select the senior team. I had been playing with the same boys for more than five years and we knew how each other played. That year it came as a shock that we did not have a trial first in the selection process; instead, we had what I call a "body check" first. The coach told us to line up and as he was walking toward the line, he pointed to people with the wrong sort of bodies for rugby, telling them to leave the team. What he said to each was, "You don't look like a rugby player." From our point of view, some of the students that were forced to leave the team were the top players over the last five years. I hope that one day I will meet my coach again and ask him what differentiates a rugby body from a normal body (meaning the body that you were born with). I need him to tell me how he knows the perfect body for rugby. What was wrong with the bodies of those whom he directed to leave?

I remember going with my mum to a shop here in Auckland once. As we went in the store, we met a lady. She appeared older than my mum, and she smiled at mum. They began kissing each other hello, but the lady's eyes were focused on me. The two women continued talking, and the lady continued staring at me. I didn't know why she was staring, but suddenly she asked my mum, "Is he your son?" and my mum said yes. In tears, she told my mum that I looked exactly like my dad, and then she grabbed me and hugged me, kissing my face and crying all over me. In fact, my father had passed away five years earlier, and this old lady had been one of my father's teachers while he was in high school. Questions remained: What does our body show to other people? How do other people see me? Is this how people saw me—that I am my father's body?

I still play rugby here in New Zealand, and one of our games was televised nationally. After the game my rugby mates met up to watch the replay. It had been a tough game and at one point during the game I got the ball and ran with it. I was hammered hard by two of the other players illegally. I felt that I needed to lie down for a minute because my stomach hurt so badly. When I felt my body was all right, I stood up and carried on playing. While I was down, the commentator felt sorry for me, judging from the way he talked, and he hurled angry remarks at the other players who tackled me illegally. The moment I stood up, the commentator knew that I was all right and he said, "Oh, luckily he is a Tongan." I did not understand why he said that. Are bodies classified differently according to our ethnicity? I think he saw Jonah Lomu as a hard Tongan man and he assumed that every Tongan who plays rugby must be similar to Lomu. I learned from this experience that my body is seen by others only through the lens of their prior associations and assumptions.

The Tongan Understanding of Men's Bodies

Susan Bordo (1999) says, "The way we experience our bodies is powerfully affected by the cultural metaphors that are available for us" (p. 38). What metaphors, then, are available to the Tongan men that they might carry in their bodies? I know that Tongan men today think differently about their bodies from the way that men did in earlier times. The core cultural bases by which Tongan men were constructed fifty years ago have been modified in the twenty-first century due to Western contact.

Tongan mythology is one of the powerful resources that affect Tongan people's way of life. Most of the stories of the past carry values and identities of the Tongan people and at the same time they impact upon the respect for and understanding of their bodies. Many Tongan myths relate to the two foundational values of our culture: respect and love through sacrifice. Respect keeps us Tongans strong and alive through the ongoing honoring of the king of Tonga, a structure of governance arising from the myth of ʻAhoʻeitu, the first Tuʻi Tonga (king of Tonga).

Tongans believe that ʻAhoʻeitu was half-divine and half-human. His father was the god Tangaloa ʻEitumatupuʻa, the Tongan sky god. His mother was Vaʻepopua, an earthly woman who fell in love with Tangaloa ʻEitumatupuʻa. In the myth, ʻAhoʻeitu was appointed by his sky god father to rule over Tonga as king, thus becoming the first Tuʻi Tonga. ʻAhoʻeitu was highly respected by the people because he carried divinity in his blood. For Tongans, one's bloodline determines one's rank in society. Carrying *totoʻi ʻeiki* (chiefly blood) elevates one to the rank of king or chief, a "power over" status in relationship to commoners. Blood relationship also dictates the class structure of respecting those who are of a higher rank. In Tonga there are many ways of showing respect, including the way in which one talks and the way in which one uses one's body.

A Tongan man's haircut displays his class and ranking. Hair styles have been classified into different types: there is a type of haircut for high school students, another for theological students, another for fathers, another for fishermen, and so on. There is even a type of haircut for criminals. Respect is thus conceived as involving all aspects of life, reflected in the regulation of bodily form and appearance. Our bodies display our identity and our sense of self. In this sense, Moltmann-Wendel (1994) is correct: "I am my body."

In pre-missionary Tonga, the harvest festival was an annual event. In this festival, different fruits and animals were presented to the Tu'i Tonga. In the ceremony, people bringing offerings were required to scoot into the presence of the king by scrambling on their backsides instead of using their feet, as a mark of respect. These people were given the name *ha'a mene 'uli*, which means "those with dirty asses." Their backsides became dirty, bruised, and scratched because of the extreme posturing of respect demanded in the presence of the Tu'i Tonga. What does it say about the Tongan body that people must degrade and injure themselves in the presence of those of higher rank? Is the body simply a tool to secure the accepted class structure? Does the Tongan body not inherently command respect?

Showing respect in Tongan culture thus has a lot to do with bodily action. How I walk portrays something about me. How I sit and look can be interpreted variously by others, and it is open for others to comment upon because my posture and mien are controlled by culture. How I dress is controlled by culture. The question remains: How can we Tongans respect our own bodies? Do we have the right to respect our own bodies, or are our bodies to be used simply to respect others? There seems to be a paradox here: Tongans seem to believe that they have a body but they are not their body, and that their bodies don't belong to them.

Mythologically, it is claimed that *kava* originated on a small island in Tonga called 'Eueiki. 'Eueiki is near the main island of Tongatapu, approximately an hour away from the capital, Nuku'alofa. At the time, the only people residing on the island were a family of three—the father Fevanga, the mother Fefafa, and their daughter Kava, who had to spent most of her time indoors because she had leprosy.

This was in the days when the Tu'i Tonga was ruler of Tonga. He had gone out to fish, but was unsuccessful. In search of food, he sailed to 'Eueiki to rest, and could see no sign that it was inhabited. Exhausted, he lay down to rest on top of a large taro plant, which was coincidentally the only means of nutrition on the island. When Fevanga and Fefafa found out that the Tu'i Tonga was on their island, they hurried to prepare a feast for him, as demanded by the custom of respect. Searching for taro for the feast, Fevanga discovered that the Tu'i Tonga was lying asleep on the only taro plant left on the island. Fevanga did not dare wake up the king to obtain the taro.

This posed a great dilemma for Fevanga and Fefafa. There was nothing to present to the Tu'i Tonga as an offering, since he was asleep on top of the only source of food on the island. The only solution was to take the life of their only daughter and offer her to the Tu'i Tonga as food. And so they did. The crewmen of the king's boats found out what had been done and reported it to the Tu'i Tonga. The Tu'i Tonga was deeply moved by the sacrificial act of the couple, and he ordered that her body be buried before he returned to Tongatapu. The childless couple laid their daughter Kava to rest in a grave on 'Eueiki.

After some time, two plants grew from the grave of the unfortunate daughter, one at the head and one at the feet of Kava. These two plants were unfamiliar to Fevanga and Fefafa. As they watched, a rat came by, gnawed on the plant at the foot of the grave, and started staggering. As the rat reached the plant that grew at the head of the grave, he gnawed on it and appeared to return to normal. Subsequently, Fevanga and Fefafa named the plant that grew at the feet *Kava*, because of its bitter taste, and the plant that grew at the head *Tō* (sugarcane), because of its sweetness. The couple harvested these two plants and took them to Tongatapu to present to the Tu'i Tonga.

Sacrifice is one of the essential values of our culture. Love is shown through sacrifice, and true love is bonded together with sacrifice. The spirit of sacrifice is kept alive in the minds of Tongans through frequent repetition of the kava ceremony. At a Tongan wedding, the kava ceremony symbolizes the love of the couple, as well as reminding those present that sacrifice is the truest Tongan form of love. In other contexts, the ceremony symbolizes different meanings, but all are bounded by the essence of love as sacrifice.

The purpose of Fevanga and Fefafa's sacrifice of their only daughter remains an unresolved question. Was it a sacrifice out of respect and love for the Tu'i Tonga, or was it a sacrifice out of love for the daughter, that she would not have to suffer any longer? Although the story is ostensibly about love and sacrifice, I want to focus on the leprous body, killed as an offering for the Tu'i Tonga. Why did these parents kill their only daughter? Was this because they needed a culturally requisite offering to the Tu'i Tonga, or was this the opportunity for the parents to get rid of her because of the leprosy that had ravaged her body? Perhaps this family moved to the island in the first place because of their daughter's leprosy. Tongans can be quick to attribute a child's disability to the sin of the parents. Removing a disabled person from the glare of social stigma, then, is one way of dealing with shame and sin.

But why kill an innocent child for an offering? If the sacrifice was to benefit either Fevanga or the Tu'i Tonga, the preferred choice would have been of a beautiful woman as the sacrifice, for the ancient expectation was that the best of one's possessions and productivity was to be offered to the Tu'i Tonga. In the end, this is a story of the murder of a female with a disabled body, in order to promote a specific relationship of recognition and honor between two men. It is, in the words of Eve Kosovky Sedgwick (1985), an act of homosociality, the use of a female to cement social relations between two men. In a similar way in Tongan culture, the young female virgin becomes a bartered commodity between two families, in order to secure privilege and prestige between male-dominated clans. In patriarchal cultures, men and their bodies need repeated recognition and affirmation.

The Strong Bodies of Tongan Men

Around the dinner table, when I lived in Tonga, I often heard the phrase, "You have to eat Tongan food in order for you to be strong." Older people needed boys to eat Tongan food because they wanted them to have strong bodies. Boyd (1995) observes that "for many men, decisions about what we eat have been made by either our mother or our wives or female partners" (p. 170). This happens in Tonga, too, but my question is what limit a Tongan man must reach before he stops eating to please others. Why do Tongan men have to be strong at all, and what does the word *strong* mean?

I think this reveals to us how the responsibilities of Tongan men to their families affect their bodies. The main sources of sustenance in the Tongan islands are fishing and farming, and it is men's task to look after the wellbeing of the family. Thus a model is constructed of a male body that is strong and that can manage hard labor. Strong, then, from a Tongan perspective, does not signify six-pack abs or an overwhelming size, but the ability to fulfill tasks that are assigned to those who are born with a penis. As Boyd (1995) puts it, "men are socialized to act as men are supposed to act" (p. 2).

Where does this understanding of a strong body come from? Our Tongan mythology contains many stories glorifying warriors from the past. The stories of Muni Matamahae, Pungalotohoa, 'Ulukalāla, and many others influence the process of growing up as a male in Tonga. These stories are passed from generation to generation, reminding Tongan men to be like warriors—to have large, strong bodies that are fearless and can do everything expected of them, including fighting, working in the plantation, and protecting their families (see Gilmore, 1990).

Understanding Tongan Male Bodies

Our bodies carry not only DNA, they also carry human history. This means that when we look at our bodies, we see values and ideals. These values and ideals are determined by what has been written by our culture on our bodies (Bordo, 1999, p. 36). Talking about my body and the way people look at me are all part of my personal history. It is clear that Tongan male bodies are constructed by our culture, and then the construct is reinscribed onto our bodies by the culture and by others. In Tongan culture, a man's body is valued primarily for what that body can do. The less one's body can do, the less one is valued as a man. But because male bodies are socially constructed, they can also be deconstructed.

Understanding my own body has been quite difficult for me, because Tongans deal with their physical bodies as if they were a tool they had borrowed, rather than as the embodiment of who they are. Talking about bodies is not acceptable in our culture. Bodies are not important, because everything that happens to the body is only seen as an outcome of what is in our spirits and minds. Tongan males understand themselves only as accidentally strong, as a product of their souls and minds.

There is a long way to go from where we Tongan males are now, to a healthy understanding of "I am my Tongan body." The heritage of Victorian Christianity, which labeled our bodies as sinful and shameful, must be rethought. Today the Tongan male embodies the confusion between indigenous and Western cultures. The connection between curse and bodily dis/ability must also be broken. To become healthy, we may also have to challenge the cultural assumption that the body of a male commoner is worth less than the body of a male chief, noble, or even the king. The cultural values of respect and sacrificial love need to be talked through again—by Tongan men in particular, and with each other—so that these basic cultural values can be performed in a way that tells Tongan men and women that their bodies are valuable because of what they are, and not just for what they can give away to others. I dream of a day when as a Tongan man, I can say "I am my body," and not feel that in saying so, I have also constructed myself as a social outcast.

References

Bordo, S. (1999). *The male body: A new look at men in public and in private.* New York: Farrar, Straus and Giroux.

Boyd, S. (1995) *The men we long to be: Beyond domination to a new Christian understanding of manhood.* New York: HarperCollins.

Culbertson, P. (2002). Designing men: Reading the male body as text. In

P. Culbertson (Ed.), *The spirituality of men: Sixteen Christians write about their faith* (pp. 165–178). Minneapolis: Fortress Press.

Gilmore, D. (1990). *Manhood in the making: Cultural concepts of masculinity.* New Haven: Yale University Press.

Moltmann-Wendel, E. (1994). *I am my body.* London: SCM Press.

Morton, H. (1996). *Becoming Tongan: An ethnography of childhood.* Honolulu: University of Hawai'i Press.

Sedgwick, E. K. (1985). *Between men: English literature and male homosocial desire.* New York: Columbia University Press.

5

Being *'Afakasi*

TINA BERKING, CAROLINE SALUMALO FATIALOFA, KAREN LUPE, AND SEILOSA SKIPPS-PATTERSON, WITH MARGARET AGEE

Tina: *I was born in Sālelologa, Savai'i, as number six of nine children. Both my parents are Samoan, and also of German and Irish descent (to name a few). I spent the first five years of my life in Savai'i and the next fifteen in Upolu before migrating to New Zealand in the early 1980s as a 19-year-old. Every Samoan parent's dream is for their children to be successful, to become a doctor or lawyer, to at least achieve beyond the parents' potential. That dream has not changed for the many generations that have made New Zealand their new homeland. The optimum is to be successful in the Western world, yet not to lose being Samoan.*

I have spent the last twelve years working in the areas of social services and education. My contribution to this essay is a reflection of my own personal experience. It is an attempt to make a connection with other Pasifika people with similar issues around identity, and especially with our children, who are our future. As a therapist, my own journey and some of my struggles along the way are paralleled by those of many of my clients, as they try to navigate the often-conflicting tides of Samoan and Western currents.

Caroline: *Nineteen-years-young in the fields of career guidance, education, and employment, I am at heart a helper, and in practice a teacher, trainer, mentor, and counselor in various guises.*

I was born forty-three years ago to parents who, like many others, traveled to New Zealand seeking a better life for themselves and future generations. My Samoan-Chinese father and Samoan-English mother produced six children of very mixed heritage, and Kiwis to boot, with me being the youngest. After twelve years in New Zealand, being taken home to Samoa to live with my grandmother for the next five years was the most life-changing and significant experience. It shaped every aspect of my life from that point forward.

My involvement in this book is therefore in tribute to my grandma Salumalo Muagututi'a, my mother Caroline Meredith, and my many other

mothers who have mentored me through life and work, including my life's work—raising two wonderful sons Rex and Michael.

The strength of character and teachings of these great women have enabled me to bless many others who have struggled to find a path for themselves. My hope is that in turn, my sons and their generation will gain wisdom from these writings—casting light onto their path and illuminating the way forward. Soifua lava, ma ia manuia.

Self-introductions for Karen Lupe and Seilosa Skipps-Patterson can be found in their respective essays.

A particular challenge facing those who work in the field of Pasifika mental health and wellbeing is the way in which significant aspects of the life experiences of many people remain cloaked in silence. This silence characterizes the way in which the community has responded to some issues that evoke discomfort or ambivalence, or attract social censure. One such challenge is the acknowledgment of those who are *'afakasi*, or half-caste. Ways need to be found to validate their life experiences and worldview, in order to support them in claiming a place of belonging.

In attempting to break the silence, we decided to come together and share our experiences and perceptions as a group of four 'afakasi Samoan women, all of whom are in our 40s and belong to therapeutic professions. This was a risky venture, audiotaping sensitive personal reflections on our life experiences, facilitated by a pālagi colleague. Because of preexisting relationships among members of the group, however, a degree of trust was already established. We had open expectations about the process and about what would emerge from the conversation, in terms of both content and the form the written account of this conversation might take.

What occurred was a wide-ranging discussion over more than two-and-a-half hours that was rich in both depth and breadth. As the tapes were transcribed, it became apparent that analyzing the material in accordance with a qualitative, grounded theory approach (Strauss & Corbin, 1990) would be most appropriate, enabling our words, as the data, to speak for themselves and to form the basis for the development of theory. A system of open and axial coding was therefore used to analyze the transcript line by line, in order to identify the emergent themes. As part of the verification process (Miles & Huberman, 1984), each member of the group read the transcript and a summary of the themes, checking the accuracy of both, according to their recollections and perceptions. Several points were clarified through this process. In presenting the themes from the discussion here, we have included illustrative quotations but have chosen not to attribute them to particular individuals, in order to protect our personal privacy.

It's about Context

For the women in our group, the consciousness and consequences of being 'afakasi have been experienced across all social and relational environments, including home and family, the workplace, with friends, at church, and so on. Intersecting with contextual factors are the influences of ethnic identification and identity development, family history, and social status and privilege, including perceived group membership, which were seen as playing out within systems, influencing interpersonal dynamics as well as intrapsychic functioning and self-perception (Atkinson, Morten, & Sue, 1998). The ways in which being 'afakasi had complicated her roles and relationships were symbolized for one person by "all kinds of extra jobs that we inherit," but the challenges seem to be both more pervasive and more complex, as the ensuing discussion revealed.

Being Held on a Pedestal: White Privilege and the Historical Context

Historically, being 'afakasi has been associated with white privilege. One group member recounted her aunt's explanation that when the white men came to the village in Samoa, villagers' daughters were given to them to marry because they were accorded higher status than Samoan or brown men. Thus 'afakasi girls were treated like princesses in the village and today there are elements of being held on a pedestal attached to both being white and being 'afakasi. She recalled community members making assumptions that she and her husband were rich because he was pālagi, and she described the way in which he was privileged at funerals by being called to the top table, ahead of some ministers, just because he was white.

It was noted that 'afakasis back in Samoa, as well as in New Zealand, tended to view others with a somewhat arrogant, "us and them" attitude. While attending high school in Samoa, one had been challenged by her full Samoan peers for choosing to spend time with them: "They asked me one day, 'How come you're different to those other 'afakasis?' and I asked, 'What do you mean?' 'Why do you hang out with us?' . . . They said, 'Oh but all 'afakasis have that . . . they think they're better than us,' and it is true." Although she was challenging these stereotypes by her actions, this exchange illustrates the effects of privilege and social stratification on both groups. Two group members had also felt uncomfortable when they had been exposed to such attitudes within 'afakasi groups of friends and acquaintances within New Zealand, where derogatory terms such as *fob* and *freshie* were used when speaking of Samoans who were more traditional.

Being on Shifting Ground

Being ʻafakasi, in fact, was described as an ambiguous experience associated with both positive and negative consequences in the lives of the group members, "sometimes working for you and sometimes against you." The capacity to move in and out of different identities and environments, and to feel at home in both at some level, could be a strength: "There is that quality, and you know it's a bit like privilege, privilege in one and privilege in the other and I think that's the positive about it." "And it's about feeling at home in both those places."

Others' perceptions and behavior could also be affirming, such as the Samoan mother-in-law who proudly told everybody that her son had married an ʻafakasi girl. The ground could shift suddenly, however, the minute one made a mistake about something: "But I also remember the minute I slipped up, 'You stupid ʻafakasi!' you know, and I remember thinking, oh, when it suits you it's good to be *ʻafa*, but when it doesn't . . ." Such abrupt switches from acceptance and affirmation to blame and humiliation leave ʻafakasis "someplace in the middle," feeling insecure about where they stand at any given time: "Just being in the in-group sometimes, and not ever being sure sometimes whether you were in or not . . . Thinking you were in but then finding that you're not actually . . . the whole dynamic of membership in and out of the group all the time." This had been experienced in all contexts within group members' lives, including both pālagi and Samoan environments.

Not Quite Belonging

As a result of such experiences, members of the group described a sense of not wholly belonging that had developed from childhood. For two of the group, this was associated with the institutionalization of privilege within the school system in Samoa: "I suddenly noticed that all the half-caste kids were put into one of two classes with a handful of pālagi kids whose parents were there on contract. And the rest of the kids were in what they called Samoan classes. And that's how it was, all the way, right up to intermediate." She described her sense of not belonging that was evoked by the reactions of her peers: "The pālagis certainly didn't see you as pālagi, and your own referred to you as ʻafakasi, so there was always the notion of, you didn't quite belong to either."

The other group member who had attended the same school in Samoa, also commented on the stratification she had observed and the effect on her when placed first with the one group, and then later, the other:

> Even in high school I noticed the top forms were the pālagis and the ʻafakasis. And because I got there really late in the school year I was put in the Samoan

> class, which was the third one down, so for me it was a different kind of experience because I came from New Zealand with the pākehās [non-Māori citizens of Aotearoa/New Zealand], defined by the system, but was put into the Samoan class, so I found it hard to adjust and actually felt more comfortable when I was put into a different class where all the rest of the 'afakasi kids were. So different sides of the same equation.

Another described feeling in the minority, both at school and at church: "I was born and raised in New Zealand and I was always put in the highest-ranked classes and very few Pacific were in there with me. And so it was the same sort of story, I didn't belong with the same members I went to church with, maybe because I'm too *fia pālagi* [behaving like a white person]."

The fourth member of the group described the rejection she and her siblings had experienced, as they were growing up, from some members of their Samoan extended family who perceived them as too white. Although there has been healing subsequently in these relationships, this has caused considerable ongoing pain associated with her sense of self, indicating the potential long-term difficulties such experiences can cause. Another group member summarized what she perceived as the need to accept the implications of not belonging:

> You don't wholly feel like you belong in either of the camps . . . for a long time, it's that notion of not being accepted and being totally Samoan or totally pālagi, and it's like coming to accept that I'll *never* be right, and there will always be somebody who will say someone is more Samoan than somebody, and it's the same on the other side. I think it's about accepting that.

You're an 'Afakasi—*That Blood Thing!*

Having one's identity and social position defined by others was a particular source of frustration for members of the group: "we're grappling with this 'afakasi thing because somebody considers you 'afakasi, you know, 'You're an 'afakasi.'" Being questioned, having one's identity dissected, and being found wanting was a common experience, as the following reconstructed exchange illustrates:

> "You're saying you're Samoan . . . you're Samoan? Full Samoan? No, no, can't be, you've got something else . . . 'afakasi . . . that sort of comment."
> "Not quite a real Samoan . . . not quite."
> "Oh, I'm sure you're not full . . ."

Being made to feel invisible was described as the cost of being discounted by others as "*only* 'afakasi . . . we're just pretend."

The whole term *'afakasi* is problematic because of the associated issue of attempting to quantify identity in terms of bloodlines. The following exchange expresses the discounting effect of "that blood thing" that is still prevalent, though outdated:

> "It is quite a problem I have with this and that's that whole blanket term *'afakasi*. I mean whether you're three-quarters or one-fifth, it's just a farce."
>
> "We could have more Samoan blood than somebody else who's perceived as full Samoan, is fluent, and has a *matai* [chiefly] title and is practicing . . . It's not about blood anymore and yet a lot of people still behave as if it is."

When her children asked questions about their heritage and attempted to quantify their Samoan side ("How much Samoan? Am I one-eighth? Am I one-fifth? . . . so how come they call us 'afakasi, 'cos that's half-caste?"), one group member told them: "You are how much you feel . . . I don't want them to have that defining us, so I encourage them to say, 'we're Samoans.'"

This kind of validation was experienced by another group member at a *fono* (public meeting) with a highly regarded matai who invited the New Zealand–born and young people to speak. He acknowledged how hard it could be to feel accepted as Samoan but spoke strongly against quantifying cultural identity: "it doesn't matter whether you've got a tenth, it's what's in your heart." Asserting that the culture was about alofa (love), he also declared that "the old people have to open their hearts." This experience was a refreshing exception to the norm, in which little seems offered to 'afakasi, or in fact to young people in general, by way of public validation by elders. Being viewed as outside rather than inside, as not fully belonging, seemed more common and seemed to have had greater emotional significance in the lives of the women in our group.

Needing to Justify Myself Professionally

In addition to the influence of quantifying cultural identity, pressure to justify oneself was commonly experienced in the workplace, with Samoan clients as well as within organizations and training programs.

Working with Samoan Clients—Walking a Fine Line

A hurtful paradox associated with being 'afakasi for some group members seemed to be the way in which clients would challenge them because they were 'afakasis working with Samoan people. As one said, poignantly: "And yet our heart is there *because* we're half-Samoan, to help our people, and yet we're being challenged about it." They felt required to explain their identity and to justify themselves to clients as to why they should work with them, yet this challenge seemed particularly hard to accept in light of their motivation and "the fact that it's our actual culture that we love and we're attached to, that actually questions us more than the European."

In addition, one group member, as a practitioner, felt that her cultural knowledge and her capacity to walk in both the Samoan and pālagi worlds have enabled her to serve clients well, without their realizing how significant these may be:

> I'm thinking we walk a fine line, because on the one hand I feel like sometimes I'm protecting my clients . . . from the system that will squeeze them into a box, without them ever knowing it. And yet I need to justify myself to them as to why I should work with them (laughing) . . . because they don't know how the system is working, and you're kind of standing in the middle, trying to mediate the system for their benefit, but also justifying that we're good to work with . . . "I try to do the best by you and yet you ask me why I'm working with you?!"

"Walking a fine line" also described the distinction between justifying yourself and locating yourself in a genealogical context to which clients could relate, in order to establish trust and credibility. One group member described establishing credibility with a community group because she was able to explain who her parents and grandparents were and what village they had come from in Samoa. The community leaders told her that had she not known those things, they would not have trusted her sufficiently to work with her. This kind of contextualizing in order to establish connections with clients had a legitimate professional purpose and was a qualitatively different experience from the kind of self-justification described earlier.

In Organizations and Training Programs

While on the one hand being challenged by clients, on the other hand, 'afakasi practitioners felt compelled to advocate for Samoan culture and to challenge Western approaches within mainstream organizations that were not in the best interests of Pasifika clients. As one stated, "It's kind of two levels in the workplace," engaging in battle on both sides.

Within Eurocentric training programs, the loneliness and struggle that group members had experienced included being required to furnish additional extensive explanation justifying a culturally appropriate intervention such as conducting a session in a client's home. When cultural issues were not acknowledged within training programs, the voices of group members were silenced in sharing their cultural perspectives and wisdom regarding both themselves and their clients.

The Questioning of Ourselves

As seasoned practitioners, some members of the group still experienced internalized conflict and self-doubt with regard to their own professional judgment:

> I know that I've taken issues to supervision because the Samoan knows that was the right thing to do in Samoa but the way I've been trained means I'm in conflict so I have to take it to supervision just to check that it was okay, but again having to justify *why* it was okay . . . the client's coming to see us specifically because you're a Pacific Islander, you're counseling in a Pacific Island way . . . and yet you're still wondering whether it's okay to do that sort of thing, 'cos it's the training that influences you . . . and yet the Samoan in me says yes, this is right, this is totally right, but that training is quite strong.

The power of the messages internalized during training can have the ongoing effect of overriding the voices of inner wisdom and cultural knowledge. This was seen as an outcome of processes of oppression, power, and control within the therapeutic professions, including the valorizing of Eurocentric perspectives over the knowledge and worldviews associated with other cultures. For some group members, the strength of their need to continue justifying themselves to themselves, as competent practitioners who could trust in their own judgment, created ongoing intrapersonal conflict and stress, overlaying other levels of internal conflict associated with being 'afakasi.

I Just Put My Culture Away: Having to Cope

In attempting to cope with such conflict and move adaptively in and out of different environments, the women in the group had found themselves operating out of parts of their identity, leaving other parts behind. Their experiences of not being allowed to be Pasifika or not being validated as fully themselves necessitated the exclusion of a part of themselves from various settings. Speaking of her school days, for example, one who was in a top academic class said: "Thank goodness there was sports, we were allowed to be Pasifika in sports . . . allowed to be Samoan, but not academic." Others spoke of censoring out part of themselves within training programs and in the workplace because of dominant attitudes of ignorance or censure.

Leaving Myself at the Door

Insight into what can occur when one moves from one context to another and leaves a part of oneself outside was provided by one group member who described the shift that she experiences within herself when visiting her Samoan aunt. In this environment her Samoan side comes forward in the form of expanded consciousness and connectedness:

> As soon as I walk in the door, my consciousness changes and suddenly my English self is left outside, somehow, and I sit differently, I relate differently, I see differently . . . my consciousness is spread out and much more connected to everybody in the room. And there's a lot more openness . . . But that changes again as soon as I walk out the door, suddenly. I gather the rest of me up again . . . it's really strange.

For some it was necessary to survive by shutting out their Samoan side within training programs: "In psychotherapy I just put my culture away in order to survive and by Jove, if you ever brought up cultural issues . . . don't ever!" Another described coping with the demands of psychotherapy training within a different organization by operating out of only one part of her self: "When I did my training I did it out of my English side because there was such a lot of information to collate and analyze, and so my Samoan side was left at the door." A third group member concurred, "We do that really well, don't we?"

In a similar vein, another felt herself to be "in different boxes" when moving between the mainstream and Pasifika departments within her workplace. It was agreed that this compartmentalizing of oneself was a familiar way of coping, and in the process, "leaving one bit [of oneself] behind" was common practice; this raises many questions about the consequences of this, and about what aspects of oneself are shut out, unavailable to oneself or others, at any given time.

Knowing How to Play the Game: Teaching Others to Cope

With clients, as well as with their own children, a valuable aspect of what group members had to offer as 'afakasi was the knowledge they had gained in negotiating the differences between the Samoan and the pālagi worlds. Knowing how to play the game and consciously teaching others the rules of engagement were seen as essential in helping them to survive within the world.

When teaching clients to cope in situations such as a job interview or a mediation, members described passing on to them the same coping strategy that they themselves were using: "Haven't you said that to your clients? When you walk through the door, behave like a pālagi and you'll be fine, and you can pick up your Samoan side as you're coming out again." One member went on to describe teaching her son in a similar way, validating this as a survival strategy:

> It's okay to know how to play the game two ways, which is much better than knowing how to play the one . . . rather than feeling incompetent and not knowing where you are and being lost in the masses really . . . consciously using those things to play the system until the system changes and they have to accept us for who we are, or until we can change it . . . so I guess it's a survival strategy.

Equipping others to claim their personal power and cope adaptively thereby becomes a way of promoting social change. Questions were raised, however, about whether this was encouraging clients to be bicultural or to split within themselves, whether splitting was in fact a safety mechanism for survival, and about the unconscious processes involved and the long-term effects of these.

The Personal Consequences

The intrapersonal consequences of being 'afakasi and coping in these ways included not only internalized personal and professional conflict, but also a range of associated painful emotions.

Having Two Different Selves

One person vividly described her experience of having two different internalized selves:

> It's finding a place outside, but it's also that I've got two different selves, and there's one self that feels and thinks like this, and there's another self that thinks and feels like this (gesturing) from the different cultural heritage, so every day when I'm in a situation, I've got two different responses. And so sometimes I feel this way and sometimes I feel that way, and sometimes I go that way, and then get sabotaged by the other side, and vice versa, and . . . I don't know whether I'm Arthur or Martha . . . but you know, I'm both . . . and it's not having a place to really be with that. It's left me with very deep feelings of existential loss which underpins my being . . . and it's almost impossible to explain that to people who don't have that experience.

This has left her with a kind of anxiety at the core of her being. For her, this was "the cost of growing up without a solid sense of cohesion and confidence at the base of myself, and that's like a constant, chronic wound."

Emotional Isolation, Loneliness, and Loss

The sense of isolation and loss here was echoed in others' descriptions of loss and sadness associated with the loneliness of being 'afakasi. One spoke of being saddened by the loneliness she felt within a group back in a Samoan village, enjoying the experience yet actually not feeling completely at home. Another described similar emotional loneliness: "Even with a whole group of people you exist in a different culture, you're lonely within that . . . The loneliness is compounded when you have children." Sadness was expressed by one mother about what her children have lost and how much more removed they are than she is herself from their cultural roots. As another said in speaking of loss, the desire is there in her children to associate with their Pasifika heritage, but without a real depth of understanding.

Frustration, Anger, and Tiredness

The lack of cultural acknowledgment she experienced within a training program left one member particularly frustrated and angry, with both herself and the program: "I'd probably introjected that a lot because I didn't know what to do . . . I couldn't actually just keep it at the gate anymore . . . oh, I was so angry . . . I was just so angry . . . I felt like I was selling myself out." Frustration and anger also came through strongly when group members talked of having to explain and justify themselves to others.

The cost of constantly having to do so was tiring as well as tiresome. As one member said, "I'd just like to walk in and say something and that's it, and not give the rationale behind it, not give the historical context for it."

Tiredness was the result of both contextual pressures and intrapersonal tensions experienced by group members. For another member, tiredness was described as a huge issue associated with the conflict between her two different internalized selves. She saw this tiredness as an ongoing cost of her life journey.

It's a Journey about Themselves and How They Fit

Members of the group perceived their clinical supervisees as seeking cultural validation in professional contexts. They also described themselves as being on a journey toward a fuller sense of belonging and wholeness. "It's a journey about themselves and how they fit" applies to both. One member envied people "who are comfortable in their own skin . . . who are integrated and more whole." Another said, "I just want to be myself all of the time . . . or most of the time would be nice." They also sought solace for their sense of emotional loneliness, and wanted "to be with people who knew that too."

Feeling Most at Home

Group members identified two settings in which they did experience a comfortable fit. Foremost among these was being with old friends from school days, with a shared history, and with whom they could relax and let their guard down. Members' children noticed a difference in their mothers when they were with these old friends, and one person articulated what this experience was about for the whole group, who were murmuring agreement throughout this part of the discussion:

> What they said to me is, you know, the language you use is different, because that's when we slip into Samoan all the time and English is our second language because your guard is down and my kids also say I just talk non-stop about historical stuff . . . there's a kind of life flow that just goes in and out of all of it and we find it all the time, just that connectedness . . . that's where I feel most at home, is with them . . . with the home base . . . your consciousness can be up there, more than anywhere else.

In response, another member described it as finding a place to rest, a respite from internal conflict: "It's like finding a place to rest, which is a place beyond that inner conflict . . . you don't have to perform . . . just being at rest somehow."

A similar educational background was an influential factor in enabling another member of the group to establish connectedness with some of her cousins who were also ʻafakasi: "As soon as they named it we could connect . . . the neat part is that we would hang out and just be ourselves."

Not Being in the System

In terms of the workplace, working outside of systems in which one has to justify oneself was a relief to one group member and had strengthened her in resisting external pressures and others' definitions of herself: "I think it's not being in the system where I have to justify myself . . . it's a huge thing not feeling like I have to do this all the time, being in our own private organization . . . Our clients come to us because they know who we are, and we don't have to justify ourselves."

Being in My 40s

As women in midlife, two spoke of feeling more comfortable than ever before with where they were in their lives at present, and being less affected by the judgments of others:

> I mean, being in my 40s, I just am past the point of caring now and I'm trying to model to my kids what I believe, that I'm as Samoan as I feel, and I just carry

> on. I mean, I feel more integrated now than I ever have previously in my life. I feel really comfortable about where I'm at . . . I mean I don't speak very much Samoan at home because my husband doesn't speak it . . . that doesn't matter to me in terms of it doesn't define whether I'm Samoan or not.

Although still seeking healing for a sense of inner isolation and woundedness, another member of the group also spoke of feeling more comfortable with herself at this stage in life: "I'm not so affected by external judgments on either side."

It's Cool to Be Samoan—Toward the Future

It seems that young people growing up in New Zealand currently enjoy an environment that is more affirming of the Pasifika aspects of their heritage than their mothers experienced. It is now cool to be Samoan and sexy to be Pasifika, something that is totally different from the prevalent attitudes when group members were growing up. One person reported that the status of her 15- and 16-year-olds was enhanced when it became known among their peers that they were part-Samoan. Another described her disbelief when she discovered that her son's social group at a very respectable school was an exclusive group of only about six couples, composed of the three Pacific Islanders at the school and the "wannabes." They were selective about who they let in, and membership was sought after.

Such an environment is likely to be more supportive of the development of a positive view of oneself than the environment had been for the earlier generation of Pasifika 'afakasi youth. There are indications that some young people are claiming their identity as 'afakasi with pride, and within the group one member commented on the fact that her daughter and niece were using "missafakasi" and "islandsuga" as their email addresses. The need to equip their children for the future, providing them with strong cultural connections, and with contextual understandings that will enable them to navigate their way through different cultural environments, raised questions and challenges for the women in the group as parents.

Conclusion

While the issues highlighted here about being 'afakasi represent the life experiences and perspectives of only four women, and it would therefore be inappropriate to generalize from this information, this has been an exploratory discussion that may contribute to the development of theory, promote discussion within the community, and stimulate further research. Some of the themes highlighted here resonate with issues identified by previous international commentators: having multiple lenses through which to view the world, and which influence decision making; moving beyond racial percentages and accepting one's identity as whole; leaving aside a part of oneself in order to succeed professionally (Clark, 2004); rejection, loneliness, anger, and struggling for connection and acceptance (Sue & Sue, 2003); the feeling of being an outsider, vulnerable to rejection; and the ongoing need to integrate the diverse elements of one's cultural heritages (Root, 1992).

In future research, the views of 'afakasi belonging to different age groups, including men as well as women, need to be sought. In addition, there are many questions to be identified and addressed, arising from the themes that have emerged here. Even before this has been accomplished, however, we would hope that this discussion of what it means to be 'afakasi will encourage others to share their own experiences and find support and validation. We also urge practitioners to be more attuned to the complexity of the stories their 'afakasi clients bring to therapy, and heighten their own capacity to hold ambiguity and pain, as well as hope, as they accompany clients on the journey to wholeness.

References

Atkinson, D. R., Morten, G., & Sue, D. W. (1998). *Counseling American minorities* (5th ed.). Boston: McGraw-Hill.

Clark, P. Y. (2004). Exploring the pastoral dynamics of mixed-race persons. *Pastoral Psychology, 52*(4), 315–328.

Miles, M. B., & Huberman, M. A. (1984). *Qualitative data analysis.* Beverly Hills, CA: Sage.

Root, M. P. P. (Ed.). (1992). *Racially mixed people in America.* Newbury Park, CA: Sage.

Strauss, A., & Corbin, J. (1990). *Basics of qualitative research.* Newbury Park, CA: Sage.

Sue, D. W., & Sue, D. (2003). *Counseling the culturally diverse: Theory and practice* (4th ed.). New York: John Wiley & Sons.

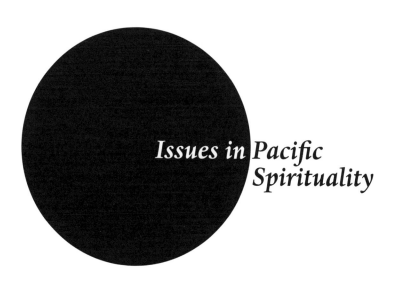

Issues in Pacific Spirituality

Editors' Introduction

The significance of spirituality and the role of religious communities for Pasifika peoples are explored in this section through widely different lenses. First, David Lui explains the integral importance of spirituality in wellbeing and particularly mental health for Pacific people. Crucial though this understanding is, spirituality and cultural perspectives have largely been ignored by Western mental health professionals, to the detriment of Pacific Island clients.

Cabrini Makasiale, on the other hand, passionately pleads for change, challenging what she perceives to be the damaging deification of culture. In critiquing the power of church hierarchies and the abuses sanctioned within these communities, she attempts to break through the silencing of dissent that keeps the needs of individual communities from being acknowledged and addressed.

Building on this theme, a survivor of abuse within the context of the church then speaks of the profoundly damaging effects of this experience on her life, from the time it occurred when she was young into midlife. The effects of the institutionalized abuse of power, including the inhibition and silencing of critique, spoken of by Cabrini Makasiale, are illustrated in this powerful and highly personal account. Here important challenges are laid at the feet of a community in which the safety and protection of the vulnerable, issues of justice, and restitution for wrongdoing have become subordinated to an ethos of not rocking the boat. This also raises questions for church communities about ways in which the role of forgiveness has become misappropriated to become a form of denial, rather than a restorative process based on an open and honest acknowledgment of injustice.

The last contribution in this section echoes themes heard in the preceding essays. Discussing the role of spirituality in preventing suicide, Jemaima Tiatia argues that spirituality is an important element in treatment plans for Pasifika young people who present as suicidal. The dramatic cries for help from participants in her research, and the inaudibility of their voices within their families, reinforce the concerns of the preceding authors. Pacific young people's need for a sense of connection and empowerment presents an urgent challenge for mental health professionals and the wider community.

6

Spiritual Injury

A Samoan Perspective on Spirituality's Impact on Mental Health

DAVID LUI

I am a Samoan of mixed heritage. My father Lui Iiga from the village of Safa'i, Savai'i, is a full Samoan. His father Iiga Kalolo was from the villages of Sale'aula and Lano. His mother was Mafina Tofa from the village of Saipipi. My mother Vera Danielson is 'afakasi. *Her father Alfred Danielson was the son of a Swedish baker Gustav Danielson who came to Samoa, fell in love with my great-grandmother Mary Hunt, and decided to stay. My grandmother Amy Purcell is a direct descendant of Edward (Ned) Purcell, an Irishman who landed at Tufutāfoe, Savai'i, and married my great-great-great-grandmother Salaevalu Siilata. I was born, raised, and educated in Samoa. I've always been proud of my heritage and considered myself a Samoan.*

I came to New Zealand in February 1975 as a scholarship student to continue my education here. I attended boarding school at Wellington College before moving south to Canterbury University, graduating with a bachelor of science degree in 1982. During my time in New Zealand, Pacific people experienced the dawn raids, the overstayer issue, and other key milestones or low points for New Zealand racial relations like the Māori uprising and forced removal from Bastion Point, the Springbok Tour 1981, and the Western Samoan Citizenship Act 1982 denying citizenship to thousands of Samoans and effectively overturning a Privy Council ruling in favor of Samoans with lawful claim to New Zealand citizenship. Some of these milestones happened during my tenure as president of the Canterbury University Samoan Students Association from 1981 to 1982. These events affected me personally and shaped me for life. After graduation I returned to Samoa to work and serve my country. I married two years later and settled into quiet family life. I returned with my family to New Zealand in 1987 to live and work.

I changed careers from marketing to mental health in 1995. I was part of the team that established the first Pacific Island Mental Health Service at Lotofale the same year. This rekindled my passion for Pacific issues and people. Religion and spirituality has been an important part of my life.

In my working career in mental health, I have observed the lack of capacity and ability of the mental health system to deal with the spiritual needs of our Pacific people. I write this essay with the hope of highlighting some of the gaps and opening the door to solutions in healing the spiritually injured.

There is an increasing acceptance of spirituality as an important part of health care among consumers, service users, community health workers, and health professionals. Even some clinicians, health care providers, and policy makers have recognized that spirituality is an important part of at least some consumers' healing and recovery process. There are now health documents from the New Zealand Ministry of Health, and especially the Mental Health Commission, which mention spirituality (see, for example, Mental Health Commission, 2004). Most policies do not exclude or forbid spirituality if it is part of a service user's recovery. Training of community support workers, health professionals, and clinicians sometimes includes the topic of spirituality. However, despite the increasing evidence from consumers and service users, family and caregivers, community workers, and people citing the importance of spirituality in the recovery process, it is still not part of routine investigations or assessments, especially clinical investigations.

My experience working in Pacific Island mental health is that Pacific consumers have a different view of, and a higher need for, the spiritual realm in their healing and recovery processes. I find that that even some consumers who may not appear to be religious or spiritual, and have not been to church for many years, express a desire to explore or include spirituality in their care plan. It is important for practitioners to understand why this is their need. My essay has been written from a Samoan perspective.

Spirituality and religion evoke different responses in different people. These responses range from skepticism and cynicism to feelings of peace, assurance, and connectedness. Questions also arise: What are spirituality and religion? Are they the same thing? How important are they? How do they relate to a person's health and wellbeing? I address these questions in the course of this essay.

The Arrival of Christianity in Samoa

It is often said that Samoans are a spiritual and religious people. It is popularly believed that Christianity arrived in Samoa in 1830, when a missionary, John Williams, landed at the village of Sāpapāliʻi in Savaiʻi. Sāpapāliʻi is an important village in Samoa. It is the village where Malietoa, one of the most prominent Samoan chiefs, resided. Malietoa accepted Christianity and paved the way for other Samoans, and indeed the whole nation, to accept its precepts and teachings, consequently transforming the fabric of Samoan society. For many Samoans, their spirituality is linked to religion and Christianity, but for others spirituality is based on a traditional view.

For hundreds of years prior to the arrival of Christianity, Samoans (and most other Pacific peoples) believed that Tagaloa was the principal god, or *atua*. A story told by a Samoan high chief, and recorded by one of the early missionaries, Thomas Powell, relates the generally held belief among Samoans in the 1830s that Tagaloa created Samoa and its people. This creation story is not dissimilar to the account in the biblical Book of Genesis. The belief was that Tagaloa made all things—the sky, the land, the seas, the fresh water, the trees, and the people. Tagaloa even made the heavens (*lagi*). In fact, Samoans believed that Tagaloa created nine heavens (*lagi tua iva*).

In fact, traditionally, Samoans had several atuas (gods); there were gods of rain, of the forest, of the harvest, of the village, and of war. One example of such a deity was Nāfanua, the goddess of war. The story goes that Nāfanua was the daughter of Saveasi'uleo, the god of Pulotu. Tired of the oppressive chiefs who ruled at the time, she led a group of warriors to battle and completely demolished the opposition. She covered her breasts with coconut palms during the battle to disguise the fact that she was a woman. Nāfanua later predicted the arrival of Christianity in Malietoa and all Samoa many years before it actually happened. In her prophecy, Nāfanua told Malietoa that his next kingdom (*mālō*) would be from the sky (*lagi*), and that this new God would be all-powerful, more powerful than the traditional gods of Samoa at the time. The arrival of Christianity is connected by most Samoans to Nāfanua's prophecy.

Today in Samoan ritual and traditions, the influences of indigenous spirituality and of Christianity are often both evident. For example, the traditional Samoan ritual during funerals, called *lagi* or *'auala* (path), usually held for *tamaalii* (high chiefs), consists of a procession of chiefs, each holding the tip of a coconut frond. They chant *tulouga le lagi* during this ritual to prepare the *lagi* (heaven) for the spirit of the deceased as a mark of respect. These rituals are still performed today, but have been Christianized. When the procession reaches the *fale* (Samoan house) where the deceased's body lies in state, each *matai* (chief) will toss the coconut frond onto the *paepae* (stones) in front of the fale before being seated. The *faatau* (oratory exchange) will then take place among the matais who took part in the 'auala. The faatau is the process of selecting the matai to speak on their behalf. The matai who is selected to represent the procession in his speech will mention *tulouga le lagi* three times (in reference to the Trinity) instead of nine, which is normal in traditional Samoa for the nine heavens created by Tagaloa.

The prediction by Nāfanua to Malietoa of the arrival of Christianity and an all-powerful God was accurate, as evidenced by the impact of Christianity on Samoan society today. According to the 2001 New Zealand census figures, more than 90 percent of Samoans in New Zealand state that they belong to a religious denomination. Similarly in Samoa, nearly everyone belongs to a religious denomination. The Samoan constitution is founded on God and on Christian principles (Fa'avae Samoa i le Atua). Given Samoa's violent history at the time of the arrival of Christianity, with wars between Samoa and neighboring Tonga and Fiji, as well as internal wars between different districts, it seems a miracle that Samoa accepted Christianity so quickly, embracing it with enthusiasm and vigor. It accepted the missionaries with open arms and put them in positions of influence. The message that the missionaries brought to Samoa is referred to by Samoans as *ole sāvali ole fīlēmū* (the message of peace).

Christianity has had many positive effects on Samoans and Samoan society. Some of the internal conflicts between warring factions were reduced, and pagan practices like cannibalism were done away with. However, its effects were not all positive. The arrival of Christianity has had a negative effect on the traditional beliefs in spirits. Tamasese, Peteru, Waldegrave, and Bush (2005) suggest that missionary influence created value judgments that spirits were evil and satanic, whereas according to traditional beliefs, spirits were to be respected, rather than feared, as they were merely guardians of the *tapu*.

Spirituality and Health

Lui and Schwenke (2003) describe spirituality in this way: "Spirituality is the feeling of connectedness a person has to the non-physical side of their being. This includes a person's connectedness to their ancestors, their land and God" (p. 176). Using this definition, spirituality is much more than just religion. It is a fundamental part of the Samoan belief system and psyche, and possibly one reason why the Samoan people have taken on religion with enthusiasm and vigor. The gospel brought by John Williams, later followed by missionaries and clerics from other religious denominations, was similar to the beliefs that Samoans already held.

How is spirituality related to mental health? A Samoan perspective on health makes the answer clearer. One view put forward by Lui and Schwenke (2003) is that health is achieved by maintaining good, safe, and balanced relationships between three elements: the person, God, and the land/environment. All relationships are sacred (tapu) and all relationships have boundaries that are defined and guarded by tapu or *sa* (p. 176). The

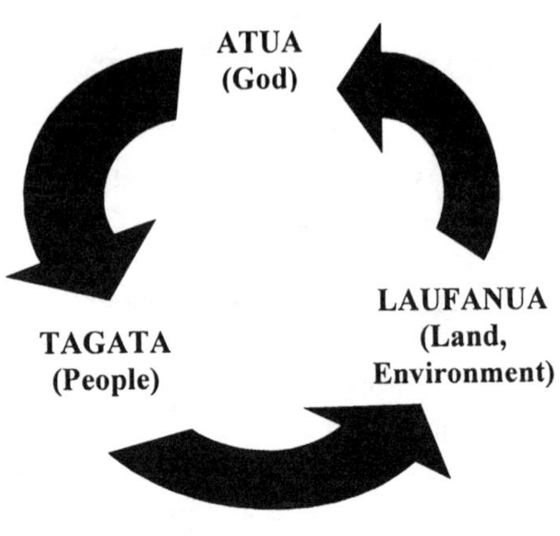

Soifua Mālōlōina Model

guardians of the tapu may be a person, a family, or a village, and in the case of the relationship between Atua and *tagata* (human beings) and between Atua and *laufanua* (land), the guardian is a spirit. This perspective I have conceptualized into a model that I have called the *soifua mālōlōina* model.

When these elements of Atua, tagata, and laufanua are in balance, a person is *mālōlōina* (in a state of wellness). When a person is in a state of wellness, she or he is able to meet his or her responsibilities and obligations to self, family, community, and God. Samoans therefore view health in a broad and holistic sense (Lui & Schwenke, 2003).

Spirituality and Our Relationship to God

Traditionally, Samoans believe that a person has two parts (*itū lua*): the physical and the spiritual (Tamasese et al., 2005). These two parts are referred to by some as *tino* (body) and *loto* (spirit or soul). Tino is the body—the physical, tangible part of a person—and loto is the nonphysical or spiritual dimension, including the soul and the mind. The two parts are integral to the whole person and cannot be separated. The spiritual part includes a person's mental dimension. Spirituality may be described as our sense of connectedness to our Atua, to the laufanua, and to our ancestors who have passed on. Samoans also believe in the existence of *aītu* (spirits) and *sauali'i* (ghosts). These can be ancestors that have passed on or spiritual guardians who guard the boundaries of our relationships with God and our spiritual realm. Spirituality is not only something that is external, but also something within us. It is an integral part of our sense of belonging, our sense of connectedness to the things that we hold dear, and it provides meaning for our existence.

Samoans believe that human beings are direct descendants of God. Traditional Samoan legend traces the origin of human beings (tagata) to the direct result of the union between *Lagi* (Sky God) and *Papa* (rock). Lagi and Papa came together to form a human. After the human was created, the spirit, the heart, and the mind were joined together inside the human to form the core (*fatu*), which in turn was joined to the earth (*'ele'ele*). This union, referred to as *fatu ma 'ele'ele* (the core/heart and the earth), produced offspring (human beings). Hence Samoan people have a strong sense of spirituality and connectedness to the spiritual realm and to God. Our spirituality is our feeling—that sense of belonging and connectedness to God and to our nonphysical realm. The Samoan term for blood is 'ele'ele or *palapala* (earth), a constant reminder to us of the direct relationship between people, God, and the earth/land.

Tapu *and Safety*

The concept of tapu (sacred/taboo) is more about safety than about a punitive measure or punishment for some wrongdoing. Tapu defines the boundary between what a person can do (safe) and what a person should not do (unsafe). As long as a person operates in the safe realm, that is, doing only those things that the tapu defines as safe, there is no negative consequence. However, when a person does things that the tapu defines as unsafe, the person then enters an area of risk. This may result in a person's being affected by a curse and perhaps being punished by the guardian of the tapu, thus possibly leading to illness. The function of tapu is to protect and enhance people's lives (Tamasese et al., 1997). Thus, relational arrangements are regulated by protocols and etiquette that define appropriate and correct behavior. Understanding and respecting tapu allows a person to stay safe and healthy—physically, mentally, and spiritually—by maintaining safe and balanced relationships with God, people, and the land.

When someone breaches a tapu, he or she then enters an area of risk that results in that person's relationships becoming unbalanced. According to Tamasese et al. (2005), such breaches place the offender outside the sphere of correct relational arrangements and thus incorrectly placed in terms of identity and sense of belonging. If the breach is of a serious nature, it may result in a person's being unwell, either physically or mentally, or both.

Mental and Spiritual Unwellness

There are several taxonomies for spiritual and mental unwellness in the *fa'a-Samoa* (Samoan way/understanding). *Fasia,* according to Tamasese et al. (1997), refers to a person who has been struck or hit by a spirit, which is normally known to happen to someone who has offended a spirit. *Sāua* is when a person is affected by the spell or influence of a spirit, usually when one has trodden upon sacred ground that is guarded by a spirit guardian. *Mala'aumatuā* and *mala'aunu'uā* refer to the condition brought about by a curse from parents or village chiefs when a tapu has been breached.

Lui (2001), in a conference presentation entitled "Traditional Healing in Modern Psychiatry," suggested that "a person's beliefs and their understanding and perception of their health and illness determine their response, their practice, and the treatment and intervention they will undertake" (p. 274). The successful treatment and healing of illness requires the correct identification of the identity of the spirit or guardian of the tapu that the person has breached. This identification is done by a *taulāsea* (healer). Lui further stated that "traditional treatment of mental/spirit illness may involve the use of herbs, massage and dialogue (talking) treatment, or a combination of all three" (2001, p. 274). The treatment is administered by the taulasea or *fofō* (traditional healer).

Spiritual Injury

A problem with modern health systems is that they are based on Western paradigms and scientific models. "These paradigms and models do not acknowledge the spiritual element. The methods of treatment available often involve use of medications and medical treatment" (Lui, 2003, p. 176). A consequence is that the models, methods, and treatments used are inappropriate, as Western medicine does not acknowledge traditional beliefs, logic, and information that lead to effective diagnosis and treatment of what is essentially a traditional spiritual illness or condition. In such cases, Western medical doctors can only deal with the symptoms, but not the cause of the illness, which is required for a full recovery of the affected person.

In traditional Samoan belief, the spirit of a person is just as important as the mind and the physical body. A person's spirit can sustain an injury in the same sense as a person can sustain an injury to the body or the mind. In the New Zealand health system and in medical circles, little is done to help care for a person's spirit (*agaga*). The spirit is not part of routine medical assessments and investigations. Yet the notion of spiritual injury applies to all people, regardless of whether their beliefs about, and understanding of, spirituality are linked to a Christian or a traditional concept.

Paradigms in Conflict

When a person sustains a spiritual injury, the mental health system is not equipped to respond to and treat such injury or condition. One reason may be that it is not acknowledged within the medical paradigm. Lui (2001) suggests that this lack of acknowledgment is because the so-called Western or European view of mental illness is based on scientific data and information, and things that can be measured with regard to an individual's body or mind or in the environment. The medical paradigm cannot easily accommodate anything that is cultural, religious, or spiritual in nature. In fact, psychiatry is often hostile to religious or spiritual beliefs, or worse, such beliefs are considered by psychiatrists to be symptoms of mental illness itself. As a result a patient often does not divulge such information to the treating physician; hence, the condition is left untreated and potentially worsens.

As already indicated, in the traditional paradigm familiar to Samoans, spirituality is an important part of a person and forms a key dimension of a person's worldview. Spiritual experiences, such as seeing or hearing deceased ancestors or other spirits, are natural and uplifting.

The Western psychiatrist, on the other hand, often discounts such experiences, or worse, may consider such experiences to be delusions or hallucinations, and a sign that the patient is "off his head." What is considered in one paradigm as normal or positive is considered totally differently in another paradigm. Hence we have the interesting dichotomy of these two paradigms.

Some of the symptoms of spirit illness are similar to symptoms of Western psychiatric illnesses. As such, traditional conditions such as *sāua, fasia,* and other spirit illnesses, are misdiagnosed by medical doctors as schizophrenia, psychosis, or other psychiatric illnesses because the symptoms may be similar in nature. A New Zealand case from the late 1990s illustrates this tension. Names and some aspects of the case have been changed to disguise the identity of the persons involved.

CASE SCENARIO ONE

A Pacific woman—Mele—was brought by her family to a psychiatric inpatient unit in Auckland because the family could not cope with her at home. The family reported to the admitting staff at the hospital that Mele had been acting differently over the past month or so. She would at times get into a state when she would be quite aggressive and appeared disoriented. During such a state she would speak in a deep voice, different from her normal voice. The content of what she said when in such a state did not seem relevant to those around her. She spoke of people and things that related to the Pacific island that she had come from, but were not related to her current environment and circumstances. The people she spoke to, in such a state, had all passed away. She also seemed to have incredible strength when in such a state. Despite her small size, a few men found it difficult to hold her down, to keep her from running onto the road and lashing out at people. These states lasted for ten to fifteen minutes. Afterwards she had no recollection of what had happened and otherwise returned to normal. Mele would get into such a state about once or twice a day, the timing of which happened randomly. The family believed that Mele's condition was a traditional one, related to a spirit or a curse, but for safety reasons the family decided to bring her to the hospital.

As a member of a Pacific service, I was asked to help find a solution to the problem. After discussion with the family, they stated their desire to seek the help of a taulāsea (traditional healer) to diagnose the illness. The family held a firm belief that Mele's illness was traditional rather than medical. The hospital, however, had a responsibility to care for Mele. The only care and treatment they could offer was from a medical perspective. I held discussions with the clinical team and the responsible psychiatrist to propose a plan. The plan involved withholding the use of medical treatment for three days while Mele was allowed to receive traditional healing from the taulāsea. Mele was granted day-leave from the hospital to receive traditional treatment and returned to the hospital each evening.

The taulāsea's diagnosis was that Mele's condition was due to a curse placed on the family by their village a generation earlier, after an incident involving Mele's father. The family was exiled from the village when Mele's father had breached a village tapu. The family's investigation of these revelations by the taulāsea confirmed the truth of what they had been told. The family found this intriguing, as the taulāsea had never met or known the family before and had no previous personal knowledge of the family's circumstances.

After the first two treatments, Mele made a remarkable recovery. She was discharged from the hospital after five days. The taulāsea recommended that for a full cure, Mele and members of her family needed to return to the Pacific island to make a formal apology to the village. This was done a month after discharge.

Due to the proper diagnosis by the taulāsea, Mele received the appropriate treatment and made a full recovery. On the other hand, had a psychiatrist made the diagnosis, the treatment prescribed would probably have been in the form of medication that might have provided relief in the short term, but would not have dealt with the cause of the illness. Furthermore, Mele would possibly have received a medical diagnosis such as schizophrenia or psychosis, and had to endure the stigma of mental illness for the rest of her life. Medical intervention, apart from not providing a cure, would have been inappropriate, because Mele's condition was not a medical one.

Lui (2001) asserts that Western clinicians are perceived by Pacific people as authoritarian and disrespectful of their beliefs, values, status, and rights.

"Many Pacific people continue to access traditional healing practices either as an alternative or at the same time as seeing a psychiatrist" (p. 276). For best health outcomes, the conflicted view of spirituality between the traditional paradigm and the medical paradigm needs to be resolved. Rather than discounting and marginalizing the traditional paradigm and the related treatment options, the mental health system can work cooperatively with it for better outcomes.

Most Pacific people who come through the mental health services in New Zealand receive a psychiatric diagnosis, which they do not question. However, investigations, and particularly appropriate interventions, can be enhanced by inclusion of Pacific philosophies, beliefs, values, ideas, and people in the decisions, treatment, and care. A look at a second case will illustrate this further. Again, names and other details have been carefully altered to disguise the identity of the person.

CASE SCENARIO TWO

Olepa came from the Pacific Islands in her late teens to stay with her family in an Auckland suburb. The family felt that Olepa would have a better life for herself in New Zealand. She might find a job to help her family back in the islands. However, Olepa was unsettled in her new environment. Her family was supportive, but she became depressed and suicidal. Olepa was admitted to the inpatient unit, where she was diagnosed with post-traumatic stress disorder and prescribed medication. She improved and was discharged, only to be readmitted to the hospital when she deteriorated again. This process was repeated a few times. The Pacific Island Mental Health Service was engaged to work with her.

Investigations revealed that she had been sexually abused by a family member in the islands when she was much younger. During our work with her over a period of several months, we felt that although Olepa was suffering from the trauma—a diagnosable mental illness as a result of the abuse—there was also another element that was hindering her recovery. I felt that she was homesick: missing her family, her friends, community, country, and the familiar environment she was used to. These are issues that are related to her sense of belonging, resiliency, and spirituality.

In this case, we had no issue with the diagnosis, but we differed from the clinical team with regard to the solution and constituent elements of her recovery plan. As a Pacific Service, we felt Olepa needed to return home in order to recover, to heal her spiritual injury and wounds, so that she might return to a condition of health that would enable her to make a full recovery, not only in her mind, but, more important, in her spirit.

After a few months, and another admission to the inpatient unit, the clinical team agreed for Olepa to return to the islands. We understand that she made a speedy recovery and has not required any medication to keep her well in the community. She is able to deal with her illness with the help of her family and health professionals. The family has also been able to deal with the abuse, and a reconciliation process was undertaken within the family as part of her healing process.

Spirituality and Recovery

Understanding the spiritual realm and the ways in which it impacts a person is vital to practitioners' understanding of health, identity, and well-being. When dealing with Pacific clients, there is a general consensus that everyone has a spirit, and the spirit may be injured in the same sense as a physical injury is sustained. For a full recovery, all injuries need to be healed. Acceptance of, and, more important, the understanding of the spiritual realm, and its inclusion in the healing and treatment care plans within our mental health system will, in my view, greatly enhance the recovery of Pacific Island mental health consumers.

References

Lui, D. (2001). Traditional healing in modern psychiatry: A Pacific perspective. In *No one is an island: Proceedings of the 11th annual The MHS Conference 2001*. Wellington: The Mental Health Services Conference of Australia and New Zealand, pp. 274–276.

Lui, D., & Schwenke, L. (2003). Soul searching. In *From rhetoric to reality: Proceedings of the 12th annual The MHS Conference 2003*. Wellington: The Mental Health Services Conference of Australia and New Zealand, pp. 175–178.

Mental Health Commission of New Zealand. (2004). A Pacific perspective on the NZ Mental Health Classification and Outcomes Study (CAOS), February 2004, at http://www.mhc.govt.nz/publications/2004.html.

Tamasese, K., Peteru, C., Waldegrave, C., & Bush, A. (2005). Ole taeao afua, the new morning: A qualitative investigation into Samoan perspectives on mental health and culturally appropriate services. *Australian and New Zealand Journal of Psychiatry* 39(4), 300–309.

7

Making Culture "God" Is Driving Our People Crazy!

AN INTERVIEW WITH CABRINI ʻOFA MAKASIALE BY PHILIP CULBERTSON

Cabrini: *In my following remarks, I do not wish to dismiss or deny the many positive and affirming aspects of our Pasifika cultures. Rather, this is an attempt to address the ways in which the shadow side of Pasifika needs transforming.*

Philip: Cabrini, at a moment in history when the whole Pacific is struggling against both globalization and the long-term effects of European colonization, to make a statement like "Making culture 'God' is driving our people crazy!" sounds pretty radical to me.

Cabrini: Earlier, I was looking in the dictionary, and it defined *crazy* in two ways: as "insane" or as "making cracks." It made me think about different kinds of cracks—unhelpful cracks in our people's living and thinking. By making culture "God," I mean something like what Erich Fromm (1959) said in his book, *Psychoanalysis and Religion,* that the deification of things is a particularly human attitude. It's normal; it's also normal for people to submit to what they want to deify. Fortunately, the balancing attitude we carry as human people is a devotion to realizing the highest principles—for example, life, love, reason, or in a Christian context, being made in the likeness of God. Fromm says this is part of our search to be fulfilled; it's part of our deepest longing. I think that what's happened for some of our Pacific people is that we have that longing for the highest principles, like any other peoples—longing to be fulfilled and to be happy. Originally we found that fulfillment in our home back in the islands, and life had a certain form, ritual, context, geography, and so forth. Now that we've come to Aotearoa/New Zealand, we've unconsciously re-created some kind of pseudo-fulfillment.

Agneta Schreurs (2002) carries on further from Fromm's theories. She says that when we deify something in our search to fill the hole of meaninglessness, we make it an idol, and that opens the door to idolatry. In the West, we have made money an idol; we deify it, and we confuse it with the highest principles of life and happiness. Pasifika has made an idol out of culture, in order unconsciously to hang on to something of what fulfilled us back home. Schreur says that we turn "a good" into "the good," and make it ultimate, and that's where it becomes idolatrous. We make the means into an end. I see culture as a means, not an end, to our faith, to our God, and the like. The display of culture, and the transaction of culture or happiness, is only the means to a higher good. It is not the end, or the higher good itself.

Philip: So culture is *a* means to happiness, but not *the* means to happiness?

Cabrini: Yes. Some of us live quite unconsciously in Aotearoa. We carry out a search for happiness using our culture from back home. But we are now on a new soil, and so a crack has been created between here and where we once belonged. Fromm argues that we need to probe the power and direction of our underlying motivation. We need to find out what's missing, in order for the crack to be healed. Pacific people already know something about enculturation, but because we are searching, all we are doing here in Aotearoa/New Zealand is reenacting old practices unthinkingly. We're in a *new* land now; we're not back home any longer. We came here because we were yearning for what this new land could provide us. We came to this country, knowing that canoes and coconuts and fishing on the reef could not give our children the education they aspired to. Now, in addition to "Pearly Shells," we need to learn to sing a new song in this new land. I don't mean that we discard or let go of tradition. We need our traditions as a base to forge something new here. We are not doing that because we are not probing, we are not critically analyzing what we are doing, why we are doing it, and when we should or shouldn't do it.

A classic illustration is what happens when we go to a *fono* (convocation, council), usually sponsored by some government department that allocates funding for a particular community work. When we turn up to this gathering, there are quite a few chiefs—*matai* (chiefs), *matāpule* (orators), you name it. The coordinator of the gathering happens to be from a particular Pacific island, so automatically we adopt the protocol of that island. We begin the welcomes, and then one hour has gone, and we are still welcoming and welcoming. The purpose of the gathering was to submit funding applications for our work, but two hours have gone by and we are still welcoming the last of the chiefs from another island group. Before we know it, only one hour is left, so who gets to present their submissions first? Those chiefs who are there with some particular project! Someone says, "But what about us? We came here to get some funding for our project!" The response will be, "Ssh, we haven't finished the welcome yet! Ssh—*fie pālangi* [you're behaving like a white person]. Keep quiet!" And then, to hurry the whole process up because we're running out of time, guess who gets the largest funding? The chief from the island or village that the coordinator comes from, because he or she has to be culturally polite to their own chief!

David Augsburger (1986) calls this gap a sacralization of culture. Here we are, singing hymns and giving offerings to the church at an exorbitant rate, all because our family name has been called out. The next day I'm sitting in my therapy room, across from a woman in the grip of anxiety and panic because she doesn't have enough money to buy groceries for her children's dinner. Why? Because her stepfather is the minister, who needs $30,000 to go to some annual meeting in some island, and I think to myself, "Where is your critical analysis?" How are we using the gospel values of justice to probe into the underlying motivation for this sort of extortion? I mean, what's happened to our ministers?

Philip: That's the single most frequent complaint that I hear from our Pasifika students. They frame the problem as an indefensible abuse of the ministerial office, and the redefinition of what it means to be a good Christian, based simply on financial donations. What do you think?

Cabrini: I think that in this process, we have deified culture to the point that the people have become comatose. People are searching for happiness, and the minister belts out this message that "God is your only happiness," and suddenly that's plastered on the top of the human process of greed, power, and position. Traditionally our chiefs were honored because they took care of the greater good of all the people. But it's become corrupt over time, even (or especially) in the ministry: "I'm a chief/minister; you are a commoner/congregant. It's your cultural/religious duty to give over your money." It's imperative that we find a way to distinguish God from culture!

Philip: I don't quite understand. Can't one stay in the church and exercise some critical skills?

Cabrini: Before that can happen, we need to help our people wake up, to make them conscious. We need programs like the liberation theologians ran in South America, designed to make people conscious of the importance of separating culture from gospel—*a* good thing from *the* good, the means from the end. We Pacific people are very spiritual. We have a great reverence for the transcendent being, which is why our souls and hearts keep on working well, but our minds seem to be asleep!

Philip: Are you suggesting that some people confuse happiness with mindlessness, or being asleep?

Cabrini: Yes—mindlessness is both soothing, and very normal. It's even easier if I am poor, or socially oppressed, or a Pasifika woman, or I have no formal education to better my lot in life. Mindlessness makes those things hurt less.

Philip: Do you believe that Pacific people are more afraid to turn on their minds than anyone else is?

Cabrini: It's very painful to swim upstream in a culture where people get their identity from the collective. It's very risky: I could be turfed out [ostracized]! Then I might not have anywhere else to go, especially if the other communities I might access all think just like the community I've just left!

Philip: My students tell me that when Pacific people walk away from the church, they lose their whole social network.

Cabrini: Yes, you start to get what David Allen (1988) calls disqualification messages: you're fie pālangi (acting like a white person); you're not a good Tongan or Samoan or whatever. You're showered with messages of shame. Because we have so identified with the collective, we have lost our ability to distinguish between uniformity and being part of a collective. Individuality is unacceptable. Yet, a healthy collective has diversity. Unity assumes diversity, but uniformity doesn't. Uniformity views difference as a threat. But if we sought unity instead of uniformity, difference and diversity would be valued and accepted, engaged and used productively. That's why we need time to reflect, as Fromm and Schreurs recommend, to probe into the underlying motivation and power of what we are doing when we do it.

For instance, in the secondary schools in New Zealand, there is a huge push to have an entire week, annually, devoted to competitive performances in cultural festivals. But we've got enough of our songs, enough of our dances. They are already well cemented, but critical thinking is still embryonic. So I suggest that we need to set aside an entire week, annually, for the critical analysis of our cultural demands and structures, in order that as Pacific people, we might find a future way of being in Aotearoa/New Zealand that will benefit us all.

Philip: But don't you think those cultural festivals are good for bolstering the students' self-esteem?

Cabrini: But what self-esteem? Is it false self-esteem, or the split one that continues to dream of the life we had back home in the islands? We are not in the islands anymore; we are in a new land. Instead, we need to be visionaries, to learn about what is best from our island homes, and best from our current home, and create something new, a new third.

Philip: It seems to me that you are suggesting that as long as Pacific peoples look backwards, toward their island homes, they will never be able to find their own sense of authority. Did the *waka* (canoe) sail before people had a chance to pack their own authority to bring with them?

Cabrini: I believe so! We need to learn to individuate because only the strong individual can make a strong community. The individual makes the community strong and the community invites and assists the individual to contribute back to it to make it stronger. There is a connection between convention and invention. Too much of one produces hysteria, and too much of the other produces neurosis. Conventional uniformity creates mass hysteria, and exaggerated individualism creates neurotic anxiety. Individuation is the path between the two: finding one's own authoritative self, while staying connected to the group.

Philip: Can you give me an example of how individuation should work with Pacific people living here?

Cabrini: Let's take, for example, the ritual of the kava ceremony with the ritual of the church. One is a cultural ritual, the other a ritual about the transcendent. We have blurred the two together, bowing to and making idols of both, but we haven't really reflected on the difference between the two rituals. So I have people coming to me for counseling concerning the fusion of culture and God, and I say to them, "Let's put up on the board a list of cultural values, and a list of gospel values." When they've done that, they say, "Gosh, they're quite different!" They've forgotten for a moment that they are in a new land; they're still operating like they're back home in the collective village. We're not in a collective economy anymore. Back home, if I don't have enough food to feed my children, my neighbors will bring me some food from their garden. But here, if I have given $10,000 to the minister's latest project and don't have enough to pay my child's school fees, my neighbors can't be expected to rescue me. Back home the neighbors might give me a pig and some taro, but here, that won't pay the school fees!

The other element that props up this crazy system of cracks, or the split between body and mind, or culture and gospel, is the traditional protocol, drummed into us from childhood, that being well-brought up means not asking questions, and allowing others to direct you. So we listen to what the pastor tells us about tithing, or the way the male is ordained to be head of the church, and we dismiss our analytical ability. Critical analysis demands that we ask questions—many difficult questions. But if you are a Pasifika child or woman, you are constantly being told, directed, and talked down to. That's how the culture is generally organized.

Philip: Who is that comment directed at, Cabrini? Surely it's culturally impossible for Pasifika children to seize the right to ask questions.

Cabrini: I'm directing it at the parents and the grandparents, and in particular to those within the system who hold the power, who hold the positions of responsibility, particularly the chiefs, the ministers, and other senior males. We must try to make changes—sustaining what is life-giving in the system and reforming what is oppressive. Structural analysis teaches us that those who are enjoying the good life do not feel the pain, and so they see no need for change. It's the people on the ground who hold up the whole infrastructure, whose backs are breaking. These are the ones who feel the pain and need the change. If I have a toothache, I am the one who goes to the dentist, not you. That's how it goes in structural analysis: if you feel the pain, you make the change. You can't sit down and say, "Oh, I wish the dentist knew about my toothache." He doesn't, nor do the people in power. We must be prepared to do education at both ends of the hierarchical structure—challenging the top and empowering the bottom—in order to bring about rebirth and renewal of our cultural values. We need to find ways that culture can give more life, here, in ways that are more real, appropriate, and productive for this new land.

Philip: It sounds like you think that the potential is there, among the young, for revolution in the Pacific.

Cabrini: Well, let's take Tonga as a classic example. People are hungry for change, and the royal family knows it. The wise ones will use the context well, but they may not have enough time before the river bursts. Again, church and culture are alike in this way. We claim to be a very spiritual people, believing that God is in everything. We claim to be a gospel people, but at the same time, some in the church are using cultural values to gain more money, mana, or position, and just plastering the gospel values over the top. In this way, people are lulled into some kind of fantasy that culture and God are one of a kind. But the gospel values I know of don't put ministers in the front row, and don't let the minister go traveling while others suffer. Sometimes I ask those ministers, "Which Bible do *you* study from?" The clever ones say, "Oh, the one we made up so that we can get those white envelopes from the people. We share those." But I've never seen those envelopes shared! They usually just vanish, and the next thing we know, the minister has a new home and two new cars and is off overseas again to attend another conference.

In the New Testament, it says that the top people should be the last to seat themselves at the table. The opposite, of course, is the Pasifika hierarchy, where the nobles and the chiefs sit at the best places at the table. I've never seen a Tongan noble say to the lame or the poor, "Come forward, come sit up here, you're really what the kingdom is about." People say, "But oh, that's our culture," and I say "Tough! Stop claiming to be practicing gospel values, because you're really just practicing some cultural traditions that I don't want to have any part of!"

Philip: Are we taking about culture, or about someone's romantic interpretation of culture?

Cabrini: Both, I think. Each one adds their stuff onto the context and structure, and some of us also project our needs onto our leaders. It makes us feel better; it makes me feel better to have you leading me, guiding me, so I project onto you: you can save me, you can give me money, you can give me a job, and I will be dependent for the rest of my life, well brought up, and won't challenge your authority. It works both ways. The best place to challenge this symbiosis is in the church. We must begin the process of critical analysis, in our sermons, family groups, and church groups, about what is inhuman and oppressive about our culture, and what is truly gospel, which means good news, which means liberation, life, freedom, forgiveness, reconciliation, and justice for all. Those are the gospel values.

It's sad how the church itself lives out the sort of splitting that I'm equating with craziness. In our churches, we are too often talked at, sermonized, yelled at, and brainwashed, but there's no reciprocity. Because there's no room for diversity in unity, pretty soon you'll have two factions fighting each other, and then one of the opposing leaders leaves with twenty families and starts a new congregation. In Tonga we have so many little churches, and they tie themselves to this or that minister, and I think it's simply a replica of the chief, the village, and the people, because that's the context they're used to. I'm thinking, why do we have to split, and continue splitting, in order to cope with our need to be different? Wouldn't it be better to do diversity inside of unity? The conflicts and the splitting are crazy-making stuff.

Philip: You've suggested that the deification of culture allows one to be soothed, to go to sleep, to give the authority over to the minister, or *faka-Tonga* (the Tongan way of life), or wherever it may reside. But hasn't that made the definition of culture so rigid that it necessitates people who police it somehow?

Cabrini: Because we believe that God is an absolute, we have deified culture as an absolute too. Rot! Culture is organic; it constantly grows and changes, responsive to the environment around it. Culture expresses the transcendent, but it is not the transcendent; the transcendent predetermines culture. The two have become blurred so that somehow, we can't raise our voices against either culture or the church. They're too close to each other, and the ministers seem to understand that they benefit from that blurring. Because there is no vox populi in the church, the people get more and more muted. We whisper in cafes and supermarkets about "the minister," and then someone says we should break away; that's how we can handle it. Or we might join a pālangi [in Samoan, pālagi] church because it's more democratic; our individual voices can be heard there. Or we might just retreat to an island ghetto, like Otara or Mangere.

Until Pacific peoples can learn to individuate—to be an individual within the collective—we have only a limited future in this new land. Conversation between the top of the hierarchy and the bottom must be encouraged. The hierarchy, whether cultural or familial, doesn't encourage it, so we go to church, and are very well brought up, and affirmed for not asking questions, and it becomes quite insidious for old and young alike. Our children take that attitude to school, so it's no wonder they come in last in the class. It's not polite to get out of your seat and go get the best book out of the library before Milly Smith gets it. I'll wait until the teacher tells me to get up, and of course, by then, the best books are gone. I can't get to 7th Form [senior year] because I will need seven others to come with me. I can't go on my own; it's in-built in us. We haven't thought through what it means to be in this new land. What was all right in the village is not all right here.

Philip: Are you saying that the lesson to sit and wait shouldn't be taught anywhere, either here or in Tonga?

Cabrini: There's a time for sitting and waiting, and a time for getting up and moving, and a time for settling down to dialogue. Somehow we just keep the needle on empty, or half a tank. You know how the needle should move according to the petrol tank? Our needle seems to be stuck on nearly empty.

We are affirmed for keeping quiet, behaving ourselves, and not asking questions. I have a Tongan relative who comes to do the gardening for the community of women I live with. He mows the lawns and then he sits down. That's good cultural protocol. Once, Patricia said, "Why is Simi sitting down?" I said, "He's waiting for our next directive; that's the protocol." So she said, "Simi, get the rake and rake up the grass clippings." "Yo!" he said. And then rake, rake, rake, and they're all in piles, and he sits down. Patricia said, "Simi is sitting again." I said, "Next order: tell him to put them around the rose bushes." So that was the first time. Two weeks later, Simi came again to do the gardening, and the same procedure: he sat. Patricia said, "Can he not deduce, Cabrini, that that's what he does from now on? Do I have to keep reiterating the directive?" "I think so," I said. So I went to Simi and said, "Simi, in this country, when you have done it once like that, then you take the initiative. You mow the lawn, you collect the grass clippings, and you put them around the rose bushes. You don't keep calling me to ask what's next." "Oh, that's fine," he said. "I shall do that."

Philip: So ever after he did?

Cabrini: Yes, he does that all the time now, but if it's a new procedure, he will start all over because that is cultural protocol. But you see, we are creatures of habit and familiarity. That's what Freud said: we have a compulsion to repeat. Once, I saw some Pacific Islanders at the bus stop where I get off in Manukau, who had been sitting for an hour. I said I'm going to do my conscientization thing, so I said to them, "I've seen you waiting; how long have you been sitting here?" "Over an hour; our bus hasn't come," they said. I said, "Do you know that there's a bus phone number you can ring?" "Oh, really?" "You can ask them if there's another bus to catch." One said, "Oh, no, I didn't think of phoning up and asking." The other said, "Oh, I don't have a phone." Two hours went by, they didn't turn up to work, and they got sacked. So I say, Think! you know, because no one has encouraged them and affirmed them and said, Go, you go Mele, you think Mele, you find out Mele, you go to the library Mele. But if Mele goes to church, and memorizes all those scripture quotations, goes home, does all the cooking for her stepmother, sweeps all the leaves off, and then starts her homework at 10 p.m., well, of course she comes last in school. We haven't translated our reality. We're still hanging on to the familiar.

Philip: But it must be very difficult to learn to thrive in a new culture, particularly when one is repeatedly misunderstood by the dominant culture.

Cabrini: Of course it is, but if we're going to thrive, instead of being crazy-split, then we must learn. And we need to find the right people to help us, those who speak to us in ways we can understand and that encourage us. A government mental health agency had been looking for a counselor for a Polynesian man who had chopped his right hand off in a factory accident. He had gone to three psychologists, but was still weepy and couldn't return to work. The employer wanted to terminate the man's counseling, and I was the last option they could locate. They granted me just one appointment with him. I quickly figured out that this man had done what so many other Pacific peoples do: conflated his search for happiness with his search for God. So I asked him, "What do you think is the meaning of this event for you, that you go and chop off not just a hand, but your right hand that gives you your livelihood, your agency?" He looked at me and said, "My right hand has fed my family. I have eight children. They've all grown up and they are well educated. I'm near retirement now and this accident has reminded me that God is my right hand. This was 'flesh' right hand, and now it is God's right hand." "Good," I said to myself, "he's separating himself and culture from the transcendent." "So," I said, "now that your physical human right hand is gone, does your faith or God have anything to say to you about the meaning of this event? Because," I said, "if you can make meaning, you will stop crying." He said, "Do you know what I think God is telling me? 'It's time for you to retire. You've delivered to your children; stop getting your business or your mana from your work,' God said. I got a lot of money from my work. It used to make me proud. 'Stop getting your meaning from what your money can buy; retire and get more spiritual.' That's what I think God is telling me through this event. I got too smart-arsed, got familiar with the machinery, and got my hand chopped off. I didn't follow the rules." "So what will you do now?" I asked. He said, "I will go in, submit my resignation, ask my boss for casual work, and I will turn my life around. I have made money, by God, because I had a lot of money in that shift work. Now I'll let my sibling and my children take on the power of supporting and feeding." And he said to me, "Do you know, I held a lot of power." "Good," I said. "Write the letter and go back to your employer. The agency will be very happy; they are only paying me for one miserable session!" And off he went. He could separate the two—what was ultimate and what was conditional. He made meaning out of it and moved on.

Philip: Karl Marx is reputed to have said something about every system containing within it the seeds of its own destruction. How can we challenge those seeds of destruction that lie within Pasifika churches and cultures?

Cabrini: For Pacific peoples, identity has traditionally been drawn from a rootedness in the land and a sense of belonging to the *kāinga* (extended family). In Aotearoa/New Zealand, we are not "the people of the land": that is the place of Māori. Also, most of us have come here within the past forty years, and in this land, that makes us relative newcomers. The challenge for us is to weave something new and fresh out of the position of ambivalence and landlessness here. The challenge is not to become less confident, but to become more reflective and creative, thinking more deeply about the sorts of highest good we can pursue here, to benefit not only ourselves, but more important, our children and grandchildren in this new land. We need to create something new to define us here in Aotearoa. If we do not do this, we will be sowing the seeds of our own destruction.

We Pacific people are a strong people, a proud people. One of the gifts of our cultures is that they have taught us to survive, in the face of hardship, by banding together. The down-side of banding together is that we immediately form hierarchies of power, turning protection into exploitation within our own ranks. And hierarchies keep many of our people immature, voiceless, and asleep. To heal the cracks, our new task in a new land is for each person to develop a sense of self that is awake, reflective, and separate, yet connected—to affirm and celebrate diversity in unity. To do that, we need to learn how to sit with paradox, because that's life: you have the universal and the local, the individual and the collective. For those who have been kept immature for too long, holding ambiguity is uncomfortable, but maybe that's the difference between being children back home, and adults in the here and now—where we now belong.

References

Allen, D. (1988). *A family systems approach to individual psychotherapy*. Northvale: Jason Aaronson.

Augsburger, D. (1986). *Pastoral counseling across cultures*. Philadelphia: Westminster.

Fromm, E. (1959). *Psychoanalysis and religion*. New Haven: Yale University Press.

Schreurs, A. (2002). *Psychotherapy and spirituality: Integrating the spiritual dimension into therapeutic practice*. London: Jessica Kingsley.

8

The Schizophrenic Church

A SURVIVOR

Samoan Christian or Christian Samoan? I remember a Samoan clergyman asking me that question when I was a young teenager. Which comes first, he asked, or is there no distinction? He said being a Christian and being Samoan are so intertwined that culture and Christianity determine each other.

I have titled this essay "The Schizophrenic Church" because the church has always been seen as the place we must go, as spiritual people, to receive spiritual blessings in order for our lives to be successful and useful to our people. At the same time if we didn't go to church we were assumed to be cursed and to bring shame on our family. We would amount to nothing and never be good for anything we set out to achieve.

For my parents, church was the central and focal point of their existence in Auckland. It represented the familiar in terms of people, language, and culture, as well as a spirituality, that ensured them a place in heaven and success and prosperity for their children and family.

Years of denial and growing up in a perfect bubble told me that God was in charge of my life. I saw clergy as the messengers of God and therefore as God's representatives. They could do no wrong; their mandate was about goodness and mercy, justice, and peace.

I look back over my life in the church and I reflect on those years. If I am to be really honest, I need to ask myself, If my parents gave me a choice not to go to church or to go, would I have gone? The answer is easy: No! I would not have gone all the time. I would have gone sometimes and I would have loved to have gone because I chose to, not because I had to. The fact that I had no choice made me resist the whole idea of church, because I never got to try out for the provincial sports teams because all the trials were on Sunday. I had a love-hate relationship with church. And it was there that, as a teenager, I was sexually abused by a newly ordained minister of the church.

The other day a relative asked me, "Have you forgiven him for what he did to you?" To say I was shocked by such a question is an understatement.

Forgiven? Forgiven? Oh my gosh—that word, that concept, that theological question was so unfair! How dare I be asked to respond, let alone consider the possibility that I had to forgive someone who had not only hurt me and violated me, but had pushed my faith almost to a point of no return? How dare I be questioned as to my role in this abuse?

In recent years I was stricken by that horrible DSM-IV diagnosis of PTSD (post-traumatic stress disorder) and depression. Occasionally, when I became a little uncooperative, then BPD (borderline personality disorder) was added to the host of letters that required my popping pills to keep me under control.

Forgive? I looked at her in disbelief. Where on earth did this damn question come from and who put those damn words in her mouth? "Unless you have forgiven him," she continued, "you will always stay sick." I felt myself drowning in a deluge of chaos and frustration.

I shouted, "Forgiveness is about accountability and restorative justice." Inside I was thinking, I'm not being defensive, I don't need to justify myself.

"That's the devil talking in you!"

"Our theologies are not the same! Your idea of forgiveness is obviously different than mine," I said.

Another relative jumped in to the defense: "Well, obviously you're still sick, so your theology isn't working is it? Maybe you need to listen to what we have to say?"

I felt my world collapse around me. All that I believed in was crumbling before my eyes. Their ignorance continued to stigmatize me and keep me in the subordinate roles of victim and patient. I cried in frustration and struggled with the dilemma: Do I sit here and continue to try and prove my faithfulness to this "holier than thou" family circle, or do I just shut up and pretend to agree? My cell phone rang, to save the day. I had forgotten that I was to meet some people ten minutes earlier, so I had to leave. I was devastated; I went to my meeting, sobbing, unable to hide my despair.

How could one family produce such diversity of theology and faith?

Prior to getting ill I had a romantic idea of culture and church. It was almost as if all churches existed side by side on white sandy beaches with palm trees swaying softly in the breeze. White hats and cardboard suits displayed our wonderful concern for purity on the outside. Our prayers of confession and condemnation of our sins ensured that our insides got washed as white as snow as well. I wrote a note to God, called "So Busy?"

> So busy trying to please God . . . playing church . . .
> Serving on committees . . .
> Walking with cardboard white suits and hats
> Lips painted on faces in the position of a smile
> Hearts hidden away to break another day.

So busy listening to God that one doesn't hear what God is really saying . . . or what the people have to say.

So busy playing church that I've forgotten why I came here in the first place.

Back in the solitude of my room off comes the cardboard suit
And the painted smile . . .

Out comes the Broken Heart.
Split in two, with no one to mend it except me and you!

There was never ever any doubt in my life that God was an ever-presence. Everything I did was done with God alongside. This was both good and bad, because not only did God hear me praying, God also heard me swearing. I knew that God had to take me as I was, warts and all, and I wished that the church could be just as accepting.

While I had once romanticized the notion that my parents' spiritual guidance was what had made me the person I am today, as I look deeper and harder, I say to myself, Be honest. Stop saying what you think people want to hear! The reality is that I feared the church as a youngster. When I think back to those days, I recall fist fights and violence like on those cowboy movies in the saloons where it was a free for all, everyone for themselves. But to be fair, yes, I got taught the values of the Christian faith, as well as the values of the *fa'a-Samoa* and the Samoan way of life and language.

At the end of the day, "if you can't beat 'em, join 'em." I was ordained as a minister. I was proud of myself. I had broken through the cultural resistance that ministry of the word and sacrament was a vocation for men only. What I didn't realize was that not only did I pose a threat to Pacific Island men in ministry, I posed even more of a threat to their Pacific Island wives. If men are the top of the invisible hierarchy and their *faletua* (wives) were second in command, would these women ministers push the wives down a notch to third place? This was the unspoken threat that manifested itself in interesting ways during my years as a student for the ministry. Despite coping with this, my years of ministry and faith had not prepared me for the living hell I was going to experience later in life.

When I got sick, I didn't want God in my life anymore. I had had no present knowledge of abuse for the first thirty-eight years of my life. It was only after the death of my wonderful father that something in my head clicked and I experienced a tsunami of repressed memories and flashbacks of sexual assault within the church. It was an explosion of pain and repressed emotions for the first time in my life.

A lifetime of stiff upper lip—being the life of the party, the clown, and the person who was always there for everyone else, but never for herself—had not prepared me for the depths of despair I was going to fall into after my dad died. His death merely triggered the inevitable. No longer could I pick up the mask, no longer could I hide behind a façade of humor and joviality. I was sprung, big time.

I struggled to work; I struggled to keep up the façade. All my daily living was consumed saving enough energy to put on a performance for my mother and my family. I didn't want them to know that I was not feeling well. I wished that I had a physical illness. I didn't want something wrong with my mental faculties. I was in denial. When my therapist said I needed to see a psychiatrist, I resisted for a number of weeks, fighting her concern with long periods of silence, stubbornness, and temper tantrums that you might see a 4-year-old have when she didn't want to go to bed.

I regressed, although I was not aware of it myself. Death was life and life was death. Death was freeing and final; life was painful and claustrophobic. I began to write more poetry to record this place in which I had found myself.

> How can I visualize the thoughts of my head and the pain in my guts that murmur and simmer waiting for a prophetic deluge of anguish and torment to vomit out of my being?
>
> I look for "that feeling," that "emotion" that suggests that if you "find it," you will begin to heal, to get better.
>
> I've searched and searched and even in the midst of despair and brokenness, it sometimes discreetly emerges, but it remains censored and wrapped up in cotton wool and apologies of guilt and platitudes of shame.
>
> I'm a controlled being, gasping to wriggle out of this human mould that I have been trapped and cast in.
>
> A puppet on a string, dancing to the tunes and miming the words of expectation and pride, success and achievement: the Dream Catcher.
>
> "We don't have words for failure and pain, no, sadness or rejection."
>
> The marionette begins to squeak from overuse and the threads separating her from the hands of her controller fray. The string snaps and my life crashes to the stage floor in front of an audience of jeering and cynical onlookers who have paid to watch and got their money's worth.

A public spectacle, fallen from her pedestal that the audience erected. "Higher, higher," they kept chanting, "See how high you can climb."

Where is everyone now? Who is left to pick up the pieces of my shattered being, my cracked ego, my fading into obscurity?

I continued to struggle. I had agreed to take some time out and let others take care of me. I thought I needed a holiday—maybe one month's leave to sort things out. One month stretched into two, three, four, twelve, fourteen months. I'm never gonna get out of this place! Suddenly I had a brain wave: "Fake it, till you make it." Yep, that's what I'm gonna do. I will retreat back to the learned behavior that got me here in the first place. What a scream! With this new plan of action I became the model patient, chairperson of the hospital community, a positive role model. Hallelujah! it worked. I couldn't believe it! This was absolutely hilarious, and perhaps there isn't a cure for madness! I felt that I had won the battle. Finally I was leaving this little microcosm of Utopia that didn't believe in culturally or ethnically appropriate treatment because we all lived in a unique culture set apart from the real world to which I was soon to return.

I still laugh about how I managed to get out.

I like what bell hooks has to say about denial in her book *Sisters of the Yam*:

> Dissimulation makes us dysfunctional. Since it encourages us to deny what we genuinely feel and experience, we lose our capacity to know who we really are and what we need and desire. Our mental wellbeing is dependent on our capacity to face reality. We can only face reality by breaking through denial. (pp. 24–25)

In retrospect, as I sit at my computer writing this story, I consider where God has been in all this and I say, "Thanks, God." During those sixteen months, I had the time of my life! It was so liberating, not having to care for the first time in my life. It was so liberating having absolutely no respect for anyone around me. It was so liberating living my teenage years again and enjoying being looked after by pseudo-parents in a clinical environment because you could slam the door in their faces and know that they couldn't hit you.

To those who asked whether I had forgiven my abuser, I say: Have I forgiven my abusers for making my life a living hell? Why do you need to know? Why do you even dare ask? Why should you be concerned about my spiritual wellbeing after all this time? What does it do for your faith to have a response to your question? How do you benefit from my answer?

Will you sleep better tonight knowing that I might go to heaven? Or will you sleep better tonight knowing that I'm not going to hell? Actually, I've been to hell, and I've survived to tell the story.

To those who overhear my accusers—whose sharp voices demand that I forgive—I say: Why do you stand silently aside while I am abused all over again by these pious bullies? Do you not understand that by failing to protect me and my own process of healing, that you are no better than those who passed by on the other side as the man lay wounded on the road to Jericho (Matthew 22:34–40)?

Postscript

After twenty-six years of silence, I decided to take a major risk to help with my own recovery. The public disclosure of my historical abuse is one of the most difficult things I have ever had to do. I had spent all these years asking: Why did I allow this to happen to me? What did I do to bring this on? I believed it must have been all my own fault.

As I began to face my fears, I knew that if taking my abuser to court accomplished only two things, it would be enough.

It would give me back my voice.

It would begin to close the door on this horrific chapter of my life.

I hoped from the outset that whether I failed or succeeded, at least justice might triumph. The fact that my abuser was the pastor of a powerful Pasifika congregation meant that many of his people would close ranks in order to uphold his position of prominence, irrespective of his guilt or innocence.

Every day during the court case, I felt like I was the one on trial. I was the one that had her life sliced open like a tin of corned beef so that others could judge my mental stability and truthfulness.

Yet I knew I had to do what I've done. For years, I could not sustain intimate relationships because I had lost the ability to trust. I could not allow myself to feel sexual because it riddled me with guilt and shame. I turned myself into a celibate so that I could focus on repairing my life through service to God. Now, however, I realize the difference between repairing and healing. Repairing got me by until the next breakdown, then someone would pull out the band-aid and we would try again. Healing, on the other hand, is a process of transformation that reclaims courage and strength from within one's wounded self. I realized eventually that the only way forward to healing was to face my abuser in a court of law.

I was a teenager when I was abused; I am now a woman ripe with midlife. I believe, at last, that I am heading in the right direction. It is important that we Pacific women find our voices to speak out against the injustices we suffer from abusers in our own community—to give sound to our silent screams. Once each of us who has suffered from sexual, physical, or emotional abuse has accomplished this courageous task, I believe that we will find our lives more full of hope, and indeed, we will want to live life to the fullest.

I can feel new wings sprouting within me. At last, I have gained new energy and vigor to live again.

Reference

hooks, bell. (1993). *Sisters of the yam: Black women and self-recovery.* London: Between the Lines.

9

New Zealand–born Samoan Young People, Suicidal Behaviors, and the Positive Impact of Spirituality

TO'OA JEMAIMA TIATIA

I was born in Tokoroa (NZ) and raised in Auckland. My father Toilolo is from Taga, Savai'i (Samoa); his father, the late Toilolo Pisa Tiatia, is from Taga and his mother, the late Folalela Stanley, from Vaigaga, Upolu (Samoa). My mother Joyce was born in Mangakino (NZ), her father the late Masuigamalie Gavet is from Siumu (Upolu) and her mother Suresa Falaniko Mauava is from Sāleleloga, Savai'i/Fusi Sāfata, Upolu (Samoa). My sisters Mary and Folalela were both born in Auckland. My name is To'oa Jemaima Tiatia.

My contribution to this book is an attempt to recontextualize youth suicidal behaviors among our Pacific young peoples with the primary objective of informing the reader to be aware, and at best, to play an active and positive role in exerting a positive impact on the lives of our young people for whom death should never be considered an option.

I am a New Zealand–born Samoan woman, interested in the improvement of the overall spiritual, mental, and physical wellbeing of Samoan and Pacific young people in Aotearoa/New Zealand, particularly in relation to suicidal behaviors. Apart from personal associations with young people who had undertaken suicidal behaviors, it was brought to my attention, through a comprehensive search of the literature, that the information available about such young people was predominantly written in the 1980s. Moreover, much of the literature regarding Samoan youth suicidal behaviors focused largely upon the population in Samoa itself. Consequently, questions arose: Are the suicidal experiences of Samoan young people in Aotearoa/New Zealand any different? Are there, in fact, distinct cultural explanations for their involvement in suicidal behaviors? This essay explores these issues primarily using a sociocultural approach within a public health perspective. It addresses specifically the concept of spirituality in relation to such behaviors, and how this concept may contribute to the improvement of health outcomes and overall wellbeing for Samoan young people.

Both nationally and internationally, public health perspectives on youth suicide (as well as the focus on risk factors for suicidal behaviors among young people) are predominantly informed by epidemiological[1] analyses of routinely collected statistical data (Coggan, 1997; Gunnell, 2000; Kosky, 2000). A growing body of literature has also recently emerged in relation to young people's suicidal behaviors with a focus on resiliency[2] and protective factors[3] (Bennett, 2002; Borowsky, Resnick, Ireland, & Blum, 1999; Forman & Kalafat, 1998; Resnick, 2000). Yet the supremacy of risk factor–based epidemiology has maintained the subordination of certain suicidal populations. For instance, there has been little research exploring suicidal behaviors and suicide prevention, not just within the Samoan community, but also among the Pacific peoples of Aotearoa/New Zealand (Tiatia & Coggan, 2001).

In response, a study entitled "Reasons to Live: New Zealand–born Samoan Young People's Responses to Suicidal Behaviours" was undertaken in an attempt to reconstruct youth suicidal behaviors in this population (Tiatia, 2003). It may be evident that New Zealand–born Samoans' beliefs, views, and practices cannot be understood or made to fit into a Western mental illness framework. Furthermore, the danger lies in disregarding the richness of cultural underpinnings in health research, which may not only skew findings, but also force alterations of data into an inconsistent framework where distinctions, overt contradictions, and other misleading interpretations may result (Turton, 1997). So it may seem that apart from anecdotal evidence, there is little known about possible suicide prevention strategies relevant for New Zealand–born Samoan young people and their *'āiga* (extended family) in Aotearoa/New Zealand.

The study included a component that critically examined young Samoan suicide attempters'[4] perceived reasons to live, with the intention that this information could contribute toward their overall future wellbeing, whether physical, mental, spiritual, or emotional. According to the Education Review Office (ERO), positive mental health is a basic requirement for the social, academic, and physical achievements of all young people (Education Review Office, 2000). The concept of "reasons to live" could be closely linked with suicide prevention, and may also raise awareness of factors that may limit future suicidal behaviors (Linehan, Goodstein, Nielson, & Chiles, 1983). This information could contribute to existing public health resources in the field of youth mental health promotion in Aotearoa/New Zealand. Additionally, factors identified by New Zealand–born Samoan young people to buffer against suicidal behaviors could potentially enable the planning and development of initiatives or services relevant for this population in Aotearoa/New Zealand, helping to minimize suicidal risk.

To address the issue of suicidal behaviors and reasons to live, every effort was made to prioritize the voices of young New Zealand–born Samoan suicide attempters. This was primarily based on the view that too often in the past, public policy has either ignored young people in general or focused on them only when their behavior has disturbed their elders (Burt, 1996). Similarly within the *fa'a-Samoa* (Samoan way), the youth voice has been somewhat covert as a result of cultural boundaries in which the young person is customarily taught to know her or his place within the Samoan structure of gerontocracy (Chun, 2000; Freeman, 1983; Mageo, 1998; Taule'ale'ausumai, 1991; Tiatia, 1998; Tupuola, 1998; Vaoiva, 1999). Furthermore, in the investigation of suicidal behaviors, it can be argued that the suicide attempters themselves are the most relevant source of information, as it is their perceptions of their experiences that are most vital (Hawton, 1986).

The research study, therefore, aimed to investigate the perceptions of New Zealand–born Samoan young people (16–25 years) following a suicide attempt. In so doing, three fundamental questions had to be addressed:

1. What are the characteristics of Samoan young people who present to Emergency Departments (EDs) in the Auckland region as a result of a suicide attempt?
2. What issues contribute to suicide attempts among New Zealand–born Samoan young people in Auckland in Aotearoa/New Zealand?
3. What are some of the reasons that young New Zealand–born Samoan people who have attempted suicide believe would enhance their options to choose life, and thus contribute toward their overall future wellbeing, whether physical, mental, spiritual, or emotional?

This essay focuses on the third question, specifically in relation to spirituality, which in the context of this essay is "defined as delving deep into the inner domain of self to connect with God," and thus becoming a subjective experience of God (Holder et al., 2000). There were twenty-seven potential participants approached by hospital Emergency Department staff during the twelve-month recruitment period, and twenty completed interviews were conducted. However, the overall objective of the main part of the research was to explore Samoan young people's explanations of what they believed contributed to their suicidal behaviors, and what they believed would work for them in terms of their future wellbeing. This was achieved using narrative analysis of in-depth interviews with this sample. Narrative analysis appeared appropriate for this study, as it has been described as enabling one to understand human motivations, perceptions, and behaviors by interpreting the stories people tell of themselves and their experiences (Riessman, 1993).

Spirituality and Wellbeing

One aspect generally unacknowledged within the Western mental illness model is the component of spirituality. Wright, Frost, and Wisecarver (1993) have suggested that health professionals interested in implementing youth programs might benefit from involving local religious and spiritual leaders. The authors argued that community churches would not only provide fellowship, but also a "purpose for living" (p. 567).

Participants in Tamasese, Peteru, and Waldegrave's (1997) study identified the importance of preventing mental illness through the strengthening of critical cultural concepts and structures. In particular, the emphasis is placed upon strengthening spiritual and relational arrangements within the ʻāiga, in recognition that the ʻāiga is the first place of relational harmony, belonging, and identity. Furthermore, the investigators suggested that in cases of mental unwellness, it is important that the church play a pivotal role in providing spiritual support and strength.

Many counselors (professional and lay), social scientists, social workers, and community workers have trained within a Western paradigm of health and illness (Siataga, 2000). Training programs often perpetuate negative stereotypes of spirituality and religious practice and beliefs within the mental health profession. Siataga further argues that "the mental health professions have tended to have a 'low' view of religious experience and spirituality" (p. 8). Spirituality is fundamental for most Samoan people and its inclusion in this research remains consistent with Samoan and Pacific concepts of health. Spirituality also can contribute to suicide prevention within the Samoan community.

Spiritual people tend to experience feelings of fulfillment and deep communion with God (Kim & Seidlitz, 2002). These experiences may provide inner strength and solace that combat feelings of anxiety and despair. Research by Pardini, Plante, Sherman, and Stump (2000) explored spirituality in relation to substance abuse recovery and its impact upon mental health benefits. They argued that spirituality's inclusion in recovery treatment is effective for those with substance abuse disorders, as it "provide[s] recovering individuals with an optimistic life orientation, greater social support, and a buffering against stress and negative emotionality" (p. 348). It has been suggested that higher spirituality is associated with increased coping, greater resilience to stress, optimistic life orientation, greater perceived social support, and lower levels of anxiety. It may be of benefit to include this view in relation to suicidal behaviors (Pardini et al., 2000). Furthermore, spiritual interconnectedness is considered an important coping mechanism for young people (Early & Akers, 1995; Holder et al., 2000; Hovey, 1999; Kim & Seidlitz, 2002).

Spirituality also is an experience that may provide internal strength and peace for an individual, thus buffering feelings of anxiety, despair, and other negative life circumstances (Kim & Seidlitz, 2002; Range et al., 1999). Furthermore, it has been argued that a strengthening of spiritual connectedness with God—particularly within the 'āiga—may be considered vital if adverse events are to be managed among Samoans (Tamasese, Peteru, & Waldegrave, 1997).

Research conducted by McGeorge (1996) with regard to young Pacific people's self-esteem found that the presence or absence of religion or spirituality in the lives of participants could have various effects: (1) Some forms of religious practice can have a detrimental effect on the self-esteem of young Pacific people because of the "fire and brimstone" approach. (2) However, a move away from religious affiliation can have a detrimental effect on self-esteem, because some Pacific young people depend on God for support. (3) A move away from religion can be accompanied by isolation from the family. (4) Furthermore, to remain in a state of disconnection would engender a psychological battle for the young person, and as a result, could directly impact upon his or her self-esteem.

While the majority of literature addressing the spiritual or religious concerns of the Samoan community appears to speak for Samoans in general, this discussion explores the relevance of spirituality particularly for Samoan young people in the context of Aotearoa/New Zealand. It is maintained that to be culturally sensitive, suicide prevention initiatives should not only facilitate pride in heritage and incorporate community outreach efforts, but also offer resources tailored to the specific needs of cultural groups such as family and church (Range et al., 1999).

The Participants

The following narratives are those of three New Zealand–born Samoan young people who had attempted suicide: Pologa, Satia, and Joe. All had presented to an Auckland Emergency Department as a result of a suicide attempt. All were brought up in religious families, and all had made an attempt on their lives as a result of interpersonal disputes. Their profiles are as follows:

Pologa was born in Aotearoa/New Zealand, is unemployed, is 19 years of age, and lives with friends. She had used a razor to cut her wrists after a dispute with her boyfriend of five months. Her lacerations to both wrists were to show her boyfriend how angry she was. Throughout her childhood and youth, she suffered physical and sexual abuse by members of her family.

Satia is employed, is 17 years of age, and was born in Aotearoa/New Zealand. She has two brothers, one older and one younger. She lives with family. She lacerated her wrists after a family dispute and wanted "to end it all." Her suicide attempt was related to high family expectations. She had made two previous suicide attempts. She considers herself to be in a serious relationship.

Joe is a 19-year-old male, born in Aotearoa/New Zealand. He lives with family and is the eldest sibling. He had presented to an Emergency Department with lacerations to his wrist. He was angry at the time and wanted "to end it all." This was his second attempt.

Findings

Research participants were asked during the course of individual interviews whether spirituality had any relevance in their lives in contemporary Aotearoa/New Zealand, and what bearing it had, if any, on their lives pre- or post-suicide attempt. After all, they had performed acts contradictory to their religious values.

Pologa had broken up with her boyfriend, and since then she perceived that her positive outlook was a result of prioritizing her spiritual life. For instance:

> Spirituality is very important. Our family is a very religious family. I didn't really believe there was a God. But ever since my breakup with my boyfriend, I go to church nearly every two days and have prayers at home every day; it has been a must for me. I've made it a priority and that has been what's picked me up again. I have chosen to live 'cos God gave me another chance to live. My faith has helped me get back on my feet, kept me busy, and helped me set goals for myself.

Pologa felt indebted to God, and as a consequence she had chosen life. This spiritual revival had given her a new sense of direction. This supports the work of Pardini and colleagues (2000), who maintained that higher spirituality increases optimistic life orientation. In addition, this also confirms the perspective of Marrone (1999), who suggested that

> the exercise of faith and the acceptance of an order beyond our control does not mean we concede our free will, or relinquish our desire to be in control. In a sense, we achieve our greatest control over our living when we choose to exercise our faith. (p. 505)

Similarly, Satia had also drawn upon her union with God which, she maintained, helped her through her ordeal. Moreover, in her response, God was likened to a friend and seen as someone in whom she could confide.

> Lately God plays a big part in my life, I always pray. I know that one thing's for sure, God is always there and if ever I'm down He'll always be there to turn to. Sometimes if I'm driving I'd just talk to Him like I would a friend and I think

> that's what's helped me get through what happened during Christmas [suicide attempt]. Last year was when things just went a bit funny and it's good I guess 'cos now it has given me time to refresh my faith and a reason to keep alive.

For both participants, it is apparent that a higher force was seen as an alternative to turn to in a time of distress. This supports claims suggesting that spiritual interconnectedness is a significant coping mechanism for young people in general (Early & Akers, 1995; Holder et al., 2000; Hovey, 1999; Kim & Seidlitz, 2002). It is also interesting to note that both deemed their suicidal acts as opportunities to renew their faith, and believed that as a consequence, God's influence in their lives had given them a reason to live.

Joe also considered God someone to whom he could turn and acknowledged that, although not a tangible presence, God was his "foundation," providing him with reassurance that he was "always there."

> It's one of the good things in my life, the bonus I have. When I've got family problems the first one I turn to is God. I still have this foundation that's always there and it's God. Even though He's not physical, at least He's always there. Praying gets me through the rough spots in life. God gives me hope and lets me know it'll be okay to value life, and to hold onto the fact that life is worth living.

It appears that when a situation in his 'āiga was problematic, Joe's first point of contact was God. Once again, consistent with other participants' perceptions, God had provided him with hope and a reason to live. Prayer was a stress release for Joe that helped him cope.

These statements highlight the vital roles that spiritual experiences continue to play in the lives of some Samoan young people brought up in Aotearoa/New Zealand. What is notable for these young people is that they perceived God as a being with whom they could connect after they had attempted to take their own lives. God seemed to be compensating for everything that had failed them or been missing at the time. God was there, was someone to talk to, providing them with hope and giving them a reason to live. Despite the small size of the sample cited here, their responses were consistent with regard to the potentially powerful roles played by their spirituality in enhancing their commitment to life and their capacity to cope.

Summary

Spirituality is often ignored in a public health approach to suicide prevention, despite research concluding that the spiritual world is considered a positive feature and should not be ignored as a potential suicide prevention resource (Kim & Seidlitz, 2002; Range et al., 1999). After all, the core beliefs and behaviors associated with spirituality have been recognized as being related to positive mental health outcomes (Pardini et al., 2000). In relation to the New Zealand–born Samoan youth experience, research findings suggest that spirituality can be of great importance in the lives of Samoan young people. These findings from the current studies reveal that in the planning and development of suicide prevention strategies, spiritual or religious components must be included for there to be any meaningful effect for Samoan young people. This information should contribute to the development of possible strategies for suicide prevention.

In the current study, it was important that participants shared what would work best for them in terms of promoting an incentive to live, and whether spirituality factored as an incentive. It would seem that their responses, in line with Jobes and Mann's (1999) argument, create opportunities to support and reinforce specific reasons to live while simultaneously helping to diminish the power of competing reasons for dying. A better understanding of factors that protect against suicidal behaviors among young people is needed in order to identify adaptive factors, and to develop culturally appropriate suicide prevention and intervention strategies (Borowsky et al., 1999). Within a public health framework, the most functional protective factors are those that are both responsive to intervention and likely to be useful and accessible to all young people, irrespective of being at risk or not, to buffer against self-destructive behaviors (Hojat & Resnick, 1998).

Spirituality is believed to sustain an individual's optimism, social support, and resilience to stress (Pardini et al., 2000), as has been the case for the New Zealand–born Samoan young people in this discussion. It is therefore most important that health care professionals address the spiritual concerns of Samoan young people in relation to their suicidal behaviors. It may be that as part of the planning of suicide prevention strategies, a standard approach to dealing with young suicidal Samoans includes eliciting information about their spiritual lives. In addition, it may be useful to include pastoral care in the help or follow-up support provided for the suicidal Samoan young person. Approaching spiritual issues requires considerable sensitivity, cultural acceptance, and the ability to be nondogmatic (Hassed, 2000), and this may be challenging for professionals in mental health services. Where possible, however, it is recommended that mental health personnel develop their knowledge of appropriate pastoral counseling services for liaison and referral of young Samoan clients, in order to strengthen the network of support around them as they strengthen their own hold on life.

Notes

1. Epidemiology is the study of the distribution and causes of disease in populations. Tracking the number of cases of disease by person, place, and time allows public health authorities to better identify who is at risk, trends of occurrence, and development of strategies for disease prevention and control.

2. Resiliency is the capacity to recover quickly from misfortune, or in other words, the ability to bounce back.

3. Characteristics of individuals and their environments associated with the increased likelihood of avoiding or recovering from misfortune or problems in the future.

4. It may be important to note that suicide attempters in this research have been defined as those presenting to an Emergency Department (ED) with an overdose, self-inflicted lacerations, or self-inflicted injury by other means. It is recognized that this definition may include individuals with varying degrees of intent to die. It may also result in underestimates of suicide attempters who present by other means, including single-occupant vehicle crashes.

References

Bennett, S. (2002). *The Risk and Resistance Project: Explorations of Pakeha/New Zealand European Young People's Suicidal Behaviours*. Unpublished doctoral dissertation, The University of Auckland.

Borowsky, I. W., Resnick, M. D., Ireland, M., & Blum, R. W. (1999). Suicide attempts among American Indian and Alaska Native youth. *Archives of Pediatrics and Adolescent Medicine, 153*, 573–580.

Burt, M. (1996). *Why should we invest in adolescents?* Paper presented at Conference on Comprehensive Health of Adolescents and Youth in Latin America and the Caribbean: Pan American Health, W. K Kellogg Foundation.

Chun, M. K. (2000). *One person, two worlds? Two persons, one world?: Cultural identity through the eyes of New Zealand born Samoans*. Unpublished master's thesis, University of Hawai'i.

Coggan, C. (1997). Suicide and attempted suicide in New Zealand: A growing problem for young males. *New Zealand Public Health Report, 105*, 1563–1570.

Early, K. E., & Akers, R. L. (1995). "It's a white thing": An exploration of beliefs about suicide in the African-American community. In L. DeSpelder & A. Strickland (Eds.), *The path ahead: Readings in death and dying* (pp. 198–210). London: Mayfield Publishing Company.

Education Review Office. (2000). *Safe students in safe schools*. Wellington: Education Review Office.

Forman, S. G., & Kalafat, J. (1998). Substance abuse and suicide: Promoting resilience against self-destructive behaviour in youth. *School Psychology Review, 27*, 398–406.

Freeman, D. (1983). *Margaret Mead and Samoa: The making and unmaking of an anthropological myth*. Canberra: Australian National University Press.

Gunnell, D. J. (2000). The epidemiology of suicide. *International Review of Psychiatry, 12*, 21–26.

Hassed, C. S. (2000). *Depression: Dispirited or spiritually deprived?* Retrieved March 23, 2005, from http://www.mja.com.au/public/issues/173_10_201100/hassed/hassed.htm.

Hawton, K. (1986). *Suicide and attempted suicide among children and adolescents.* Beverley Hills: Sage Publications.

Hojat, M., & Resnick, M. D. (1998). Protecting adolescents from harm. *Journal of the American Medical Association, 279*, 353–355.

Holder, D. W., Durant, R. H., Harris, T. L., Daniel, J. H., Obeidallah, D., & Goodman, E. (2000). The association between adolescent spirituality and voluntary sexual activity. *Journal of Adolescent Health, 26*, 295–302.

Hovey, J. D. (1999). Religion and suicidal ideation in a sample of Latin American immigrants. *Psychological Reports, 85*, 171–177.

Jobes, D. A., & Mann, R. A. (1999). Reasons for living versus reasons for dying: Examining the internal debate of suicide. *Suicide & Life Threatening Behavior, 29*(2), 97–104.

Kim, Y., & Seidlitz, L. (2002). Spirituality moderates the effect of stress on emotional and physical adjustment. *Personality and Individual Differences, 32*, 1377–1390.

Kosky, R. (2000). Perspectives in suicidology. *Suicide & Life Threatening Behavior, 30*, 1–7.

Linehan, M. M., Goodstein, J. L., Nielson, S. L., & Chiles, J. A. (1983). Reasons for staying alive when you are thinking of killing yourself: The Reasons For Living Inventory. *Journal of Consulting & Clinical Psychology, 51*, 276–286.

Mageo, J. M. (1998). *Theorizing self in Samoa: Emotions, genders, and sexualities.* Ann Arbor: University of Michigan Press.

Marrone, R. (1999). Dying, mourning, and spirituality: A psychological perspective. *Death Studies, 23*, 495–519.

McGeorge, T. (1996). *Self-esteem in New Zealand raised Pacific Islands young people.* Auckland: Health Research Council of New Zealand.

Pardini, D., Plante, T., Sherman, A., & Stump, J. (2000). Religious faith and spirituality in substance abuse recovery: Determining the mental health benefits. *Journal of Substance Abuse Treatment, 19*, 347–354.

Range, L., Leach, M., McIntyre, D., Posey-Deters, P., Marion, M., Kovac, S., Banos, J., & Vigil, J. (1999). Multicultural perspectives on suicide. *Aggression and Violent Behaviour, 4*, 413–430.

Resnick, M. D. (2000). Protective factors, resiliency, and healthy youth development. *Adolescent Medicine: State of the Art Reviews, 112*, 157–165.

Riessman, C. A. (1993). *Narrative analysis.* Beverley Hills: Sage Publications.

Siataga, P. (2000). The church and alcohol related harm. In T. Gibbs (Ed.), *Pacific issues workshop report: Alcohol and Pacific People.* Auckland: Target Education and Management Consultants.

Tamasese, K., Peteru, C., & Waldegrave, C. (1997). *O le taeao, the new morning:*

A qualitative investigation into Samoan perspectives on mental health and culturally appropriate services. Auckland: The Family Centre.

Taule'ale'ausumai, F. J. (1997). Pastoral care: A Samoan perspective. In P. Culbertson (Ed.), *Counselling issues and South Pacific communities* (pp. 215–237). Auckland: Accent.

Tiatia, J. (1998). *Caught between cultures.* Auckland: Christian Research Association.

Tiatia, J. (2003). *Reasons to live: NZ-born Samoan young people's responses to suicidal behaviours.* Unpublished doctoral dissertation, University of Auckland.

Tiatia, J., & Coggan, C. (2001). Young Pacifican suicide attempters: A review of emergency department medical records, Auckland, New Zealand. *Pacific Health Dialog: Journal of Community Health and Clinical Medicine for the Pacific, 8,* 124–128.

Tupuola, A. M. (1998). *Adolescence: Myth or reality for 'Samoan' women? Beyond stage-like toward shifting boundaries and identities.* Unpublished doctoral dissertation, Victoria University, Wellington, New Zealand.

Turton, V. L. R. (1997). Ways of knowing about health: An aboriginal perspective. *Advances in Nursing Science, 19,* 28–36.

Vaoiva, R. (1999). *New Zealand born Pacific Island youth: Identity, place, and Americanisation.* Unpublished master's thesis, University of Auckland.

Wright, L., Frost, C., & Wisecarver, S. (1993). Church attendance, meaningfulness of religion, and depressive symptomatology among adolescents. *Journal of Youth and Adolescence, 22,* 559–569.

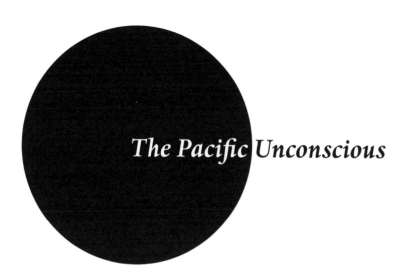

The Pacific Unconscious

Editors' Introduction

The following five essays address ways in which the unconscious—in the form of symbol, metaphor, mythology, and intrapersonal dimensions of being—serves as a rich resource in the world of Pacific identities, relationships, and healing. First, Cabrini Makasiale discusses the significance for Pacific Island people of the symbolic inner world and its expression in metaphor and relationship. In her essay she not only addresses these aspects of cultural awareness, but also provides a rare glimpse into the cross-cultural therapeutic process.

Developing the focus on working with clients as well as the incorporation of mythology in therapeutic approaches, Karen Lupe explores the culturally determined ego structure of Pacific people. This discussion of therapeutic geography and process illuminates a further aspect of cultural awareness, casting the lens in particular on the *vā*, or psychological/spiritual space between client and counselor.

Seilosa Skipps-Patterson uses Petruska Clarkson's analysis of the different types of relationship between therapist and client as a framework for discussing the relationship between the personal and the professional in Pasifika therapeutic relationships and process. In doing so, she develops themes introduced in the previous two essays, but she grounds her discussion in the constructs of psychoanalytic psychotherapy, in contrast to those of analytical psychology and psychosynthesis reflected in Karen Lupe's work.

In Fia Turner-Tupou's account of her work with a Samoan woman whose response to grief had been diagnosed as mental illness, the value of an holistic, *mea-alofa*-based approach is sensitively illustrated. We are invited to consider questions about the validity of mental health diagnoses when the cultural context and the client's story are not taken into account. This case study also serves to echo Cabrini Makasiale's voice in questioning earlier commentators, such as Sia Figiel, who asserted that in collective, Pacific culture "I" does not exist. As a consequence of social change brought about by immigration, living in multicultural societies, intermarriage, and increasing numbers of people with complex cultural heritages, identity is far from static, but needs to be recognized instead as dynamic and frequently complex. Ambiguity associated with identity and relationships can be hard to articulate, and similarly, finding ways of providing "safe holding" for clients in acknowledging and managing "both-and" rather than "either-or" in their lives presents a great challenge to the therapeutic community. These are also themes that appear in the essay, "Being *'Afakasi*," in the first part of this book.

A strikingly different therapeutic process is illustrated in the final contribution in this section. Peta Palalagi's sequence of poems bears testimony to her journey of healing from the cycle of domestic violence, and is indeed the therapeutic means through which she finds her own strength and way forward in her life. She illustrates not only a powerful example of therapeutic writing, but also the way in which a therapist is able to care for herself.

10

The Use of Symbol and Metaphor in Pasifika Counseling

CABRINI ʻOFA MAKASIALE

My name is Cabrini ʻOfa Makasiale, of Tongan and English ancestry. I live with a community of Christian women with religious vows in Auckland. To date, I have worked in South Auckland-Manukau City for close to twenty years; for twelve of these I have worked as a counselor/psychotherapist, tutor, supervisor, and spiritual director.

Reflecting on my training and work, I realize, more and more, that the impact of certain cultural, traditional beliefs and practices on Pacific peoples is past its "use-by" date. In the case of many women and children, the impact is oppressive, abusive, and harmful. Some Pacific peoples will not agree with what I write. That is understandable.

I write with the aim of bringing about further discussion, deeper understanding, and continuing growth to our evolving Pacific identity in Aotearoa/New Zealand. We need to continue the work of synthesis with courageous analysis.

Within the helping professions, theories of human development that inform our understanding of human nature have been associated with Western counseling theories and therapies. Today, however, there is a movement to recognize the validity of cultural perspectives that are other than Western. There is also a challenge, I believe, to uphold both the Western and non-Western models of human development as of equal significance.

I wish to introduce a term that carries with it an inner attitude and dynamic that I believe to be essential in any cross-cultural interaction. The term is *interpathy,* coined by Augsburger (1986, p. 27). He maintains that interpathy is the ability to

> enter a second culture cognitively and effectively, to perceive and conceptualize the internal workings of that culture into a dynamic inter-relatedness, and to respect that culture with its strengths and weaknesses as equally valid as one's own. This interpathic respect, understanding, and appreciation make possible the transcendence of cultural limitation. (p. 14)

It is precisely the experience of this dynamic that motivates my writing of this essay. I am a Pacific Islander/Tongan who has received much from being brought up among Fijians, Indians, Part-Europeans, Europeans, and Chinese; I was later nourished at the tables of formal Western educational schools. I have never felt anyone articulate my internal cross-cultural experiences as well as Augsburger has done. Augsburger has presented the following comparison of sympathy, empathy, and interpathy (1986, Table 1-2, p. 31).

Sympathy	**Empathy**	**Interpathy**
In sympathy, I know you are in pain and I sympathize with you. I use my own feelings as the barometer; hence I feel my sympathy and my pain, not yours. You are judged by my perception of my own feelings. You are understood by extension of my self understanding. My experience is both frame and picture.	In empathy, I empathically make an effort to understand your perceptions, thoughts, feelings, muscular tensions, even temporary states. In choosing to feel your pain with you, I do not own it, I share it. My experience is the frame, your pain the picture.	In interpathy, I seek to learn a foreign belief, take a foreign perspective, base my thought on a foreign assumption, and feel the resultant feelings and their consequences in a foreign context. Your experience becomes both frame and picture.

This essay is about some of my learnings in the interpathic dynamic of "to-ing and fro-ing" between my Pacific Island world and the Western world, with specific focus on the counseling/psychotherapeutic context.

The Psycho-Spiritual World of the Pacific Island Client

We are not human beings having a spiritual experience;
we are spiritual beings having a human experience.
(Teilhard de Chardin)

For the Pacific Islander, the psyche and the spirit are inseparable. Hence, a spiritual perspective has a profound impact on the personality development of such a client. The two aspects are interwoven and if there is to be a hierarchy, then the spirit element, in theory, takes precedence.

Pacific Islanders believe in the transcendent, and include in this belief an understanding of the role of good and evil in daily living and universal happenings (Augsburger, 1986, p. 55). While it is true that critical theologizing has been happening over several hundred years, and that religious belief is humanly generated, most Pacific Island people hold the traditional view that truths come from above. These truths are often seen as unchangeable and beyond criticism.

The spirit is, therefore, the "someone" out there, namely, God, who will provide moral guidance over our thinking, behavior, and feelings, and can act independently of us. This theoretical perspective also relates to intangibles, such as thoughts and feelings of enlightenment, harmony, inspiration, conscience, and understanding (Richards & Bergin, 1997, p. 77).

These spiritual maxims are similar to those contained in the other major monotheistic traditions, with a significant leaning toward the Christian tradition. They cover the themes of transcendence/deity; human nature; the meaning/purpose of life; mortality (life and death); morality and values; and the organization of the universe (Cornett, 1998).

The following general notions of the Christian tradition form a foundation for Pacific Island spirituality:

1. Harmony with someone beyond this known reality (God) is possible.
2. The human person can choose to relate or not to relate, to act or not act, that is, has free will.
3. There are laws which we should seek out in order to live in peace.
4. There are paths that lead to personal and social peace, growth, and happiness.
5. Material prosperity is a sign of God's approval.
6. Physical death is not the end, only a transition into life with or without God.
7. Through grace God offers an unfailing and steadfast love to each human person and faithfully upholds the uniqueness and wellbeing of each one to the end. (Richards & Bergin, 1997, pp. 76–78)

One can see, then, how a theistic, spiritual perspective has a profound impact on how the Pacific Island client views growth, development, and healing. In my psychotherapy training, however, spirituality was left outside the door. For me, as a Pacific Islander, it was like being asked to leave an essential part of me out in the corridor. It is this experience that strongly motivated me to complete my psychotherapy studies and to experiment with the undoubted belief that the Pacific Islander's view of life and the world is well suited to counseling and psychotherapy.

To a large extent, the Pacific Island client truly believes in the motherly/fatherly love of God. We believe that it is God's presence, God's being, that makes all the difference in anything human.

In the human development process of the Pacific Islander, a similar attitude exists. God as father, as the force guiding the universe, is unavoidably equated with the parents (Cornett, 1998). The baby's total dependence on the parents, and particularly the mother, facilitates the baby's seeing mother as Godlike. For the baby, mother is interchangeable with God. The baby is totally dependent on the parents for food, shelter, protection, and emotional sustenance (Cornett, 1998). It is true to say, too, that the reverse happens, that parents facilitate the child's imagery of God and the child's developing spirituality. In the early life of the child, Pacific Island parents are generally very affectionate and attuned to the child's all-round needs. Later, though, from close to school age onwards, punishment and denigration are often acted out. There is rarely a word of praise and the child has to work very hard (Morton, 1996).

Every human being has dimensions that are universal (all the same); dimensions that are cultural (like some others); and dimensions that are unique (like no other) (Augsburger, 1986). The matrix or milieu in which all of the developmental stages take place differs markedly for Pacific youngsters from the Western taxonomy of human development. Within the cultural context, the Pacific Island child is trained by a large number of persons —mother, father, aunts, uncles, grandparents, older siblings. The parenting figures discipline the child predominantly by threats of rejection or punishment (verbally or physically). (On the religious and spiritual abuse of children, see especially Capps, 1995.)

Consequently an externally referenced personality emerges. This aspect is significant in the client-therapist relationship, which I describe later. The child is, then, unlikely to interject internal superego functions since control is directed by the expectation of others (Augsburger, 1986). When there is misbehavior, shame begins to form, and where there is misbehavior and ensuing shame, the sense of belonging and one's identity are threatened. Identity is particularly threatened because the Pacific Island child is reared by many significant others, an extended family system. In the Western context, the child is usually reared by two or one parental figures.

In a Pacific Island context, the child, the young adult, and even the adult are under constant observation by the older ranking members. External authority is always present in every sphere of life, with God being the authority par excellence. Crucial to the therapeutic relationship is a cultural understanding of the development of the Pacific Islander's self in relation to external authority, group belonging, and hierarchy. It is crucial because the therapist needs to have some understanding of the power she or he holds in the relationship, and how impactful the words of the therapist are because the images of God, parents, elders, and other authority figures are transferred to her or him. We learn a language, a religion, a system. Culture-specific, intrapsychic organizations influence how one processes and experiences the world (Tseng & Streltzer, 1997).

Pacific Islanders identify with the collective and when they individuate, they incorporate a collective identity. With this collective self, they experience a sense of solidarity, which contrasts with the Western emphasis on a distinct, individual identity. Through a self that is based on family and community, the Pacific Islander embraces the group ideal ego as a guiding principle, and conformity and cooperative affiliations are held in high regard. With conformity and cooperation, acceptance and belonging are undoubted rewards. Values are relational, rather than objective and intrinsic (Augsburger, 1986). The positive end of the continuum of this self-development based on communal solidarity generally brings about harmonious and unified relationships. Deviation from these dimensions brings social judgment, distress, violence, and cultural excommunication. The negative end of the continuum can, therefore, escalate rapidly to uncontrollable violence, a topic warranting further investigation.

Therapeutic Relationships with Pacific Island Clients

When the Pacific Island client enters the consulting room, she or he is likely to walk in carrying the wisdom and groundedness of a theistic believer. The client generally trusts that the counselor/therapist will be benevolent, God-like, parent-like, and unconditionally giving. The Pacific Island client may be hurting like a child, and may believe that the therapist will listen, care, and guide her or him to a place of peace, healing, and forgiveness. This attitudinal stance is potentially gold in the hands of the therapist, yet such openness and trust can also lead to further abuse, manipulation, and the arrogant invasion of the vulnerable inner world of the client.

It is the trusting, open stance of the Pacific Island client, combined with the gracious love from the therapist, which makes therapy so disturbing, warm, human, and healing. Right here in the therapy room, the gratuitous love that God offers the human person is incarnated in a limited way. This is the wisdom gift that the Pacific Island person brings: a warm simplicity that makes the counseling relationship both humanly tender and demandingly responsible on the part of the therapist. "The relationship *is* the therapy" (Kahn, 1997, p. 1). In my years of experience in counseling cross-culturally in South Auckland, it is the Pacific Island client who comes with the big heart, the warm heart, and the wounded heart. This does not discount the inner stance of other clients. But the Pacific Island client's heart is easily visible, trustingly bared. With other clientele, generally speaking, much more work is needed to defrost or melt down the protective covers. So the relationship is built up slowly but nonetheless surely. I believe that this is the edge that the Pacific Island client brings to the counseling room, the innate quality and gift of being warm and humane.

As early as the 1940s, Carl Rogers, the American psychologist, proposed that the therapeutic heart required empathy/interpathy and unconditional positive regard for the client (Kahn, 1997). Perhaps Rogers carried some unconscious knowing of the heart of the Pacific Islander. In the Christian belief system, warmth, love, and respect have always been among the core tenets of a relationship with God, others, and self. The emphasis on being in the presence of God and in the presence of the other with love and attunement has been ever present, to a greater or lesser degree, in the spirituality of the theistic traditions. Western therapy schools are still struggling today to include the concept of spirituality in their models of learning.

There are many subtleties in the counseling relationship, awareness of which has been identified as perhaps the most powerful tool (Kahn, 1997). For the Pacific Island client, the protocol of metaphorical conversation and storytelling is one of the most potent therapeutic tools, incorporating both spirituality and subtle nuances of meaning within the therapeutic relationship.

The Cultural Protocol of Metaphorical Conversation

The way we language reality in Pacific Island cultures conforms to certain protocols. In special events, the protocol used by the Pacific Island person is a manner of speaking in metaphors and similes, and the use of story. It would be akin to using Shakespearean language in daily mainstream life. I use the term *conversational* to differentiate the oratorical context from the counseling context. The term *conversation* is also used to highlight the importance of reciprocity—sharing of thoughts and feelings—which does not happen in the field of oratory. It includes the notion of a personal meeting between the parties involved.

The use of simile, metaphor, and story in dialogue is inbred in the Pacific Island person. We hear it from birth to death. The Pacific Island person learns this protocol primarily through *experience*, by attending formal and informal ceremonies and participating in the rituals of significant life events—births, baptisms, and other rites of initiation from childhood to adulthood. The use of metaphorical conversation, and more precisely, the symbolic language used in the conversation, meets the Pacific Island client where she or he is "at home." Being "at home," the client is doubly at ease and can describe her or his inner and outer worlds with openness and confidence. When the client experiences that the therapist is also attuned to this symbolic manner of speaking, then mutual understanding is deepened and expanded.

The Pacific Island person is born into a world (first family) that communicates in a "talking picture" manner, not a "pen picture," as is the case in the Western context. Many Western people believe that they are to polish things up, and speak from the head, whereas the feminine in the Westerner would proclaim that she too, speaks from the heart and expresses affective distrust in metaphoric terms. Thus the feminine in the Westerner is in touch with the elements: the sea, the tides, the wind, the moon, and the cycles of nature (Kearney, 1997). The Pacific Island client would nod knowingly and warmly to the language of the feminine goddess.

In using this metaphoric form, the Pacific Island client experiences what Augsburger (1986) terms *interpathy*, that is, the nonjudging and "being with" stance that the therapist enters into with the former. In much the same way, I interpathize with someone who comes from a Western background, but my language style would be different: more linear, less circular, sometimes direct, and less symbolic.

In the Pacific Island context, direct expression of feelings and thoughts about another is considered rude. It is not protocol. For example, when a person walks into a room and I hold that person in high regard, I would not say, "I really like you." I would not give such a direct message particularly in the presence of others. Rather, I would couch the message in a simile that says, "When you walk into the room, it is like the sunrise, warm and bright." So when the therapist engages in metaphoric dialogue with the Pacific Island client, the latter feels met where she is. When this meeting takes place, there is some hope that the client will experience the confidence to move to a new place of understanding and action. "Meet me where I am before you invite me to a new place" is a saying I have used to illustrate such an encounter. To ask a Pacific Islander a question such as, "Can you tell me what happened?" may not be as culturally inviting as, "I wonder what it is like for you today? Is there rain or sun in your world? Which part?" and so forth.

Case Examples to Illustrate the Counseling Dynamic

In my South Auckland practice, I have discovered that metaphorical language is pure common sense. How else can one communicate with another unless one speaks the other's language, verbally or nonverbally? Here are two examples from my work experience.

CASE ONE

A young Tongan woman was referred to me from a South Auckland medical clinic. She was 18 years old and a recent migrant to Auckland. I will call her Kita. According to the doctor, Kita needed counseling, as there was no physical data to show that Kita's migraines were medically based.

In our first session, Kita and I exchanged stories about where we came from, which island group, parents, and kinship. This is the Pacific Island way. I offered some relevant information on the working parameters of our agency, what we offered, and how I would work in the counseling process.

Then there was a pause, a silence, and Kita lowered her head markedly. Rather than directly mentioning her presenting medical issue of migraines, I tentatively approached her apparent world of pain:

Therapist: I feel as if there is rain in your soul, heavy rain.
Kita: Yes, there is, heavy rain like in the islands (voice is almost inaudible).
Therapist: Is it raining everywhere, inside of you, or only in some places?
Kita: Only in some (silence).
Therapist: Tell me some more, only what you want.
Kita: In other places, there is only cloud and no rain. In another place there is a little sun. Another part, there is only hard rock and no water. And in another part there are rocks and the waves are hitting the rocks over and over again.
Therapist: (Feeling as if it's heavily raining in me too). Where, which place do you want us to go to today?
Kita: Where it is raining, heavy rain.
Therapist: (Glancing at Kita, I notice tears dropping onto her lap. In the Pacific way, we look up and away to lessen the anxiety or intensity that may be present in the interaction. Then the encounter is not so direct, not so linear, and more circular, so to speak). Is there a story to the heavy rain?
Kita: Yes (tears rolling down her face).
Therapist: Tell me about the rain, the heavy rain.
Kita: My story is so long, so full, so heavy in my head.
Therapist: I'm ready. I'm listening. We'll be together there and we'll get wet together. That may not matter because you won't be alone.

Sobbing profusely, Kita tells of how her mother left the family in Tonga four years previously. Kita was 14 years old. She is the only girl in the family of seven. Her mother had cancer and was to seek help in Australia, and then to return after four weeks. Kita took on the role of mother in the family, but her mother never returned. She stayed away for two years. She died in Australia, and had no intention of returning, as Kita's father was busy having love affairs with other women. Kita's sobbing intensified as she told of her unmet longings to see her mother, her feelings of betrayal and anger with her mother for not returning and with her father for his love affairs.

Therapist: I see the rain, so much rain. I feel the rain with you . . . so much rain, so much pain.

(Silence)

Kita: (Raising her head slowly). My head is not so heavy. I feel light.

Therapist: We might do what we usually do back home, dry ourselves (offering her paper tissues).

(Silence)

How will you take care of yourself during the week if more heavy rain falls on you?

Kita: I will see you beside me and then I know I won't be alone and I will come back and tell you my story.

Therapist: (When a Pacific Islander participates in a meaningful event, she usually leaves with something, some object, some memento.) What then, will you take away with you from our time together, something that will keep you dry and safe?

Kita: I will take you in my heart and your voice in my head. That will keep me dry and safe.

In this case, the language in metaphor and story was the key to opening the heavens within Kita. She took up the cue of my metaphorical questioning like a fish takes to water. Kita opened up and responded with her tears and poignant story. In the sessions that followed, Kita did lead me to the other places, in particular to the "place where there are rocks and no water." This was the place where she vented her anger and despair toward her parents.

I assume that if I had taken the tack of directly asking Kita about the frequency of her migraines, and when and where the headaches took place, I might have gone down a long, distracting route far from the place of "heavy rain." Knowing the protocol of another, or the *tika,* as Māori say, can facilitate an effortless, meaning-filled, cost-effective encounter. Knowing another's protocol can be a point of contact, a point of entry into and alongside the world of the other.

CASE TWO

My second example involves a Samoan man in his early 40s, whom I shall call Tia. Tia was referred from the courts because he had struck his wife violently. Tia was reluctant to see a counselor, but the thought of going to jail propelled him to see one. This was not easy work for me. I'm also a woman. Culturally, the help is meant to be the other way around. Tia was resistant, proud, and highly defensive.

After the usual Pacific Island protocol and acknowledging how difficult it is to receive assistance from a woman, I opened the dialogue.

Therapist: I have the feeling that your anger is like a covering, like a blanket (Samoan: *ufiufi*), protecting something very tender. I wonder what might be there under this protective cover.

Tia: (Sits silent, tapping his fingers on his lap, looking out the window). Maybe.

Therapist: If we were to lift up the cover, what might we see underneath?

Tia: (Whispering) A little boy.

Therapist: What does this little boy need right now?

Tia: (Gulping back the tears). The little boy needs his mother and father.

Therapist: What will we do to make this happen?

Tia: The little boy is running and running through the plantation. It's me (sobbing). I am running and my parents are getting into a truck to go back to Savai'i. I have to go to school in Apia—stay with my grandparents. I turn and run and run and I fall to the ground and cry and the truck is gone. (There are no more words, only sobs.)

(Period of silence and a sense of being met)

Therapist: Tia, there is a story in the pālagi culture that says that when something really, really happy or sad happens in the past I can relive this happening in the present. How is the little boy's story, your story connected to your anger?

Tia: That is the only time I hit my wife. This is my first time. I love my wife, but when she is late coming home, like she will say that she will come home at 6 o'clock and something happens in the factory and she only comes home at 8 o'clock, I feel worried. I feel she will not come back. I will watch the clock and watch the clock and walk up and down. But this time she wanted to go to a factory do [social event] and I ask her "please come back early." But she can't because it will be rude. So I ask her "please don't go." And still she wanted to go. I feel so silly but I am going out of my mind. I feel like my little son. I want to hang on to her.

Therapist: Going out of your mind like . . .

Tia: Like I am a little boy running and running in the plantation or a little boy hanging onto his mother's dress. (More tears and shaking of the head.)

(Silence)

That is why I hit her that night. All these years I didn't

know I have this little boy inside me. Today I find my little boy. Today I find myself.

Therapist: So your anger is like a protective cover for your fear of being left behind.

Tia: Yes. All this time I never know.

Therapist: I'm happy with you. I'm sad with you too. Such a sad thing and a frightening thing to happen to you when you are little. The pālagi story is true.

Tia: So true. So good to know.

Therapist: What is our next step?

Tia: I will go to court and tell my story. I will go home and talk to my wife and tell her my story and say sorry. I think a lot of our men feel the same as me.

Therapist: What or how will you take care of the frightened part of you when your wife has to stay out late?

Tia: I will look after my little boy inside the same way I look after my own son. I will sing to myself. I will watch a happy video or I will read a nice story or listen to my island songs. I will not blame my wife anymore.

His session ends with my connecting him to a psycho-educational program in anger management. But Tia leaves with a deep-seated relief in expressing his fear-filled feelings and story that he had so successfully protected outside of his awareness over the years.

In this example, the Pacific Island protocol of the use of simile—anger being like a protective cover and that of storytelling—proved to be an effective tool in facilitating Tia to trust and further explore the power that the past had over his present. This dynamic usually takes a long time to build up to in the therapeutic relationship (Kahn, 1997). With Tia, the use of simile and storytelling seemed to have provided a more direct route that enabled him to bring to the surface some of the buried principles that had been governing his expressions of anger. Time and time again in my experience, the use of these language tools has not failed me.

I liken this catalytic therapeutic tool to a time when I first arrived in New Zealand. I was walking along Remuera Road in Auckland, when I heard a person speaking in Tongan. It had a magnetic effect on me. It gave me a sense of kinship, belonging, and connection, a piece of home away from home.

Some Comments on Using This Methodology

I believe that it is my capacity to cross over and come back between the worlds of the Fijian, Tongan, and European (mainly) that has facilitated a cross-cultural attitudinal stance within me. Furthermore, because this process developed in me from a young age, I have come to normalize something of its complexity. When one is located within a mono-cultural environment, this process can prove difficult, or even daunting.

Furthermore, any technique remains ineffective unless it is in the hands of a humble, genuine practitioner. The tools that I have identified and applied in the illustrative examples do not come to life unless they are finely honed to weave a pathway between the two worlds of the client and the therapist. In fact, these remain crude, or blunt, if the therapist has not developed a cross-cultural ground or soul. It is this sacred ground of the therapist that facilitates the client to discover her own sacred ground, and then look into her own chaos and find some life-giving form emerging. When the therapist becomes familiar with the world of the Pacific Island client, it is knowledge of these two protocols and the art of working with them that holds the secret to the healing process.

Some other guidelines to keep in mind are:

1. Frequent exposure to interacting and working with Pacific Island clients is paramount in formal and informal settings.
2. Engaging a Pacific Island supervisor who is bilingual helps to provide an environment for clinical discussion, analysis, and theological dialogue.
3. Taking Pacific Island case studies to cross-cultural study group settings enables knowledge of other cultural therapeutic tools to further sculpt and refine one's own learnings and discoveries.

This takes time and practice. The art of using metaphor, story, and simile in the therapeutic relationship is not the sole prerogative of Pacific Islanders; any cross-cultural therapist has the ability to use these therapeutic tools. The other dimension is the depth of spirituality that the cross-cultural therapist embraces. This calls the therapist, in the words of Augsburger, "to embody grace, to incarnate agape, to flesh out the steadfast love of God" (1986, p. 38).

In conclusion, it is important to note that any tool used beyond its point of effectiveness and out of its context loses its potency. In the therapeutic relationship, these tools that I have described and applied can easily become therapeutic obstacles. In the first dimension of indigenous wisdom, where the Pacific Island client is highly trusting of the therapist or elder and shows little defensiveness, an unhealthy dependence can develop on the part of the client. This can diminish the client's initiative and sense of confidence. The parent-child cultural dynamic is compounded, and enmeshment can follow.

Second, in using metaphor, storytelling, and simile the Pacific way, the therapist can become stilted and too preoccupied with the tools. The relationship then becomes more artificial, more of a performance, and less genuine.

Third, where the Pacific Island client can access her affect readily and easily, she can also be prone to losing herself in her feelings and get stuck in the mire.

Fourth, the protocol of using metaphor, simile, and storytelling can lead the Pacific Island client to deflect her hidden, real feelings and/or use the oratorical protocol to cover over or defend against her pain, fear, rage, or any other associated affect. Culture is then used as a mask or camouflage (Culbertson, 1999).

To conclude, it is precisely because I have traveled between cultural worlds, crossing over and coming back between the Western and Pacific Island worlds in the field of healing, that I have happened upon the learnings described in this essay. To know only one culture can mean that I know no culture. In knowing a second and a third culture, I discover the enriching wisdom of paradox: things assumed to be universal are also specific, things absolute are relative, things simple are also complex (Augsburger, 1986).

The Pacific Islander believes that all healing is grounded in grace and the therapist or the elder is the healing touch of God in human form. The Pacific Island clients who have graced me with their trust and poetical language in the therapeutic relationship will never know how transformational their presence has been and still is for me. I honor them in this essay.

References

Augsburger, D. (1986). *Pastoral counseling across cultures*. Philadelphia: Westminster.

Capps, D. (1995). *The child's song: The religious abuse of children*. Louisville: Westminster/John Knox.

Cornett, C. (1998). *The soul of psychotherapy: Recapturing the spiritual dimension in the therapeutic encounter.* New York: Free Press.

Culbertson, P. (1999). Listening differently with Maori and Pacific Island clients. *Forum: The Journal of the New Zealand Association of Psychotherapists 5*, 64–82.

Kahn, M. (1997). *Between therapist and client: The new relationship*. New York: W. H. Freeman.

Kearney, C. (1997). *Face of the Goddess: New Zealand women talk about their spirituality*. Auckland: Tandem.

Morton, H. (1996). *Becoming Tongan: An ethnography of childhood*. Honolulu: University of Hawai'i Press.

Richards, S,. & Bergin, A. (1997). *A spiritual strategy for counseling and psychotherapy*. Washington, DC: American Psychological Association.

Tseng, W-S., & Streltzer, J. (1997). *Culture & psychopathology: A guide to clinical assessment*. New York: Brunner/Mazel.

11

An Ocean with Many Shores
Indigenous Consciousness and the Thinking Heart

KAREN LUPE

Currently I am a psychotherapist working in private practice in Auckland. I trained at the Institute of Psychosynthesis in both counseling and psychotherapy. Born in Auckland, I was raised in a mixed-race family: my mother Daisy Felix was from Western Samoa and father Francis Aldom was from England. As part of the great Pacific migration wave my mother left her village of Togāfu'afu'a, Apia, for New Zealand in the 1950s. Some thirty years before, my grandmother Akenese Pereira left the Tokelau Islands to attend boarding school in Western Samoa. It was there she met my grandfather, Vave Felise Levai, from the chiefly Levai line of Savai'i. As my grandmother was not Samoan-born my grandfather's family did not approve the union. Nevertheless my grandfather, being the man he was, did not bow to family pressure. They married and were blessed with thirteen children! The high chief's title of Meleiseā was later conferred upon him.

This essay is dedicated to the memory of my grandfather, whose guiding spirit I have often felt close by in the process of writing this work. I also wish to respectfully acknowledge the involvement of Sauma'iafe, a Samoan aītu, in writing this essay. Her many testings have strengthened my will and helped to create the endurance so necessary to give birth to the following words.

I must confess to borrowing the words of my title from Jorge Ferrer's book *Revisioning Transpersonal Theory.* "An ocean with many shores" sounded so Pacific that I could not resist. Ferrer's metaphoric ocean is the vast field of human spirituality where there are not many pathways to a single destination, but rather, many pathways to many destinations. The metaphor is well suited to the purpose of this essay.

About ten years ago, I began to realize that there were different streams of human consciousness, and that the Western form was merely one of those streams. My subsequent research into depth psychology, mythology, religious symbolism, and, more recently, transpersonal theories has confirmed my earlier intimation of different streams of consciousness. In this essay I use the word *culture* to refer to the collective matrixes from which these streams of consciousness emerge. Culture, in this sense, is more than a vehicle to carry forward traditional beliefs and rituals—the way we do and see things. Culture is a living force within the psyche (soul) of each person and an energy field that binds people together.

A Matter of Heart

Carl Gustav Jung, a psychiatrist from a conventional middle-class background, left Switzerland in the 1920s with the desire to meet people from non-European cultures in their own environment. His travels took him to Africa, Central America, and India. These journeys had a profound impact on the formulation of his theories, which later came to be known as depth psychology. The following quote from Jung's autobiography, *Memories, Dreams, Reflections,* records a conversation between Jung and a Pueblo Indian elder. It was out of this meeting that a rather remarkable friendship developed.

> "See," Ochwiay Biano said, "how cruel the whites look. Their lips are thin, their noses sharp, their faces furrowed and distorted by folds. Their eyes have a staring expression; they are always seeking something. What are they seeking? The whites always want something; they are always uneasy and restless. We do not know what they want. We do not understand them. We think they are mad."
>
> I asked him why he thought the whites were all mad.
>
> "They say that they think with their heads," he replied.
>
> "Why, of course. What do you think with?"
>
> "We think here," he said, indicating his heart. (Jung, 1993, p. 276)

This conversation conveys not only a meeting between two men from different cultural backgrounds but also a meeting between two different streams of consciousness. Jung embodied Western egoic consciousness and Ochwiay Biano carried what I loosely term *indigenous consciousness,* a stream of consciousness that is qualitatively different from Occidental or Oriental consciousness, though closer in nature to the latter. From personal and clinical experience I have found that thinking from the heart is also true of Pacific peoples.

In the West the mind has long been associated with thinking and the heart with feeling. To imagine a thinking heart is a strange concept for many people. Yet recent scientific studies in the field of neurocardiology (the study of the heart's neurological systems) have revealed that 60 to 65 percent of the heart is comprised of neural cells, the same type of cells found in the brain (Walker, 1998). Another finding is that the heart has its own nervous system separate from the rest of the brain/body, named by medical researchers as the "brain within the heart." Such findings provide scientific credence to the notion of the thinking heart, perhaps more correctly called heart intelligence.

Different Consciousness

Extensive colonization and migration in the Pacific have resulted in the overlaying of indigenous consciousness by a foreign mentality—the Western mind. This change has occurred in a relatively brief span of time and I will not dwell on the outer manifestations of colonization, as these have been well documented elsewhere. It is evident that collective cultural trauma occurs when a culture is separated from its deep roots. The Sioux holy man Black Elk spoke from a place of deep pain when he said that the hoop of his tribe was broken and the sacred tree was dead (Neihardt, 1961, p. 276). This tragic state of affairs leads to what ancient peoples recognized as soul loss, where the animating spark within a person that gives meaning to relationships and to life itself is gone. It is this very soul loss, in its multiple manifestations, that has been diagnosed by modern medicine as mental illness. What is missing from this paradigm, however, is the awareness of the suffering of the heart and injury to the spirit.

The devastating losses of homeland, native language, traditional knowledge, and rituals have all contributed to cultural trauma. There is another factor that is as harmful as the other losses, and perhaps more insidious because of its invisibility—the phenomenon of psychological colonization. The early missionaries zealously set about not only to Christianize but to "whiten," a process identified by Fanon (1986) as lactification. The rationale behind this was the widespread and erroneous belief that native peoples were less (humanly) developed than Europeans and therefore needed help to make the transition from primitive to civilized dwellers on the planet. The best remedies considered to achieve this aim were school and church. What was not understood then, nor to a large extent in today's world as well, is that these cultural differences are not a question of development, but rather a difference in consciousness, with its own historical, geographical, psycho-biological, and therefore archetypal foundation.

The failure to appreciate the psychological differences of another culture leaves them as the alien other, in essence unknown and hence targets for shadow projection. The process of lactification subtly continues in the mainstream education system. From primary schools to tertiary institutions, teaching programs have been designed to develop rational cognitive faculties in order to absorb and critically analyze massive amounts of factual information. This approach to learning is, I believe, foreign to those who do not have a Western ego-structure, and its imposition over a period of years leads to an inner separation from one's own psychodynamic pathway, and hence, one's self. I suggest here that this mainly intellectual approach to learning has also resulted in a serious collective imbalance in the Western psyche, as the wisdom of the heart is derided as irrational emotionality. Albert Einstein, one of the greatest western minds of the twentieth century, was quoted as saying: "We should take care not to make the intellect our god; it has, of course, powerful muscles but no personality. It cannot lead; it can only serve" (Lewis et al., 2000, p. 32).

I intend to explore the notion of different consciousness by examining the foundations of the Samoan psyche. Initially I will demonstrate this difference by comparing Samoan and Western ego-structures. It is my premise that Samoans (and other Pacific peoples) have historically developed an ego-structure that, in contrast to the Western ego, emerged from matriarchal consciousness. As Western psychological development has generally been assumed to be the norm, there is a dearth of information about the inner-life processes of non-Westerners.

The Samoan ego, I propose, having emerged from matriarchal consciousness, has a structure that is intrinsically different from the Western ego. Psychodynamic processing of the former is mediated by a body/heart pathway that differs from the Western ego's central core of mental-field activity. The Western maxim, "I think therefore I am," could be equated with a Pasifika maxim, "I feel therefore I am." I am not saying that Pacific people do not think and Westerners do not feel—this is obviously not so. What I am referring to are primary modes of perception and inner processing that profoundly affect one's relationship to nature, other human beings, and God. Recent scientific research (again from the field of neurocardiology) has discovered that the heart produces an electromagnetic field that radiates about ten feet from the body (Childre & Beech, 1999, p. 33). It is significant that this field is holographically identical to the earth's energy field. It is discoveries like these that reinforce the body-heart-earth connection of indigenous peoples.

The Western ego emerged from out of a patriarchal consciousness that had its beginnings in Europe. This type of ego, as it developed, separated out from nature, the unconscious, and the divine realm. I use the word *unconscious* to denote that vast area of the psyche that lies outside normal waking consciousness. The personal level of the unconscious contains all the biographical information (experiences and memories) belonging to a person's life. Beyond the personal unconscious is the family unconscious, a level that is shared by each member of a family. New understanding of the family unconscious suggests that this level itself is extensive and reaches back into the past for up to five generations and one generation into the future (Bynum, 1999). Each movement downward into the depths of the psyche becomes increasingly collective. The deepest layer of the unconscious is closely connected to the body and the natural world and, as such, the life-death processes. Indigenous cultures traditionally lived close to this deep level of being. Their immanent spiritual worldview is an expression of this particular relationship to the world: matter, body, and earth as divine substance.

Unlike the Western ego, the Samoan ego does not completely separate from the unconscious at maturity. Each type of ego-structure has its strengths and limitations. The Samoan ego, which continues a relationship with the unconscious, is enriched by that relationship, although the problem here is the risk of being engulfed at times by contents from the unconscious and/or very strong emotion. The Western ego enjoys unparalleled freedom of intellectual thought. However, the problem arising from too long a separation from the unconscious is the risk of deadening psychological and/or physical entropy.

I suggest that the type of thinking associated with the Samoan ego is of a more reflective and comprehensive nature, whereas the Western ego has developed a thinking style that could be described as abstract and conceptual. In *Multicultural Issues in Counseling*, Courtland Lee describes the traditional African perception of reality as "field sensitive." He gives an example of a quiz given to children of the Nigerian Ibo tribe to test their perception of reality. One question is, "There are 100 birds in a tree and a hunter shoots one; how are many left?" The correct answer is "none." The Ibo child is expected to factor in other realities beyond the numerical one, which is that the natural behavior of birds is to fly away if one is shot. This is a clear and lovely example of indigenous thinking, "where processing reality tends to take into consideration the interactions between and among objective and subjective realities as well as the consequences or implications of such interactions" (Lee, 1997, p. 74).

The archetypal foundation for the Western ego is the masculine Christian Trinity of Father, Son, and Holy Spirit. In a natural human trinity of father, mother, and child, the child and father are united by the body of the mother. However, in the Christian Trinity, the uniting factor is the Holy Spirit, which therefore removes not only the feminine element, but also the physical body from the Godhead. This form of spirituality is known as transcendent spirituality (in contrast to immanent spirituality), where God is separated from the earth and humanity (Kawai, 1996, p. 162).

The belief that the Western ego is the peak of human development pervades the field of psychology. This is not surprising since the field of psychology itself emerged in late nineteenth- and early twentieth-century Europe. Pathologies arising from the Western ego-structure required their own special medicine, and that medicine is known today as psychotherapy.

If this is so, then how do psychotherapists transmute "white man's medicine" into a universal elixir? I suggest that the solution is to be found in the heart; that the language of the heart is that universal elixir. The term *psychotherapy* is derived from root meanings that translate into "care of the soul" (Moore, 1992, p. 5). The inclusion of heart would bring psychotherapy to the brink of its original purpose and potential; the field of psychotherapy finally coming-of-age. I look further at the importance of the heart in the final part of this essay, which addresses the therapeutic relationship.

Myths and Folktales

I have chosen to engage in a kind of psychological archeology by examining myth and folktale to illuminate aspects of the Samoan psyche. The ancient material under consideration consists of two creation myths and two folktales of Samoan origin. I suspect that some of the mythic themes contained in the creation myths were already ancient knowledge by the time they were carried to the Pacific by the original wave of travelers. Myths and legends of a particular culture are the collective dreams of that culture and, although this information may not be known consciously, remain alive in the unconscious of its members. Joseph Campbell speaks about the importance of myths for the development of humanity: "These bits of information [myths] from ancient times, which have to do with the themes that have supported human life, built civilizations, and informed millennia, have to do with deep inner problems, inner mysteries, inner thresholds of passages" (Campbell, 1991, p. 2).

There are two types of creation myth: the evolutionary type, describing the development of the cosmos and the gods, and the creative type, describing a specific creative act by a deity or deities. I have included one of each type. In one version of an evolutionary myth, the original primal pair, or *ur-couple,* are two rock formations that unite to produce the earth. The family tree continues by including a variety of natural phenomena, as follows:

Male	Female	Progeny
The high rocks	The earth rocks	The earth
The earth	High winds	Solid clouds
Solid clouds	Flying clouds	Confused winds
		Quiet winds
		Boisterous winds
		Land-beating winds
		Dew of life
Dew of life	Clouds clinging to the heavens	Clouds flying about

Male	Female	Progeny
Clouds flying about	Clear heavens	Shadow Twilight Daylight Noonday Afternoon Sunset
Quiet winds	Beautiful clouds	Cloudless heaven
Cloudless heaven	Spread-out heaven	Tagaloa

It is interesting to note that in this genealogical sequence all the feminine elements were preexistent. The masculine elements were created by subsequent unions and the only preexistent male was the high rocks in the primal pair. The elements of this myth reflect a matriarchal consciousness, where the matrix of existence was basically female and the male element provided the creative impulse for new growth.

Tagaloa appears in the following creative myth in the context of the principal god of the Samoan pantheon. His epithets include The Creator, The Immeasurable One, and The Maker of Miracles.

> In the beginning was Tagaloa, who resided in the Illimitable Void. Brooding over the boundless sea, he saw a rock in the water. He brought back this rock which he shaped into a woman and inspired her with life. The woman became his wife. She then gave birth to a daughter in the form of a tulī bird. When she was ready for the journey, Tagaloa sent his daughter to the world below. Finding unending watery horizons and no place to rest, she complained to Tagaloa, who promptly threw down a rock. This rock was to become Manu'a, the main island of the Samoan group. The tulī bird then complained to her father that there was no shade on the rock. He sent down a vine to provide shelter from the hot sun. So rapidly did the vine spread that it threatened to smother the whole island. At his daughter's behest, he sent grubs to devour the vine. From underneath the remnants of the decaying vine emerged large, healthy maggots that moved about in the sun. Tagaloa came down and gave the maggots limbs and heart and soul. Thus the first human-beings were created.

The creation of human beings from maggots is an unusual mythic motif. With the imagery of the maggots, there is the underlying ethos of life emerging from death and decay, congruent with a worldview of immanent spirituality. A later addition to the myth of the creation of human beings from maggots was that only the common people came from maggots. Ingenious and complex family trees linked the chiefly family lines directly to a divine ancestor. The first supernatural being in these genealogies was always a demon mother.

Returning to the creation myth, what is significant is that at the point of Samoa's coming into being with the island of Manu'a, there is a divine family comprised of Tagaloa, his wife, their daughter, and the Illimitable Void, who could be described as the grandmother. In Greek mythology, she was called Chaos, the dark silent abyss from which all things emerged. Perhaps it is no coincidence that the most influential member in a Samoan family system is the grandmother. Although Tagaloa is the creator god, he is in effect an agent for the Void, who is the primal ground of existence. The daughter has the task of making a journey into the unknown, supported by Tagaloa from a distance. Again we have a feminine universe—however, with matriarchal consciousness at a more developed level than the first creation myth. My tentative hypothesis is that the archetypal foundation, or trinity, for the Samoan ego is Grandmother-Son-Granddaughter.

Fāgogo (folktales) were traditionally told at night by a storyteller to groups of adults and children in the home. My mother recalled with pleasure such evenings when her aunt, a traditional storyteller, would recount many tales to the family. Not surprisingly the scariest stories were the most popular. Storyteller and Jungian analyst Clarissa Pinkola Estés speaks of the natural healing function of stories:

> [Stories] have such power; they do not require that we do, be, act anything—we need only listen. The remedies for repair or reclamation of any lost psychic drive are contained in stories. Stories engender the excitement, sadness, questions, longings and understandings that spontaneously bring the archetype back to the surface. (Pinkola Estés, 1992, p. 14)

Loa and Sina

In the Samoan tale of Loa and Sina, I found an interesting parallel to the Western story of Rapunzel. These two stories contain similar themes. However, it is precisely where the tales differ that important cultural factors are revealed. Rapunzel is an adolescent girl who is kept prisoner in a high tower by a witch, who is her guardian and stepmother. Rapunzel is isolated from other people, and only sees the witch who brings her food each day. A wandering prince hears Rapunzel's singing and is enchanted. He observes the witch as she calls Rapunzel, who then unravels her hair as a ladder for the witch to climb up. Of course the prince does learn to climb her hair too: boy meets girl and they fall in love. With a slip of the tongue, Rapunzel reveals the prince's visits to the witch. In a fit of rage, the witch cuts off Rapunzel's hair and takes her to the desert, where she is left. The witch then tricks the prince with Rapunzel's hair. The distressed prince jumps out of the tower and is blinded. Both broken-hearted, Rapunzel and the prince are eventually reunited after several years of suffering in the wilderness.

In Loa and Sina, we also have a mother and daughter pair who live in an isolated manner. Loa, we are told, is part-human and part-ogress with cannibal tendencies. When she goes out hunting and fishing for their food, Sina stays home. (The implication, though not expressly stated, is that Sina is human.) Sina is also an adolescent girl who is a prisoner to her mother and kept away from other people. The signs that Loa is returning home are peals of thunder, flashes of lightning, and torrents of rain. One day a young male, Fitilo'ilo'i, ventures onto Loa's land and meets Sina. Again, boy meets girl and they fall in love. Each time her mother is away, Sina calls him with an elaborate song ritual. Soon enough, Loa suspects a male visitor, which is vehemently denied by Sina. After a time, Loa is certain her suspicions are correct. She tricks both Sina and the young man, and, with Sina out of sight, Loa swallows him whole. Meanwhile Sina, who has been calling Fitilo'ilo'i for most of the day, becomes very weak. It is apparent to Loa that Sina is close to death. Feeling pity for Sina, Loa vomits up the young man, who is still alive and intact. At the end of the story they live together, *all three of them!*

What are we to make of the ending which is so unlike a Western fairytale? In Rapunzel, the witch plays no further part in the story after tricking the prince. The reign of the mother has ended. In Western psychology, the ego must free itself from the "mother world," which is the realm of matter, the instinctual/emotional body, the natural and supernatural worlds. The prince began that process when he left his parents to undertake his journey. Sina, however, is not separated from Loa. Instead, Loa, Sina, and Fitilo'ilo'i set up family together. On one hand we could say that this story reflects the Pacific Island extended family system, or, on the other hand, indicates a lower level of ego development from the Western perspective. I suggest that both are superficial interpretations, and that there is a deeper meaning conveyed in this story.

Rapunzel is presented as a naïve young woman who is initially afraid of the prince. Although they fall in love, it is the prince who has chosen Rapunzel for his bride. The prince, as active masculine principle belonging to the outside world, symbolizes the ego in search of the feminine soul. This is necessary because the outer world of Europe is patriarchal and the nature of the ego (for both men and women) is masculine. The feminine element therefore is missing from consciousness and must be discovered and married (integrated) for psychological balance. (When using the terms *feminine, masculine, matriarchal,* and *patriarchal,* I am not referring to gender, but to tendencies, qualities, values, and systems that apply equally to men and women.)

Fitilo'ilo'i, we are told, comes not from the outer world but from the underworld. A mutual attraction grows between him and Sina. Although not explicitly stated in this tale, the implication from Sina's inconsolable grief is her awareness of Fitiloʻiloʻi as her *mānamea*. In common usage, the word *mānamea* means a special friend; however, in the context of the fāgogo, the deeper meaning is that of one's beloved soul mate. A recurring theme in Samoan folktales is that a beautiful young woman rejects many suitors, as she is waiting for her mānamea whom she does not yet know but will recognize when he appears. The young man comes not from the outer world but from the underworld. In other words, the new masculine element emerges from the unconscious and enters matriarchal territory.

The witch and Loa are both associated with the natural world. Rapunzel's name is taken from the dark green spinach-like vegetable that her birth-mother craved from the witch's garden. Loa's relationship to nature is reinforced through the story by the peals of thunder, flashes of lightning, and torrents of rain that precede her arrival. The world of nature is not associated with warm feelings, as there is in nature a relentless life-death-decay cycle that continues outside the human sphere. For example, the natural forces that create an earthquake do not have feelings for the people killed or made homeless.

What is surprising is that Loa feels pity for her daughter, who is close to death. This point in the story holds the key for the final positive outcome. Here Loa's heart has been touched by Sina's suffering. The vomiting up of Fitiloʻiloʻi is an action stemming from her heart response. We can imagine that this is not the usual modus operandi for a part-ogress with cannibal tendencies. By this act, Loa in fact becomes more human and thus a potentially destructive mother complex transforms into a positive one that supports the possibility of new life.

In Rapunzel, there is no equivalent response of pity from the witch, who abandons a distressed and pregnant Rapunzel in the desert. The witch remains outside of normal human life, negative and untransformed. At the end of the Samoan story, the matriarchal structure is maintained and invigorated by the new masculine element. Without Fitiloʻiloʻi there would be no future for the mother-daughter pair. At the end of Rapunzel, the patriarchal structure is maintained and infused with new life by Rapunzel and the children.

The Snake

There are many stories of a young woman named Sina in a variety of circumstances and roles. She is the universal Samoan maiden. In the story "The Snake," she is the third daughter in a poor family that has no food. The parents know of a well-off family with a son who is available for marriage—the perfect solution to their food crisis. However, the catch is that the available male is a rather large snake. The older two daughters both offer to marry the snake, but these attempts fail as they are afraid of him at first sight. However, Sina bestows great affection on him from the first visit. In the story, the reason given for her patience was due to her love for her parents. I suggest here that Sina is able to perceive the snake's true nature and recognize him as her mānamea.

The snake, out of love for Sina, changes into his human form. They marry and live with his mother. Sina gives birth to a baby girl and after a time wishes to visit her family with the baby. As she approaches her family, she seems to lose her perceptive abilities and does not foresee the tragedy ahead. On the path, one of her sisters abducts the baby from her father's arms. Her husband is sure that it was her sister that took the baby, but Sina disagrees and they argue. After searching for the baby, Sina lies down to rest in her parents' house. Her sisters, in a jealous rage, beat her to death. Her husband knows that something terrible has happened to Sina. He changes back into his snake form and, upon returning to the house, finds her dead body. Grieving and outraged, he avenges Sina's death by killing her sisters. He then finds where his baby daughter is hidden and takes her back home to his mother.

This is certainly not a "happily ever after" story. Sina's parents are prepared to sacrifice their daughters to a snake in order to satisfy their hunger. They represent a complex that is driven by power, not love. The fact that they have no food indicates symbolically that this is a family that does not have enough nourishment for its children—in fact, a negative mother complex. Because of the strength of the feminine in a matriarchal culture, this form of mother complex is particularly dangerous to the developing ego, manipulating cultural injunctions such as "always honor and obey the parents" to control. Sina's baby was abducted by her sister, and later that night, Sina was beaten to death by both sisters. The sisters can be seen in this story as extensions of the negative mother represented by both parents. By contrast, the mother of the snake is presented as a positive mother figure, generous and gracious. I contend that the Samoan ego is represented by Sina in both interpretations of "The Snake." Sina's capacity to perceive the true nature of a person or situation, coupled with courageous love and devotion, reflect a level of consciousness that is imbued with heart intelligence. Although the story ends tragically, there is hope contained in the baby who is the new Sina. The ending maps the movement into the future for a stronger ego-structure and I believe that future is *now*.

The Therapeutic Relationship

These understandings of indigenous consciousness and ego-structure have significant implications for personal and professional cross-cultural relationships. In this essay, I am focusing particularly on the therapeutic relationship.

When engaged in conversation with my aunt who is a *fofō* (traditional Samoan healer) about my working with Pacific Island clients, she simply advised me to "be yourself." These wise and reassuring words have stayed with me and have also reinforced my training, that the self of the therapist is the catalyst for the therapeutic process. Lewis, Armani, and Lannon, the authors of *A General Theory of Love,* describe therapy as "the ultimate inside job." And indeed it is so. A vital thread at the core of the therapeutic relationship is the therapist's ability to emotionally attune to the inner life of the client, to perceive and feel the essence of the other. The therapist must be able to step beyond the parameters of her world to meet the client in his or her own world. The task, then, is to discover and maintain an often precarious balance of what is perhaps best described in the metaphor of "one foot in and one foot out" of the client's inner world. With "two feet out," there is no emotional relationship built, and with "two feet in," the therapeutic space has disappeared into an enmeshed unconsciousness. Neither is much use for the client.

When we wish to work cross-culturally, the question arises whether it is truly possible to meet a client from another culture in her or his own world, given the differences in physical appearance, language, and upbringing, as well as in the interior world of consciousness itself. I believe that this is possible, with one major proviso: that the therapist is conscious of the connection with his or her own heart and is willing to listen to those heart messages. Without this heart connection, it is not possible to step beyond one's own culturally created super-ego constructs to genuinely meet the other. This is even more difficult if the client is from a culture where the heart is the primary center of thinking.

When a therapist and a client are sitting together in a room, there is an interpenetration of both their hearts' electromagnetic fields. This field of the hearts is the physical space where the therapeutic relationship is created—the third place that is beyond the body of the client and the body of the therapist, yet connects and contains them both. It is through this electromagnetic field that our hearts pick up information about another person or situation. At the same time that a therapist is picking up information about the client, the client is also picking up information about the therapist. The degree to which this information filters into awareness depends on the level of conscious connection to one's heart. A therapist without such a connection, sitting with a Pasifika client who is already tuned into his or her heart, will not be able to navigate the relational, intersubjective space.

In Samoan culture there is already an understanding of *the sacred space between two persons.* This is known as the *vā*. I believe that if the vā of a therapeutic relationship is receptive and creative, there is the possibility for genuine meeting and unfolding of the other. I recall working with one of my earlier Pasifika clients who saw (in an inward sense) a group of her ancestors standing behind her in the room. Her ancestors appeared on several occasions, always the same group, each dressed in their own distinctive clothing. Mostly they remained silently in the background as a comforting presence for my client. I did not initiate these occurrences by using any of the imaginal processes that I am trained in. The ancestors were able to appear, I believe, because the vā was open and receptive.

The sharing of dreams was a normal occurrence in traditional Samoan society. I encourage therapists to be willing to work with their Pasifika clients' dreams. Dreams provide a rich source of unconscious material that is invaluable for the therapeutic process. A dream is, in fact, a series of images that symbolically represent the flow of psychic energy in the dreamer, the deep story of the dreamer. They are veritable treasure troves containing clues about wounds from the past, conflicts in the present, and the pathway to the client's future potential.

My final suggestion may seem out of context with the rest of this essay, yet I feel it is not. Consider offering your Pasifika clients a cup of tea or coffee at the beginning of the session. This simple gesture brings bodily concerns into the equation as well as engendering a sense of *us*—two people in a room sharing a drink together and having this conversation.

I have chosen to end with a Samoan blessing:

> *Le Atua i le tatou vā:* God in Our *Vā*

References

Bynum, E. (1999). *The African psychological lineage on dream states, family dynamics, the unconscious and beyond.* Boston: University of Massachusetts Health Series.

Campbell, J. (1991). *The power of myth.* New York: Random House.

Childre, D., & Beech, H. (1999). *The HeartMath solution.* San Francisco: Harper.

Culbertson, P. (1997). *Counselling issues in South Pacific communities.* Auckland: Accent.

Dixon, R. B. (1964). *The mythology of all races.* New York: Cooper Square.

Estés, C. P. (1992). *Women who run with the wolves.* London: Random House.

Fanon, F. (1986). *Black skin, white masks.* London: Pluto Press.

Ferrer, N. F. (2002). *Revisioning transpersonal theory.* New York: SUNY.

Jung, C. G. (1993). *Memories, dreams, reflections.* Glasgow: HarperCollins.

Kawai, H. (1996). *The Japanese psyche: Major motifs in the fairy tales of Japan.* Putnam, CT: Spring Publications.

Kramer, A. (1999). *The Samoa Islands.* Auckland: Pacifica Press.

Lee, C. L. (1997). *Multicultural issues in counseling.* Alexandria: American Counseling Association.

Lewis, T., Armani, F., & Lannon, R. (2000). *A general theory of love*. New York: Random House.
Moore, T. (1992). *Care of the soul*. New York: HarperCollins.
Moyle, R. (1981). *Fagogo*. Auckland: Auckland University Press.
Neihardt, J. G. (1961). *Black Elk speaks*. Lincoln: University of Nebraska Press.
Walker, C. (1998). Waking up to the holographic heart: Starting over with education: an interview with Joseph Chilton Pearce. Retrieved August 7, 2005, from http://www.ratical.org/many_worlds/JCP98.html.

12

Hawaiki-Lelei
Journeys to Wellness

SEILOSA SKIPPS-PATTERSON

For some time I have described myself as a New Zealand–born Samoan. On my journey to know myself I have realized that I had forgotten the island ways, but as I have reflected on my life, particularly with motherhood, I recall that during my pregnancies all I craved was raw fish and taro—food that I detested as a youngster growing up in central Auckland in the 1960s. I'd never been massaged, but after two difficult deliveries I sought the traditional healing arts of the Samoan fofō, which resulted in my only natural birth. I considered myself Westernized, and with my pālagi husband was perceived as such.

In Samoa, I identify myself as a New Zealander. However, the older people see my facial traits and identify my Chinese-Samoan line almost immediately. For most of my life, I have struggled to know where I fit in as a Samoan. I was raised in an area where few brown faces lived, and at church I was teased because I did not speak Samoan. Yet my father was a son of a fisherman from the village of Puipa'a and my mother came from a more affluent area, Lotopā. My mother's family is Lotu Mamona and contributed generously to the church. The land on which the Mormon Temple stands was once our family land, and the most repeated and favored family story concerned my great-great-grandfather's conversion to the Church of Jesus Christ of Latter-Day Saints.

I have worked in the social services field as a family support worker, social worker, and counselor. More recently I became the first Samoan graduate of the AUT Master's in Psychotherapy Program. It was one of the hardest journeys of my life—one in which I often felt lonely and marginalized. I hope that I am pioneering a way forward for our people to train in mental health, particularly in paradigms that appear privileged, such as psychotherapy. My ancestors sacrificed much for my parents to have a better life, and so it is with our generation: to better ourselves, to provide adequately for our family, to have those privileges, and to leave a great legacy for our family.

> *I haere mai ahau, i hawaiki-nui, i hawaiki-roa, i hawaiki-pamamao.*
> I came from the great Hawaiki, from the long Hawaiki,
> from the far distant Hawaiki.
> (Sutton, 2001, p. 140)

Hawaiki is the name often used by Māori to identify their ancestral homeland, before their migration to Aotearoa/New Zealand. Some believe that Hawai'i is the original Hawaiki in the Pacific. Tahiti is another possible Hawaiki; Rarotonga another; and we might also include Samoa, as it has an island named Savai'i (Hawai'i) (Sutton, 2001). I would include Tonga, Niue, Tokelau, and all of the Pacific Islands as other Hawaikis. Like Sutton, I have chosen Hawaiki in my essay title to inspire our Pacific people to a proud remembrance of their heritage, *whakapapa* (genealogy), ancient traditions, and legends.

I grew up in an area where few Pacific people lived, so my relationships with Māori have filled the cultural connections that my soul pined for. I am grateful for the *tuakana/teina* (older sibling/younger sibling) relationship they have offered me, and for my identity as a New Zealander, as will be reflected in parts of this writing. *Lelei*, in Cook Island Māori and in Tongan, is a manner of wishing each other "well life." In Samoan, it means "enough," and I can't help thinking that the connotation of "enough" is one of timing, of "the now." Let us journey into "well life" less oppressed, with insights to heal and nourish the crippled parts of ourselves and our people. Let us honor the journey taken by our ancestors, and in so doing, honor our present journey by saying "Hawaiki-lelei," meaning "Journeys to Wellness."

This essay tracks some of my own journey as a psychotherapist in training with Pasifika *whaiora* (clients). Motherhood has been my greatest learning tool as a psychotherapist, and I use both object relations (Winnicott, 1965, 1993) and attachment theory (Bowlby, 1979; Karen, 1998) to underpin my approach. Winnicott's (1965) idea that "there is no such thing as a baby" resonates with the Polynesian collective identity. Figiel (1996) states, "'I' does not exist. I am not. My self belongs not to me because 'I' is always 'we,' is part of the *'āiga* (family) . . . a part of the *nu'u* (village), a part of Samoa" (p. 135). The Western style of individuation runs contrary to Samoan cultural protocols.

The Fonofale Model (Pulotu-Endemann, 1995), which originated with Pasifika mental health professionals and is endorsed by the New Zealand Ministry of Health, begins with the family as the foundation. (Paiheretia and Tapa Whā, developed by Durie, 1998, are equivalent models for working with Māori.)

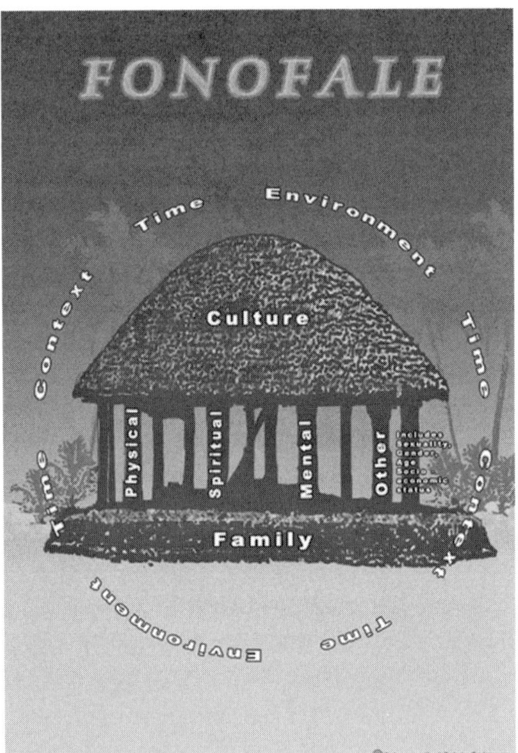

Interpretation of the Diagram

- The roof provides protection from the elements, including rain, wind, and storms. Thus culture provides protection from the world's view. Pasifika culture is a shelter for life. Culture is comprised of philosophical drives and attitudes. It can also include systems of belief, which might incorporate traditional methods of healing, a Western method, or both.
- The foundation is the nuclear and extended family, ancestral and genealogical links that form the fundamental basis of social organizations for Pasifika people, and is an important source of strength. The family provides the base, which supports the four posts and the roof.
- The spiritual post is the sense of wellbeing that stems from a belief system that can include Christianity, traditional spirituality, or a combination of both.
- The physical post is the biological wellbeing of the body, which can be measured by the absence of illness and pain.
- The mental post represents psychological wellbeing, including the health of the mind.

- The "others" post includes variables such as gender, employment, sexuality, age, and the like.

All of these aspects of health exist within the context, environment, and time period relevant to the individual. In addition, variables such as age, status, village, island of origin, age on arriving in New Zealand, contact with extended family, and place of birth (New Zealand or Pacific Islands) are interrelated.

Makasiale and Culbertson (2003) inform us that five major issues define Pasifika identity: hierarchy, obedience, family, land, and spirituality. "Caught between two worlds" (p. 121) is their description of Pasifika clients who are trying to live out their cultural identity in the midst of European dominance. They encourage us to assess the client's unique developmental stage in the process of learning to live in these two worlds. They also suggest, from clinical experience, that the most effective therapeutic modalities for Pasifika clients include family systems theory, narrative counseling, object relations theory, and psycho-educational or behavior modification methods.

Self Psychology (Kohut, 1971) is a pālagi therapeutic modality that emphasizes mirroring, validating, and empathically attuning. Empathy and unconditional positive regard were earlier identified by Carl Rogers as core conditions of therapy, and characteristics inherent in effective client-centered practitioners (Raskin & Rogers, 2004). As a Samoan cultural therapist, I prefer to name this type of connection *alofa* (love), one of the basic emotions in the Fonofale Model.

Winnicott (1987) was in awe of a mother's intuitive ability, distinguishing between two types of maternal function: knowing and learning. Knowing is what a mother intuits, simply by virtue of being the mother of her infant, as opposed to learning what to do. Winnicott argued that knowing and learning were as far apart as the east and west coasts of England, a distance that resembles the cultural difference between some therapists and their clients.

As a psychotherapist I work best when I am intuitive and when I privilege connection. Theories that override my thinking make it feel as though I am colonizing the client, and they intrude upon our relationship. Welcoming Pacific people by a culturally appropriate embrace, or by speaking in their respective Pacific language, allows clients to bring their cultural selves into the room, and to cooperate in building a working alliance.

Enculturating Clarkson's Theories of Psychodynamics

As a developing psychotherapist, I have found Petruska Clarkson's (1990) classification of five types of therapeutic relationship to be particularly useful. These are:

- The Working Alliance
- The Transference/Counter-transference Relationship
- The Reparative/Developmentally-Needed Relationship
- The I/You Relationship
- The Transpersonal Relationship

Clarkson's relationship categories provide a helpful perspective when integrating cultural aspects into the therapeutic relationship.

The Working Alliance

Belonging and identity are key issues in psychotherapy. McGoldrick (1998) writes:

> The goal is to create a world we can each call home—a place where we will each have a voice, where our flowing sense of group identities gives more sense of boundaries that include than of divisions that exclude. The notion of culture is almost a mystical sense of connection with all the threads of which our human community is woven. (p. 8)

McGoldrick (1998) describes the importance of experiencing connection within a world we can call home; it is equally vital that the client can experience connection and find a place to belong within the therapeutic relationship. One way in which Pacific people join others is via symbolism and metaphor (see Makasiale in this volume). A Fijian client saw an ornament from Fiji on my table, and instantly began talking about her childhood memories of growing up there. The symbols in my room invited her to do so.

An effective working alliance is vital to any therapeutic relationship, but is not always easy to achieve. Holmes (1992) critiques therapist-patient misalliances and therapists' overreliance on ego-supportive approaches when white therapists work with African American clients. Though Holmes is speaking of a specific cross-race dyad, I would argue that a same-race dyad can also be experienced as though it were a cross-race dyad. I am a brown therapist using critical white theory; a brown client may therefore experience me as a white therapist, or as highly colonized (Fanon, 1968).

A Samoan female, Mahana, came to see me. She reminded me of a minister's wife. I felt that she perceived me as a white therapist because of the way she spoke in a very intellectual manner to me, not allowing her more-relaxed, real Samoan self, and her emotions, to show. I intentionally adopted *whanaungatanga* (culturally sanctioned ways of connecting) as a method to ally with her, including my cultural knowledge of family and God, in responding to her:

C 1 You know, there must be a reason. I just got my diploma last month and I planned to keep going. I don't know, am I supposed to give up? and I said to my husband, maybe there must be a reason, and I will see what I can do.

T 1 Sounds like you love coming to school and sounds like you put the Lord first.

C 2 Yes (Quiet response; facial display of sadness and dismay)

T 2 So, it sounds like—it's more about what you believe the Lord wants you to do.

C 3 That's why (crying), you know, that's me. You know, I don't know what others believe. But you know, I just believe in what I believe. You know, I try to balance it all out. You know, just like mum. She was really happy when she found out that I'm having a baby.

T 3 Your mum?

C 4 Yeah, but she is a sick person and she really can't help out. Yeah, she came here when my youngest son was born, and she now has her permanent residence and is staying with me.

T 4 Hmm (softly).

C 5 But she was really excited when she found out that I was pregnant and said, "Oh thank God. Oh, we should thank God for what He's giving. You know you still haven't got enough babies!" And I said, "What? Four children is enough!" and mum said, "No, you should have five or six at least," and I said, "No, four children is enough here in New Zealand. This is not Samoa. You have to rely on money and you have to go out and work to feed your babies."

The empathic cultural matching I offered to her facilitated the development of our working alliance. As Clarkson (1992) says, "The therapeutic alliance is the powerful joining of forces which energizes and supports the long, difficult and frequently painful work of life-changing psychotherapy" (p. 296).

The Transference/Counter-transference Relationship

Sione, a Samoan-born male, migrated to New Zealand when he was 11. As an adult, he came to therapy seeking a "cultural match" (his words); previously he had seen two different pālagi therapists, but left dissatisfied. In our initial session, Sione embraced me with a culturally appropriate kiss on the cheek and a simultaneous handshake, which then recurred at the beginning of every session. I engaged in this protocol because Sione initiated it each time. In session 28, we discussed the embrace, and he acknowledged that there were times when he experienced me as one of his aunties, so that the embrace was offered out of obligation. We were able to speak about transferred feelings this way, and Sione gained insight into other transferences, both positive and negative, which occurred in our work together.

In the first session with Sione, I made a strong mental connection with the biblical Parable of the Prodigal Son and his return home. Sione had been severely abused—sexually, physically, and emotionally. His diagnosis was complex, and I knew to be careful with interpretations. On reflection, I understood that Sione's excitement was generated by his desire to go home to his parents, especially to be accepted by his father. In a similar way to the parable, I was his father in an idealized transference. By keeping our focus on the culturally appropriate ways of relating, we formed a connection outside of the pathologizing realm, and our therapy relationship continued over seventeen months.

"The transference relationship is an essential part of the analytic procedure as the analysis consists of inviting the transference and gradually dissolving it by means of interpretation" (Clarkson, 1993, p. 27). My counter-transferential remembrance of biblical stories and metaphors helped me to culturally match Sione, who comes from the world of symbolism.

Sione proved unable to remain substance-free during therapy, however, and this often blocked our relationship. My naiveté as a beginning therapist added to the cultural collusion. My relationship with him was blinded by the avoidance of further cultural explorations, particularly in monitoring his substance abuse. I became aware of my collusion through supervision, understanding how I over-identified with Sione. Unresolved issues around my own father's substance abuse prevented my seeing how often Sione was stoned, and why I was unable to be fully present for Sione. Cultural transference and counter-transference (Seeley, 2000) for nonwhite clients are affected by the collective self and the symbiotic attachment that is culturally appropriate.

Kitayama and Markus (1995) illustrate the difference between an independent construal of self (a more individuated self) as opposed to an interdependent construal of self (those who are socialized to adjust themselves to an attendant relationship). Many non-Western cultures neither assume nor value the overt separateness of the independent construal of self. The primary cultural task is, rather, to adjust oneself to fit in and maintain interdependence among the group. I kept asking myself, "How do transference and counter-transference work culturally, especially when the construal of self changes in relationship?"

Sione and I talked several times about his feeling that, in order to be intimate with someone, he had to be stoned or drunk. I used the transference to explore whether he had thought of me sexually, which he then admitted. I felt flattered, but scared at the same time:

T 1 It would be hard to hear anything when you're . . .
C 1 (he interrupts and finishes my sentence) . . . boozing or drugging and sexing all the time.
T Sounds like, too, sexing is, is like boozing, and drugging.
C 2 Yes, yeah it is. Yeah, I can't believe I'm actually saying these things to you. It's really neat.
T 3 Yeah it is.
C 4 It's like it's really honest and I kind of—yeah, it's good, it's empowering. I don't have to do devious things to, like, you know, you can just talk about it, you know, it's okay.
T 5 Cause, yeah, I felt like last week I was wondering if you were doing devious things to me, cause you had said to me, that you know my values, and I kind of thought, "How the heck do you know what my values are?"
C 5 Yeah, yeah.

My pālagi supervisor at the time, who works primarily from psychodynamic processes and has little Samoan cultural knowledge, felt that my intervention at T 5 was shaming, controlling, and leading. In reevaluating my response, and my counter-transference as a Samoan matriarch, I felt as though I had been breastfeeding Sione, and when "the baby bit me," I had immediately removed him from the nipple.

Although unsure whether my pālagi supervisor was correct, I believed my interventions had come from a nurturing place of knowing (Winnicott, 1987). I was left wondering how a pālagi supervisor, carrying an independent construal of self, could know how a Samoan female therapist, carrying an interdependent construal of self, could work with the transference of a Samoan male client who also carried an interdependent construal of self.

The Reparative/Developmentally Needed Relationship

Sione had not attended therapy for two weeks because he had not been substance free. On arriving for his final therapy session, he announced, laughing, that he'd been naughty. I invited him to talk about his substance abuse and to think what the consequences needed to be. He acknowledged our verbal contract to remain substance free, and he acknowledged his choice of marijuana over therapy.

The intentional provision I offered to Sione was for him to choose to acknowledge and accept the consequences of his drug use. When he chose to remain with his substance abuse, I did not respond with a hostile or punitive reaction, though I'd thought I would. Instead, I believe I represented his *'āiga* (family) and his *nu'u* (village). I believe I was acting out Clarkson's

(1992) description of "the intentional provision by the psychotherapist of a corrective/reparative replenishing parental relationship (or action) where the original parenting was deficient, abusive or overprotective" (p. 299).

My main task during the last session was for us to part on good enough terms, allowing Sione to continue to feel loved. Sione's previous relationships had always ended in violence and abuse. Seventeen months of therapy had now passed, and at session 62, this was my cultural intervention:

> Therapist: I, um (fumbling, nervous), I'm going to sing you a song and this is my gift for you as you go away and it's really short and it's just about love. And if you're needing something—maybe you can remember this: "Te aroha, me te rangimārie, tātou tātou e" (Love and peace be with you always).

Tears streamed down Sione's face; this was a sacred moment in the therapy room for both of us. After some time, he gathered his composure and spoke, telling me how suicidal he had been when first arriving for therapy. The use of a *waiata* (song) was not like the terminations he had experienced with his previous pālagi therapists, and he felt he had achieved his original desire to be culturally matched, and thereby fully met.

The I-You Relationship

"The I-You relationship is characterized by the here-and-now existential encounter between two people" (Clarkson, 1993, p. 33). This quality of here-and-now, profoundly meaningful connection was evident in the concluding session with Sione, described above. It also occurred with Huia.

When I first began to meet with Huia, a Cook Island client, my therapy room was part of a Pasifika counseling center in an academic institution. The history of the land and building was significant in working with this Pasifika client. Like all Pacific people, she held certain beliefs around land and place, yet she also had an unfortunate history of being discriminated against at school. The building where my office was located had once been the asylum unit for a psychiatric hospital, but prior to that, it was a Māori battlefield. The abuse of Māori youth was also part of the building's history. Other clients had mentioned feeling spooked around this site. I was aware that Huia also sensed the conflicted cultural history of the building where we met at first, and that this would be affecting our therapeutic relationship.

Huia often had trouble making it to her appointments. Eventually, due to her financial hardship and regular car problems, I arranged to meet her for a session in her home. I experienced Huia as being more empowered when we met in this new location. It seemed that my act of removing my shoes when I entered her home allowed her to let me in internally. She opened up with her dreams, speaking freely and honestly. Her dream of a lion waiting outside her home, and having to stay inside for fear of the lion outside, was a beautiful metaphor for how hard it was for her to allow me to enter her internal world. Huia needed me to come to her safe place, as opposed to having to come to me. Practical considerations aside, I believe my instinct to meet her in her home, rather than my office, arose from a cultural knowing that is appropriate in a relationship of alofa (love).

The Transpersonal Relationship

Grof (1985) defines transpersonal experiences as involving an extension of consciousness beyond usual ego boundaries and the limitations of space or time. When Clarkson (1995) discusses the transpersonal, she references the theories of Jung, arguing for an appreciation of all things spiritual, and acknowledging a deeper level of interconnectedness between us all as human beings. "[Interconnectedness] implies a letting go of skills, of knowledge, of experience, of preconceptions, even of the desire to heal, to be present" (Clarkson, 1993, p. 37). For Pasifika people, the transpersonal can also include experiencing the presence of their deceased loved ones.

In my last year of psychotherapy training, at our annual *noho marae* (overnight, experiential training in Māori culture), our *tuakana* (older sibling) group began an experiential training session—a group therapy session. Chairs were placed in a circle, the same setup as if we were on campus. A number of students complained, advocating that the chairs were culturally inappropriate for inside the marae. Without joining into the discussion, I went to get a mattress and sat on it on the floor. Upon doing so I said, "I don't mean to show disrespect, but this *whare* (Māori meetinghouse) holds me here in this process, not you (looking at the facilitators), and I am going to sit here with my great-grandmother, just like I used to sit with her under the coconut tree, because that is what feels right for me."

Strengthened by my great-grandmother's presence, I claimed my *tūrangawaewae* (cultural place of belonging) in a way that I had never done before. This was a culturally reverent moment in my training and I understood what I have always known: that I carry my ancestors within me. My behavior may have been interpreted as rebellious by others there, but I knew it wasn't, because I felt guided by *tūpuna* (ancestors). In my most desperate times during training, when I believed I could no longer carry on, I often felt my great-grandmother close by, lifting and supporting me in the dark times.

Cross-Cultural Issues in Supervision and Training

As a psychotherapist I am required professionally to be fully supervised. Of course I have chosen a supervisor to whom I am able to take my cultural issues and my cultural self. My supervisor is also fully supervised, by someone else who is supervised, and so on. In this way I am supported by many others, reminiscent of belonging to an extended family and village. This reminds me of reciprocity and of the circle of life.

Having worked with both pālagi and Pacific clients, I find working from a culturally centered approach to be more challenging, because I am working not only with the Pasifika clients who sit before me, but also with the families and heritage they carry with them. Usually they are in therapy because of some trauma in their lives, and often they are unable to integrate the different identities and attachments with their multiple family figures.

Cultural assessment within supervision is crucial. Foliaki (1993) described the case of a Tongan man who had severe migraines at the same time every day, but no physical cause for his illness was discoverable. The man was admitted to the hospital, but no relief could be found. Meanwhile, some relatives visited their grandparents' burial grounds, where they found that roots had penetrated through the grandparents' bones. When the grave was cleaned and the bones wrapped in tapa cloth and reburied, the man's severe migraines stopped. This illustrates the cultural belief that ancestors maintain constant communication, spiritually and physically, with those still alive. Cross-cultural supervision requires that non-Pacific supervisors are capable of honoring this way of seeing the world.

Cross-cultural supervision may demand that the supervisor work outside the dominant supervision paradigms of Western theory. Waldegrave (1998) discusses an example of cultural intervention in a therapist's work. The therapy session occurred in a clinic, in a room with a one-way mirror. Behind the mirror stood a Māori cultural consultant, alongside Waldegrave, in his capacity as a psychologist. At one point in the session, the Māori consultant interrupted the therapist, bringing him behind the mirror in order to inform the therapist of critical information about Māori values that the therapist was overlooking.

This cultural perspective changed the therapist's approach. Waldegrave realized that he and his colleagues had never been taught the things that the Māori consultant was pointing out. He began to wonder how often in the past their work with nonwhite clients had been culturally uninformed because cultural knowledge had not been seen to be significant in clinical work. Since then, as a result of this experience, Waldegrave has advocated for the inclusion of cultural knowledge in New Zealand training programs.

Similarly, Abbott and Durie (1987) had earlier advocated for the inclusion of cultural knowledge and cultural appropriateness in psychology training programs, in the hope that such sensitivity would increase entry into the profession by Māori practitioners. They pointed out that the applied psychology disciplines were probably the most monocultural, in terms of Māori representation, of all New Zealand professions. Both training institutions and mental health providers had been found wanting in their capacity to equitably serve Māori needs, and it was evident that the steps that had been taken to embrace *taha Māori* (the Māori way) needed to be amplified significantly.

While much progress regarding these issues pertaining to Māori has been made in the last twenty years within some professional bodies and training institutions, others lag behind. Additionally, in training programs for helping professionals, less attention has been paid to the need to include Pasifika cultural awareness, information about issues pertaining to Pasifika communities and clients, and to teach culturally appropriate ways of working, as there is no statutory or regulatory requirement to do so.

Conclusion

As we strive to strengthen the wellbeing of our communities and our clients in their journeys to wellness, we ourselves are also undertaking our own journeys of healing, strengthening, and growth. Who we are is at the heart of what we do—the personal and the professional are inseparable. In finding our way and moving forward as helping professionals, we have rich resources to draw from and to support us: our cultural heritage of Pasifika history, traditions, spirituality, and processes; Western ways of working that we find effective or can adapt; a developing knowledge base that can inform our practice; and increasingly, the voices of Pasifika practitioners and researchers in sharing our understandings and wisdom. Supporting and empowering each other in this way, we can tackle the obstacles in our pathways to wellbeing, the professional and personal challenges we face. Let us strive for Pasifika success in our own Hawaiki-lelei!

References

Abbot, M., & Durie, M. (1987). A whiter shade of pale: Taha Maori and professional psychology training. *New Zealand Journal of Psychology, 16*, 58–71.

Bowlby, J. (1979). *The making and breaking of affectional bonds*. London: Routledge.

Clarkson, P. (1990). A multiplicity of psychotherapeutic relationships. *British Journal of Psychotherapy, 7*(2), 149–163.

Clarkson, P. (1992). *Transactional analysis psychotherapy*. London: Tavistock Routledge.

Clarkson, P. (1993). *On psychotherapy.* London: Whurr Publishers.
Clarkson, P. (1995). *The therapeutic relationship.* London: Whurr Publishers.
Culbertson, P. (1999). Listening differently with Maori and Polynesian clients. *Forum: The Journal of the New Zealand Association of Psychotherapists, 5,* 64–82.
Durie, M. (1998). *Whaiora: Maori health development* (2nd ed.). Auckland: Oxford University Press.
Fanon, F. (1968). *Black skin, white masks.* London: Granada.
Figiel, S. (1996). *Where we once belonged.* Auckland: Pasifika Press.
Foliaki, L. (1993, November). *Tongan illnesses: Akafia.* Pacific Islands Mental Health Meeting, Wellington.
Grof, S. (1985). *Beyond the brain: Birth, death and transcendence in psychotherapy.* Albany: State University of New York Press.
Holmes, D. (1992). Race and transference in psychoanalysis and psychotherapy. *International Journal of Psychoanalysis, 73,* 1–11.
Karen, R. (1998). *Becoming attached: First relationships and how they shape our capacity to love.* New York: Oxford University Press.
Kitayama, S., & Markus, H. (1995). Culture and self: How cultures influence the way we view ourselves. In D. Matsumoto (Ed.), *People: Psychology from a cultural perspective* (pp. 17–37). Pacific Grove: Brooks/Cole.
Kohut, H. (1971). *The analysis of the self.* New York: International Universities Press.
Makasiale, C., & Culbertson, P. (2003). Mental health and Polynesian clients. *The GM Resource and Referral Directory, 2003,* 121–122.
McGoldrick, M. (Ed.). (1998). *Re-visioning family therapy: Race, culture, and gender in clinical practice.* New York: Guilford.
Pulotu-Endemann, F. K. (2001). *Pacific mental health services and the workforce: Moving on the blueprint.* Wellington: Ministry of Health.
Raskin, N. J., & Rogers, C. (2004) Person-centered therapy. In R. J. Corsini & D. Wedding (Eds.), *Current psychotherapies* (7th ed., pp. 128–161). Stamford, CT: Wadsworth Publishing.
Seeley, K. (2000). *Cultural psychotherapy: Working with culture in the clinical encounter.* Northvale: Jason Aronson.
Sutton, B. S. (2001). *Lehi: Father of Polynesia: Polynesians are nephites.* Orem, UT: Hawaiki Publishing.
Waldegrave, C. (1998). The challenges of culture to psychology and postmodern thinking. In M. McGoldrick (Ed.), *Revisioning family therapy: Race, culture and gender in clinical practice* (pp. 404–413). New York: The Guilford Press.
Winnicott, D. W. (1965). *The maturational processes and the facilitating environment.* London: Karnac Books.
Winnicott, D. W. (1987). *Babies and their mothers.* Boston: Addison-Wesley.
Winnicott, D. W. (1993). The location of cultural experience. In P. Rudnytsky (Ed.), *Transitional objects and potential spaces: Literary uses of D. W. Winnicott* (pp. 3–12). New York: Columbia University Press.

13

Using *Mea-alofa* in a Holistic Model for Pasifika Clients

A Case Study

FIA T. TURNER-TUPOU

I was born and raised in Samoa, and my parents are from the island of Upolu. My father is Misa Mu from Matāutu and my mother is Avasa Taefu from Si'ufaga, though she lived most of her life with the Tuivaiti family, her relatives in Levī, Falelatai. I enjoyed my childhood, and most of my teenage years were spent at the pastor's house, helping coordinate activities for youth and serving in general.

I am the mother of four children and grandmother of two lovely grandchildren. I spent twenty-two years at home caring for the family, then studied psychology and counseling part-time for the next six years. For the past seven years, I have worked in the community as a counselor, gaining wide experience advocating for families. Currently I work part-time at tertiary institutions as a counselor for Pasifika students, and also run a private practice providing counseling services for the family court, government departments, and the prison service. I also offer supervision, mediation, and facilitation.

My passion is simply to make a difference in people's lives, empowering families by using a culturally sensitive and holistic model based on the traditional Samoan concept of mea-alofa.

This essay grew out of my belief that when mental health problems occur with any Pasifika person, one treatment method is more effective than all others. When the client is dealt with in a culturally sensitive manner, working preferably with someone of her own culture, who speaks the same language, is of the same gender, and knows the cultural/spiritual values and beliefs of that client, then chances are that the treatment will be more successful in the end, than if she were seeing a counselor of another culture. It is vitally important that the initial assessment of the client be done in a similarly sensitive manner. This should minimize any misunderstanding of the client's situation. The integration of cultural, spiritual, and therapeutic frameworks is also necessary in order to address, in a holistic manner, not only the needs of the person, but also of the family and the wider community.

Passing Down Intergenerational and Intercultural Mea-alofa

Throughout history, our forebears taught the generations that followed the significance of passing down gifts, or mea-alofa, of their own traditional culture, from one generation to the next. In a conference presentation, Seiuli (2004) remarked:

> In a broad Samoan interpretation, mea-alofa is a love offering, a precious gift, a valued treasure, a legacy, a heritage, a call, and an object of adornment. This mea-alofa is likened to a heritage and when you inherit this mea-alofa heritage, it then becomes part of you and also who you are, whether you realize it or not.

He went on to say:

> Mea-alofa can therefore be seen as a foundational component in the make-up of the Samoan person, as it brings together their physical, emotional, familial, and spiritual attributes. Thus, mea-alofa represents a unique way of understanding and relating to Samoan people. It encompasses the totality of the Samoan being, especially in relation to counseling.

In her research on indigenous approaches, Webber-Dreadon (1999) stated that these gifts, or mea-alofa, are handed down from and by our ancestors. Anae (1999) emphasized the importance of continuing this journey of our ancestors and of having close ancestral connections. Both of these writers bring to our attention the fact that this concept of a cultural approach, implemented by people of the same culture by passing down gifts from our ancestors, has been around for a long time. It is not a new concept.

Putting these mea-alofa-based approaches into practice in a culturally safe and sensitive way, and witnessing the successful results with Samoan families affected by mental health problems, validate my own experiences as a counselor. Understanding the processes of the passing down of these mea-alofa is significant in determining good outcomes when working with Pasifika families.

The following case study describes how supporting a client within the mental health system was done by a counselor of the same culture. Throughout the journey with this particular client, the culturally appropriate model was carefully interwoven into the process with a solution-focused approach, so that by the end of the counseling sessions, the person was well physically, emotionally, mentally, spiritually, and socially, and was able to function as a normal person again. Furthermore, this culture-specific approach helped to identify gaps, to clarify related issues, and to address them in the client's language and protocols, enhancing and empowering her within, as she became well and independent again.

It is worth noting that this model needed to be integrated with a clinical approach, forming a holistic model for the wellbeing of the client concerned. Finally, support by family members, friends, community networks, and government agencies involved in the case, in collaboration with others, needed to be put in place to provide on-going support for the client in the future.

Pasifika people live in a communal network of relationships. Any counseling that occurs, therefore, needs to take place within the context of the family. The formation, structure, and bonding of the family are strongly knit together, in that when one member is affected, the whole family is affected. In addition, a Pasifika family consists of parents, children, grandparents, grandchildren, uncles, aunties, nephews, nieces, cousins, and so on. They share with one another their time, faith, possessions, finances, and burdens. Each member plays a vital role/responsibility in the construction and wellbeing of this family. Therefore, it is equally important for them to come together when the need arises, and also to challenge each other when appropriate. Children are expected to honor their parents, however, and young people to show respect to their elders.

The same applies to counseling: it has to address the individual in the context of the family. It is important to know the age, place, role, and responsibilities of the person involved within the family, as this information is crucial in determining how counseling can be implemented in the most effective way. Furthermore, assessing the most suitable time for other family members to join the client in family therapy depends on the progress of the counseling process. It is vital for the family members to be aware of their roles in supporting the ongoing healing and restoration of the client before counseling is completed.

Therefore, with permission given by the client, who was referred for counseling four years ago by a community agency, it is a privilege for me to share this particular counseling process as an example of a successful case. The success was due to implementing, in the client's language, the traditional gifts handed down from our ancestors, along with traditional and Christian values and beliefs, using cultural protocols in a safe environment.

Background to the Case Study

Mele was a Samoan single mother in her mid-30s, intelligent and articulate, raising her young son and living with her father and brother in the family home. She had given up work to be a full-time mother, caring for her child. She was born and raised in Samoa; therefore, she spoke very little English but was fluent in Samoan. Her husband and her mother had both passed away not long before we met, and she was still grieving these enormous losses in her life. She had particularly requested a Samoan counselor, as she had been to a pālagi counselor before and was frustrated because she felt misunderstood as she struggled with the English language. She also felt that her case was handled inappropriately according to her culture, so she requested that the agency concerned refer her to a Samoan counselor who knew her language and culture. It is important to clarify that she was referred to a pālagi counselor first because (1) there was a lack of qualified Samoan counselors, and (2) the pālagi counselor lived in her area. At the time, there seemed to be no choice but to refer her to the pālagi counselor, who had done her best to help.

The Initial Assessment

In order to establish a successful counseling relationship with Mele, I had to spend sufficient time building rapport with her—getting to know her, her situation, and her environment. This first step needed to be thorough and, while this was taking place, I had to proceed carefully, using counseling micro-skills and reflective listening with open questions, so that I could get the information I needed to assess her situation. I used a form of storytelling or narrative approach, starting with her history, which included her birthplace, family (nuclear and extended), health, education, career, and personal life. I also needed to explore her current situation, as well as her plans and goals for the future. The beginning of this process was handled delicately, according to the appropriate cultural protocols, by way of respecting her and her home. By this I mean knowing her family name and status, so that I prepared myself to address her in the proper customary way to gain her respect and openness to therapy.

Mele greeted me at the door with open arms, as if she had been expecting me for weeks. I greeted her, in return, in the proper Samoan way, using the right words and tone of voice. Likewise, I dressed appropriately, wearing the traditional clothing, as these all counted in the initial meeting. The outcome of our first meeting would surely determine the nature of the following meetings. I took off my shoes outside, while waiting for her to answer the door. When she first appeared, Mele looked tired, but offered a big smile and open arms to welcome me into her home. She immediately noticed I had slipped off my shoes and said, grinning, "It's okay; leave your shoes on." I left my shoes outside anyway, as I knew she was just being polite. She led me inside, straight to the kitchen, where the tea was already prepared on the table for us. We both sat down and briefly introduced ourselves to each other. She asked me to pray before we started counseling, which I immediately agreed to do.

The Sociability of the Samoan Self

Figiel (1996), in her exploration of Samoan identity, concluded that interpreting the Samoan self is very important in understanding how Samoan people perceive themselves: "'I' does not exist. 'Myself' does not belong to me because 'I' does not exist. 'I' is always 'we.' 'We' is part of the 'āiga, the village, the church, the youth group, the school" (p. 135). Samoan people are therefore knit together with this sense of "we" and not "I," which also creates closeness as they live and relate with one another in their location, relationship, or status in their family, village, country, and the church.

I was fully aware that it was not only Mele that I needed to consider, but also her whole family, which consisted at the time of her father, her younger brother, and her son. As I commenced counseling with her, it was therefore important to include the whole family during the process, each approached according to status, age, and gender, and with great respect. I also believed that Mele had to be present when I talked with her father and brother later on, as they were males and it would not be wise for me to address certain issues without a female present, apart from getting the whole picture by putting together all the stories. This protocol I had learned from my father as I grew up in the village.

Note that the pālagi concept of counseling is still foreign to most Pasifika people. In our cultures, conversations about one's wellbeing normally take place in the home, where the family members gather and share stories or problems, for traditionally, these are to be solved within the family. Therefore, Pasifika people do not readily attend counseling, even when referred. In addition, because we live communally, confidentiality is an unfamiliar concept. We are closely related to one another, so how and with whom information is shared is also of concern when it comes to counseling.

Building a Relationship with Mele

I knew I had to be skillful during this first meeting with Mele—the kind of questions I asked and how I asked them—so that she would be open and honest with me, and especially, trust me to keep all her personal information confidential. In addition, I had to choose my tone of voice and the words I used carefully, as there are Samoan words that convey deeper meaning, the use of which would soften her heart and make it easy for her to open up. For her to be at peace and relaxed during our sessions, I had to make sure she understood certain ethical issues and the professionalism of my work; I also needed to assure her of the boundaries and rules I would be protecting.

I asked Mele, "How are you today?" She replied, laughing, "Well, you must have heard that I am mental!" She then went on to say, '"I am *not* mental," several times, as if trying to convince me that she wasn't. I then said, "Well, I am here to be with you and listen to your story. Is that okay?" She quickly replied, "Thank you. I am ready to tell you my story because it seems no one has listened to me in the past." I asked, "What do you mean by that?" She replied, '"My father rang the hospital to come to get me because I was out of my mind, and the counselor who saw me before agreed with my father, without listening to what I was trying to tell them." I asked, "And what was that?" She stated, "I said to them that I was not mental; I was missing my husband and my mother who died not long ago." I asked her, "So are you mental?" Quickly she laughed, saying, "No, no, no, I am not mental. I just miss my husband and my mother." We ended up laughing with each other for a while, and all this was happening while we enjoyed the tea and food she prepared for us.

Food and drink are very much part of counseling in the Pasifika way. This relaxes clients, allowing them to share more openly, as did the home environment here, in contrast with the usual pālagi counseling setting, which is private, in a separate room, focusing solely on the client and being mindful to keep conversation to a one-hour maximum. In the Pasifika way, it is rude to look at the clock and to worry about finishing on the dot. The counselor needs to close the session in a respectful way, usually with prayer, and not be seen to be rushing because of time, even if a session takes more than an hour.

Before Mele continued her own story, I had to introduce *myself*, which included naming my family, village, island, school, job, and other significant parts of my personal history. This is mandatory protocol, and gave her some idea of who I was, which would help her in deciding whether to trust me and to carry on with counseling. Samoa is a small island with a population of approximately two hundred thousand people, so we all tend to know one another or have had contact with each other before coming to New Zealand. It goes without saying that if one had a good reputation in Samoa, then one is readily accepted. If not, then the counseling relationship might be hampered from the outset.

Equally important was Mele's introduction of herself, similar to mine, in order for me to make connections, which are usually already there. Sure enough: her older sister went to the same high school I attended and I remembered she was smart and had a good reputation. Mele also came from a very respectable family in Samoa. We immediately made connections and from there, things flowed smoothly, with lots of laughter and tears of joy. Toward the end of the session, as is our custom, we again prayed together.

I am asked again and again why Pasifika counseling should take place in the home. My answer is simple. In the home, I am able to assess the client and her situation in a more holistic way, using all my senses as I observe, listen, communicate, and feel how the client interacts with family members, and how she responds to interruptions, whether a phone call, a family member interfering, or people visiting the home. As I listened to Mele, I observed her physical movements and experienced the condition of her environment, her presence, and the other aspects of the whole situation. Furthermore, Samoan people would rather talk face to face, as this is showing respect for one another. Safety is important for both counselor and client, so this was also assessed as we continued to meet at home. In addition, like some other Pasifika people, Mele had no car, nor did she drive. Such complications could easily prevent a client from attending counseling when it takes place away from the home.

Mele's Story

Mele told me that her father had called the community mental health agency to come and get her, as she needed help and that she was out of her mind. I asked her why, what had she done that made her father call the agency? She answered that ever since her husband and mother had passed away, she was completely lost. Every time she looked at their photos, she cried uncontrollably, especially for her mother, who had shared everything with her; they did almost everything together. She also added that, in her grief, she sometimes locked herself in her room for days, neglecting her son. She would not talk to her family for weeks. She did not have any energy and felt listless. In addition, she would put on dresses that had belonged to her mother, trying them on in front of the mirror, then wearing them around the house. This behavior went on for weeks, causing great concern to her father and brother. Both felt she was mental and needed medication.

The medical professionals came to her home. When she tried to explain what had happened, they did not take time to listen. They had already heard a story from her father, and assumed there must be no other story. She needed help and it was time to go to the hospital. Other people also needed help, so they needed her to cooperate with them. All this was done in a hurry and before she knew it, she was in an isolation unit, where she strongly felt she did not belong.

I questioned her about the counselors that she had seen previously, and their kind of support at the time. She responded that they had agreed with her father that she needed help from medical professionals, and that it was a good idea for her to get help from a mental health institution. She disagreed; she felt she was not being heard or understood. According to her, all she needed was someone that listened and acknowledged her, and would support her through the grieving process. In addition, she needed time to grieve in her own way, without being ridiculed by her family. I felt the urgency of listening to her well; acknowledging and understanding her story was vital. My process with her took some weeks, and sessions were sometimes as long as three hours.

I had met her just after she came home from the isolation unit. There, she had been forced to take medication and, because she refused, was tied to the bed and injected. During her time in the hospital, she tried to point out to the staff that she was not mental, but no one acknowledged her. Her experience in the hospital was like a nightmare that wouldn't end. She was outspoken, including using strong language, which worked against her, as the medical professionals deemed her a nuisance. She believed that she was misdiagnosed and the treatment given her was unnecessary and harmful. She seemed to get worse on the medication; the side effects included sleepiness, lack of energy, anger, and loss of a sense of reality.

As I listened to her story, several thoughts came to me. (1) Had she been misdiagnosed? (2) Many of her symptoms were typical of loss and grief. (3) She needed a culturally appropriate counselor with knowledge of language, protocols, culture, values, and her belief system, and even gender matching, for safety purposes. Over six sessions, trust was gradually built in our relationship, and I shared with her my own thoughts and feelings, acknowledging her and her story, looking for a strategy to help her, focusing on a solution for her healing emotionally, psychologically, mentally, physically, and spiritually, and finding a way forward.

The Middle Phase of Our Counseling Process

The counseling was undertaken in the Samoan language, in which Mele was fluent. This allowed us to use words with deeper and richer meanings than we would have been able to do in English. She felt safe to tell me, woman to woman, how our work together was empowering her to share her feelings regarding her family and her situation, her experience and learning from the whole incident, and her ability to cope in the midst of all that happened to her. The more she shared, the better she felt. It was like emptying herself of all the frustrations held within, gaining back her strength and power.

Her values and beliefs were somewhat challenged, for though she respected her father and other authorities, she also felt misunderstood and mistreated by all of them. She held onto her great faith in God, and in fact, her faith was strengthened. One of the tools she used at the time was prayer, sometimes with deep groaning, as the pain was too much to bear; at other times, she prayed out loud, sharing her anger with God. God seemed to be her only hope; no one else believed in her. She shared that when she prayed in the hospital, she became less agitated. She could then concentrate on getting well, with the clear intention of getting out of the hospital. She was released when she stopped arguing with the medical staff and began cooperating with them.

One of the areas we needed to explore was the structure and dynamics of her family. As an adult, and more so as a single parent raising her young son, she felt that her father treated her like a little girl. She felt no power of her own, being expected to listen to and obey her father, as this was part of her culture, especially since the family home belonged to him. She could find no private space to grieve the loss of her husband and her mother. Instead, she was expected to be strong and to attend to the daily needs of the family. Also, with the loss of her mother, she seemed expected to replace her, taking up the role and responsibilities of caring for the family. Furthermore, she was lost without her husband, who had supported her and her son financially, without having been given time to grieve for him. She was trying to cope with her own pain at the same time as meeting the expectations of her family. Her world had been turned upside-down and she had no control of circumstances around her. Yet she still believed that had she felt heard, acknowledged, and understood, with culturally appropriate support in place to give her insight into her strange new world, she would have been able to cope.

Mele felt the burden of caring for the men in her family: her father, younger brother, and son. She had wanted to move to her own place with her son, but because of her father's expectation that she would take care of him, such a move seemed impossible. However, she had to make a decision, and finally decided to stay home to care for the family. This was when everything started to fall apart and she had no idea what would happen. It was a long and painful process while trying to cope with daily duties at home. She was naïve, believing she could cope easily and move forward. Little did she understand that the loss of both her husband and mother had left such a huge gap in her life and there was a need to grieve her losses intentionally and well.

This is, it seems to me, an example of a clash of cultural perspectives regarding a client's diagnosis. Because the family had not known how to help her, out of frustration and concern they reported her to mental health professionals as a family member who was out of her mind. According to these professionals, she had a medical problem: bipolar disorder. Yet, according to Mele, it was just a matter of her being given space to grieve two huge losses in her life and being supported through the grieving process. She was crying out to be heard, understood, and supported appropriately in her time of need.

The Last Phase of Our Counseling Process

Toward the end of my six sessions with Mele, in her presence I spent time with her father and brother to hear their stories. This was a long and emotional session, and it was quite obvious that they, too, were hurting because of the loss of the mother and the husband. They felt helpless themselves, and according to the father, he had not meant to hurt Mele by calling the hospital for help. He felt guilty about his part in what had happened to her. Both men, in turn, shared their pain and explained how they had tried to cope with it. Their doing so was of great significance within this family, as Pacific Island men do not usually express their feelings overtly. This opened up communication between them at heart level. For the first time they were able to express their sincere apologies to Mele, asking her forgiveness for what they had done. In response, she also broke down and cried tears of release and relief, experiencing for the first time their understanding and acceptance of her, both regarding past wounds and the current pain she had been experiencing. Their hearts were now connected.

This process of healing and reconciliation between herself and her closest family members was a crucial part of the client's journey to wellness. It also benefited her son; he became happier and more settled, and he was able to focus again on his school work and his own interests, and get on with his own life.

As the counseling process progressed, changes were evident in the way Mele was coping in daily life, resuming the activities she had managed before. She would make sure her son attended school, making his lunches, being home when she was needed, and being fully present for him. She was able once again to take care of him and take care of herself in practical ways.

Postscript

Beyond the formal counseling process, ongoing support was vital for Mele as she undertook a computer training course. Her father had told me she was smart, and though there were many times she doubted her capacity to cope, Mele persevered and graduated, with strong encouragement from me through telephone contact as well as in person. Together we celebrated her success. Mele then found the courage to apply for a job, for which she had to attend an interview in another city. She secured a regional position as an advocate for Pasifika mental health.

As I walked alongside Mele throughout her journey, I knew that ongoing support was necessary, beyond the initial six sessions. My role with her changed over time, but underlying our work together was the constancy of my commitment to her, an ongoing faithfulness that reflected my belief in her capacity to change and grow.

For Mele, a Pasifika woman who had been diagnosed with a mental illness, relief and restoration to wholeness became a reality when she was able to engage in a counseling relationship with another woman of the same culture, who spoke the same language and used the same cultural protocols. These reflected the mea-alofa, the traditional cultural and spiritual values and beliefs, integrated effectively within a holistic model of practice. At all times I attempted to be fully present for her. The complete acceptance the client experienced through this quality of relationship enabled her to build trust in me as her counselor, and therefore to relax and express her thoughts and feelings more freely than she had ever done before. Meeting with Mele in her own home, an environment where she felt free to be herself, as well as eating, drinking, and sharing prayer together, contributed significantly to the safety she experienced in our therapeutic relationship and thereby to her healing process. Our prayer together in every session was also a source of spiritual strength for Mele.

The involvement of the immediate members of Mele's family was a further powerful element in the therapeutic process that was consistent with the holistic nature of this mea-alofa-based approach. Even though she would need support in the future as she faced further challenges, the rebuilding of the heart connection between Mele and the other important people in her life enabled her to move forward in her journey to wholeness with renewed strength and assurance. And together, we celebrated her success every step of the way.

References

Anae, M. (1999). *Born in New Zealand*. Paper presented at the Pacific Vision International Conference, Auckland, New Zealand.

Figiel, S. (1996). *Where we once belonged*. Auckland: Pasifika Press.

Seiuli, B. (2004). *Mea'alofa, a gift handed over: Making accessible and visible Samoan counselling in New Zealand*. Unpublished manuscript, University of Waikato, Hamilton, New Zealand.

Webber-Dreadon, E. (1999). He taonga mo o matou tipuna (A gift handed down by our ancestors): An indigenous approach to supervision. *Te Komako: Social Work Review, 11*, 7–11.

14

"Keep Your Doughnuts to Yourself"
Using Poetry in Pasifika Professional Practice

PETA PILA PALALAGI

My name is Peta Palalagi. I am a New Zealand–born Niuean/Māori/pālagi ethnic fruit salad! I was born in Auckland and raised by a Niuean couple, Henry and Favavau Pila. I was attracted to the helping professions in 1996 after my marriage ended. I then began my counseling training as a single parent in my 40s, seeking a new direction. My children were preschoolers, yet my work ethic instilled in me from my father caused me to gain a counseling qualification for the future.

Training as a counselor has made me reflect deeply on what I hold onto as a Pacific Island woman and what I wish to let go of. What part of pālagi culture nourishes or harms me? What part of being Māori do I wish to keep? All is yet to be discovered! As I was raised strictly with Niuean customs and protocols, that exploration is still in process.

I have worked in South Auckland for four years, running groups for Pacific Island parenting, women's anger, and co-gender stopping violence. My own background with family violence has led me into this work. I am committed to no longer being victimized or oppressed. My desire is to assist Pacific Island men and women who are violent to find nonviolent ways of coping with anger. The work is demanding, challenging, and fulfilling. What undergirds me is a strong faith in God and writing poetry.

In my training as a counselor, and now in my work as a counselor and group facilitator, I have repeatedly encountered clients in a great deal of emotional, personal, and relational pain. Being so constantly exposed to others' pain inevitably resurrects the ancient hurt that any counselor carries around, left over from old wounds. In the pālagi world, this is sometimes called identification; at other times it is called the counselor's transference, and it is seen as contributing to parallel process. Poetry helps me process my pain by making meaning of it through writing.

I began writing poetry in 1996, while I was in a training program at Manukau Institute of Technology. As I was being stretched and turned upside-down and inside-out by my studies, a friend said to me, "You're learning so many things. Why don't you write about them in poetry?" I was sure I couldn't, and certainly, no one had ever suggested to me that I could write. Those first tentative steps toward writing poetry assisted me in my journey to self-awareness. I saw my own beauty, and the beauty around me, in a way that I hadn't seen before, in part because I was so consumed with the pain and hurt in my own life.

More than three hundred poems later, I have found my voice. My poems are a summary of my observations about my clients' journeys—individually, in couples, or in a group process. Other poems are about what I'm learning about myself and others, in various ongoing pālagi training sessions. These poems capture special moments, helping me make sense of what I'm going through at the time, either inside myself, or in response to my clients. These are the ways I make meaning in my life and the lives of others. Poetry forms the narrative of my journey.

These poems are like my own children. They are birthed inside of me, awakening and deepening my consciousness, and making me more aware of myself—both who I was then and who I am now. Poetry flows from all my life experience—inside myself, outside, and all around me. In my work, poetry is my way of honoring and capturing the therapeutic relationship, a way of making meaning of experiences, and always there to access. It never leaves me. Poetry unlocks parts of myself that I never knew before. It asks questions that in the past I didn't have enough nerve to ask myself. In the past it was unsafe for me to speak. All I knew how to do was to yell and scream, in order to survive. The voice in and of my poetry can now ask questions of life and have no fear. Poetry restores my ego strength and enlivens my soul.

Writing is still difficult. Sometimes it hurts me. I write in the vernacular because that is how I express my passionate Pacific nature!

Editors' Note: Because Ms. Palalagi's poetry is undated, the editors have chosen to arrange the poems so that they make their own story, a fictional parallel with what might be happening with a female Pasifika client as she recovers from an abusive past. This arrangement has been approved by Ms. Palalagi.

You Hit

My father hit my mother:
My mother hit me.
I learned hitting, not talking,
sorted out conflicts between
others and me.
My father hit my mother:
My mother hit me.

I learned being strong, not
weak, and saving face is what
I learned from watching my family.
My father hit my mother:
My mother hit me.
I went to school and
hit other children,
then no one wanted to play
with me.
My father hit my mother:
My mother hit me.
When I was little I wanted
to run away because they
scared the shit out of me.
My father hit my mother:
My mother hit me.
Now I hit my children,
and the cycle is being
repeated through me.
My father hit my mother:
My mother hit me.
I had to have power over others
to hide the fear and powerlessness
in me.
It's not easy, this process of
choice and change.
Yet I have to ask myself the
Question: What will I hand on
to the next generation?
Do I choose to hit?
Or do I choose to quit?
It's time to take a long hard look
at how I behave and what I believe,
For I now know I am responsible,
I am responsible for me.

Black Room

I'm sent there when I'm naughty.
I'm not allowed out to play.
I feel mean and nasty
stuck in the black room all day!
I feel cut off, neglected,

I feel put away.
When I'm allowed out I
scare everyone to death.
Would you expect anything less
of a willful child that is me?
Black room has no light;
Black room breeds contempt!
Black room of seething emotions:
'Out of sight . . . out of mind!'
How come adults always send
you there? When the black in
you comes alive?
They duck and run for cover
when they see the willful child
on the rampage!
I want to learn not to
resist the black pearls of existence
in the black room of my life.
Black room . . . don't say Why
bother and pass me by!
Come and get to know me;
You could be surprised!

Someone

Someone else's thinking
shaped what I believe
about me.
Someone else's bidding
I followed and never
questioned whether it
was right for me.
Someone else's culture
influenced
who I would be.
Someone called mother
and father made me
feel like meat in a sandwich,
ready to meet their need.
Someone comes across my path
who appears different
can seem pretty
threatening to me,

for they mirror what I
haven't got, and lack wears
the face of fear.
Someone comes and
someone goes, in and
out of my life today.
Somehow I'm learning how
to live my life as
someone who now knows
how to listen to my own
inner knowing and become
someone who is unafraid to
grow.

P. I. Boy

I tell you my story,
haltingly, what
I haven't said.
Suicide and murder come rolling off my lips.
Just like a stick of liquorice out comes what is twisted in me.
I tell you my story in little and
big bits;
I tell you stuff
I've stuffed away.
I feel safe and warm inside
when I talk to you, all
I wish I could
take you all, home,
where I am a misfit.
I tell you my story,
you tell me yours,
and together we will
learn . . . to listen . . . and begin to hear . . .
everything inside ourselves
that has been unclear.

You and I

You and I are different,
yet you and I are the same.
You and I are poles apart

in thoughts, feelings, and ideas.
Is it any wonder I struggle with
getting closer to you?
You and I are meandering on
a path that has so many unknowns
it kind of frightens me where it is
all going to go.
You and I fight
and react at things that happen
like it is a fact.
You and I have barriers that we
have built to keep each other safe.
It's difficult dismantling those barriers
in between you and me.
You and I need time to consider
how we are going to get from
A to B.

Hammer, Hammer, Hammer

Hammer, hammer, hammer:
Your words would flow
like a nail into me,
blow by blow.
Hammer, hammer, hammer:
on and on you would go.
How it hurt and caused a pain in me to grow.
Hammer, hammer, hammer:
It feels like death.
You were merciless in your action;
you showed no regret.
Hammer, hammer, hammer:
From long ago.
You appear to me in authority at times
with a striking blow.
Hammer, hammer, hammer:
I feel like a child with you.
Hammer, be gentle:
Hammer, go slow:
Hammer, harmless,
no longer frightened by
what the future bestows.

Warriors of Flesh

We fight each other
till there is no breath.
We fuck each other
Like warriors of war,
the past in the background to reminisce
how we nearly clubbed each other
to death.
We are strangers, yet familiar;
We touch each other's skin,
starved remembrance as our bodies connect.
We torment each one's will, battle
together as our emotions plumb
the hidden depths.
We pour into each the unexplained:
Hurt, anger, rage, passion, longing,
Loving?
We come together the best we can;
the old and new merge, together,
mysterious . . . no understanding,
yet with no regret.
The old me is gone forever;
I hold on no longer to any
past in me.
I feel peace; a tentative hope
is being born in me.
I'm not afraid anymore;
I feel my connection with me
in a deep place of abiding
where I am not hiding me,
and I know only God will make clear
what the meaning of this is for me!

A Man's Pain

A man's pain
a woman carries
until she feels it
is her own.
A man's pain
is not static;
it touches every

surface of a woman's life.
A man's pain
is never hidden
to the wife by
his side.
A man's pain
runs into her
life heart like a
gushing blood stain.
A man's pain can drive a
woman insane
if left unchecked.
A man's pain
I now relinquish
so all that remains is my
growing sense of
relief.

Joey

Joey was my husband, Joey was my sex.
Joey was my addiction that left me dependant
and hooked so I wouldn't get to know me.
Joey and I have children,
two of the best.
Joey wants to come back to me.
I'm not sure.
He fucked too many sluts which
killed my love and respect.
Joey, I want friendship, not sex
with you! Passion only leaves
me ending up screwed!
Joey, you are a good man;
Joey, you are kind;
Joey you are gentle; it is
still in you.
Why do you act like Mr. Macho?
You cover so much
of you? You want to get in my
knickers; you think
that will fix it for us.
Trouble is, I've changed and
sex is not enough!

I want a man who listens
and respects my NO!
If he won't listen he can
go to hell and leave me alone!
Joey, I will take a step
to you. It is the step of
friendship, not sex, I can give to you!

You Gave Me

You gave me flowers that definitely weren't
from Foodtown and had a wonderful style.
You gave me perfume that was expensive and rare.
You gave me a window into a man's soul,
shared so deeply that I could receive untold
treasures that made me whole.
There will be a cadence as I walk to my
future, more assured.
We sharpened each other for the journey
that now draws us apart,
secure in the knowledge that we are all that
there was; nothing wasted in the time we had.
We spurred each other on to realize our potential.
We gave each other space to stretch and grow.
We matched each other's pace with thought,
provoking ideas.
Dark places we had journeyed, where there was
brokenness and fear,
we overcame by believing in ourselves;
in each other's company letting go of our fears.
It's hard to give up something that felt so good.
We've both taken a different direction, stepping
out into other roads.
What we learned together has prepared us for
the change.

Goodbye

It doesn't matter anymore
if you contact me or not.
I waited and wondered, was
vulnerable
along the way.

I believe I'm getting closer
to letting go of you a little more.
I feel peaceful and am mending
the what-could-have-been in me.
Goodbye to a time that
was scented with heaven's sweetness.
Goodbye: the past lingers with no regret,
just a treasure trove of memories
which have not all been spent.
Goodbye: there have been so many in my life,
yet even though letting go of the old opens
up the abattoir of goodbye again,
cruel as it may be!
I don't feel passive or indolent.
Goodbye: I am just now ready
to accept it in me.

I Wanted You

I wanted you to love me unconditionally;
I now know you don't even know what it means.
I wanted you to talk and hold me in your
tender embrace;
I now know you have no idea.
I wanted you to soothe every hurt and take away
my pain. I now know
I wanted you to be superman,
always at my beck and call.
I wanted you to love the unlovable me;
I now know you have to want to see to believe.
I wanted and expected so much
of what you could never be.
I now know I have to take responsibility
for my own unmet needs.
I still don't know what that means:
wanting you to fulfill in me what
I need to do myself.

May I

May I be like fallow
ground
as the wind of your

Spirit runs through me,
like a plough.
As you toss and turn me,
I'm reminded,
God, you are tilling me
so I can become
holy ground.
May your Spirit help me not to
wallow in mistrust, unforgiveness,
and fear.
For the path of the righteous
follow Jesus who is ever near.
May I be mellow as you
deal with me.
May I not run away.

To Journey

What can I say about the gift of your friendship?
However it's to be I count myself as richer for
the privilege of journeying with you.
I feel safe, supported, accepted—just a few
pearls I've received along the way.
Out of the broken places we have journeyed,
there is a place of beginning again.
The acceptance of the old and celebration
of the new.
Thank you for reflecting to me that I am okay.
I know as a friend I want to do the same for you.
So wherever you may journey in the days to come,
pākehā man with a māori heart!
always let your aroha, mana and integrity surround
you like a cloak.
Dare to rise up and seize the shadow and
light part of your being.
Believe in your potential and be true to yourself.
I wish you well as you journey.

My Son and Daughter

I watched today
as Nana squirted your
brown pint-sized bodies with the hose.

Your gleeful laughter filled the air
and mischief danced on your
faces.
Little feet running to and fro,
bodies racing,
hearts pumping,
feet jumping,
rushing round and round
the clothesline you go.
Prickles under feet—
Ouch!
Laughter and fun is
hard to pass up.
How much joy
it is to play.
If any two can play
with enthusiasm and joy,
it's my son and daughter.

Silence

Silence: you scare me.
Silence: you are too loud.
I want to escape your presence.
I feel swallowed up.
Silence: you are too much for me.
Maybe I'll evaporate into nothing—
boring, boring, uncomfortable unease.
Silence: you lengthen
something short in me.
Silence: you are unnerving
something inside that doesn't
feel deserving.
Silence: I reserve the right
to preserve my thought and
my feelings in a way
that works for me.
Silence, selective, silence, selective.
Silence: in me.
Silence: I sure never expected
you to sound like a
megaphone in me!

Tangata Pasifika

Tāngata pasifika, who are you?
Tāngata pasifika: is your anger
hidden or does it come out unbidden?
Tāngata pasifika: your strength
is your culture, your people your way.
Tāngata pasifika: has it ever occurred to you?
As a pacific people we are good at 'We',
yet we know not 'I'.
Maybe its time to
learn the pālagi's way before
'I' can take care of 'We'.
'I' need to take care of me.
Tāngata pasifika: violence kiss the
floor argument finished. Yet hurt, misunderstanding
and conflict still remain, for a knock-out never
changes anything.
Tāngata pasifika: won't you reconsider your
position? Take time out for you . . . so you
can think about what the next step will be.
Tāngata pasifika: pride of the pacific
Is now not the time to ride out the old
and ride into the new?
For your women, sons and daughters are
influenced by all you do!
Tāngata pasifika: take your
anger and choose not to allow it
to hurt others.
Is it not time for a change?
Tāngata pasifika:
Take pride in you.

Black Beauty

I'm black and sassy
with a spirit unbridled from
the dark side of me!
Black Beauty bursting pulsating
with passionate playful energy.
I need lots of space to run about,
explore all around me!
Black Beauty, straining at the bit!

When expectations of other people
hold me back from me!
I kick, I fight, I trample to protect
the real me!
Black Beauty who is wild and racy,
dancing, prancing, running free,
threatened, frightened
doesn't stop me.
Canter, gallop, lightening pace takes me
to any place I want to be!
Black Beauty with a feisty stallion
spirit, captivating, charismatic,
gentle . . . yet so in tune with me!
Black Beauty, you beauty of
royal pedigree,
you are a new breed born to shine.
The trail you blaze is a freedom
journey for a stallion
of symmetry.

Pararaha River Adventure

Down the river I sauntered through
greeny bush,
across slippery watery rocks,
up cliff faces through the bush track.
Some parts are tough,
swampy smelly mud underfoot,
Yucky . . . mucky . . . made me
stinky, that's for sure.
I think I'd rather hurry through this bit.
Tramping along I canoe to a clearing.
My eyes feast on black sand and
grey sea beckoning me to
come and see
Pararaha River adventure,
like my life, full of the unexpected.
Sometimes little surprises along
the way keep me guessing
and entertained.
A day in the bush
has stirred in me
a spirit of adventure,

exploration, fun and play,
appealing to the natural
child in me!

Xena Warrior Princess

You are a woman with beauty and wit.
You break the balls of men who are condescending.
I like the way you stand ready to do battle!
Agile . . . alert!
You are intelligent and shrewd;
you handle every situation with tactical cunning.
You are a warrior princess,
a subtle blend of passion and gentleness
woven into the core of your being,
velvet over steel.
You embody all the qualities
of a strong
woman that is positive to me.
You call to my Warrior Princess to rise
up and never give my power away!
You capture my imagination
to be Bold! And to be Strong!
The legacy of Xena Warrior Princess is . . .
Dare to be different!
Dare not to conform!
Challenge false assumptions!
Don't be afraid anymore!

I Love You

I love you, Peta!
I surely do.
I love you simply
because you are you.
I love the way you
laugh out loud
and hold the hand
of those who cry.
I love the warmth
that flows through you,
touching lives with your
vibrant smile.

I love your girlish playfulness
that's so alluringly feminine.
I love the pensive expression
on your face and how you question
almost everything.
I love the Warrior Spirit
in you which forges a way
that works for you.
I love you simply because
You are you.

Rosie, Rosie

Rosie, Rosie,
keep your doughnuts to yourself.
It is a time to dine in
and be mended,
not give away your wealth.
Rosie, Rosie,
be gentle with yourself!
Especially when you are
dismantling old patterns
and bringing in the new.
Rosie, Rosie,
you came home to be
revitalized and renewed.
God is trying to do a
makeover when it comes
to you!
Rosie, Rosie,
you are confident in God.
Now comes the tough bit,
to be confident in you!
Rosie, Rosie,
there are challenges ahead.
Don't look to the old ways
to sort it out for you!
Rosie, Rosie,
when the path ahead is
blocked with old baggage
which spoils the view,
remember it's important
to believe in you!

It's a very special season;
there is so much to do!!
You really must be gentle with you.
Rosie, Rosie,
keep your doughnuts
To yourself.
In time you will understand;
then, when you are ready,
you can give away your wealth!

To Know

The year has nearly ended:
A few more hours to go.
I am reflecting on how
I've grown and it feels
good.
To know I have lived
my life open to experience
the new.
To know I am choosing
friendships that are healthy
and safe.
To know I can express my
opinion with thoughtfulness
and care.
To know I can do hard
things well brings a smile
to my lips.
To know I give and can
say no without feeling bad.
To know whatever happens
in my life, I feel assurance
of soul that God is designing and
rearranging parts of me;
and the future can only
be brighter as I am
sensitive to the Spirit's
guidance in me.

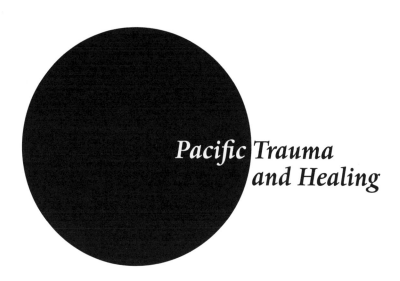

Pacific Trauma and Healing

Editors' Introduction

Each of the contributions in this section of the book addresses a specific mental health issue within the South Pacific context, including depression, abuse within families, substance abuse, fetal alcohol syndrome, and gambling. Keawe Kaholokula highlights the significance of historical trauma and contextual influences on mental health in his examination of the relationship between colonialism, acculturation, and depression among the *Kānaka Maoli* of Hawai'i. This brings into sharp relief the painful contrast between two, coexisting worlds: in the words of Paul Theroux, "not all is rosy in the happy isles of Oceania."

Themes of traditional values, transition, and conflicting agendas are also evident in Karanina Siaosi Sumeo's discussion of the abuse of children and of domestic violence within family and village structures in Samoa. Her voice echoes those of authors in earlier sections of the book in raising questions of accountability and challenging both Pasifika and the mental health communities.

In addressing alcohol abuse, Aukahi Austin examines further the consequences of colonization in the Pacific. Alcohol abuse in this context can be seen as a way of coping when indigenous people leave their native culture or have it taken away from them by the overwhelming power of colonialism. When imposed or consequential disruption to natural support systems occurs, ways of coping may be adopted that are self-destructive or damaging to individuals and communities.

The consequences of such abuse, in the form of alcohol use during pregnancy, then become the focus of the following essay. In a passionate voice, Suia Simi calls for the Pasifika community to address this issue and prevent the devastation caused by fetal alcohol syndrome.

Finally, Yvette Guttenbeil-Po'uhila and Sione Tu'itahi echo themes of earlier contributors to this section in discussing contextual factors influencing problem gambling within the Tongan community in Auckland. Immigration, social change, and the collapse of the *kāinga* system, as well as traditional beliefs and values associated with perseverance, good fortune, and appropriate conduct, contribute to exacerbating this growing and destructive problem within the community. As researchers investigating the influences that seemed to be supporting Tongan gambling, the authors employed a methodology based on Tongan cultural values. The results of this study provide valuable understandings and indicators of ways forward for mental health professionals working with Pasifika clients for whom gambling has become a problem.

15

Colonialism, Acculturation, and Depression among *Kānaka Maoli* of Hawai'i

JOSEPH KEAWE'AIMOKU KAHOLOKULA

My father, Lawrence Pauahi Kaholokula, Sr., was born in Pā'ia, Maui, and was raised in the area of Pu'uhale, Kalihi, on O'ahu. My mother, Beverly Leilani Lyons Kaholokula, was born in Honolulu, O'ahu, and was raised in Hilo, Hawai'i, and Honolulu. I am their second child of three and their eldest son, Joseph Keawe'aimoku Kaholokula. We are descendants of the Pahukoa and Kaloi ancestral lineage—the union of two moku *(islands), Maui and Hawai'i, respectively. I was born, raised, and live in Honolulu, O'ahu. I am of Hawaiian, Chinese, and Caucasian ethnic ancestries. I am the first in my immediate family to earn a college degree and, more so, a doctoral degree (PhD in psychology). I am a member of the Halemua o Mauiloa and Halemua o Kūali'i. I am a Kānaka Maoli (Hawaiian) —this is my* mana.

Through my personal and clinical experiences I have come to learn that the return to traditional Hawaiian values, beliefs, and practices is vital in repairing the damage that American colonialism and exploitation have done to our 'āina *(land) and our* Lāhui *(the Hawaiian race). Once an industrious and healthy people, we contemporary Hawaiians have the poorest health and social status when compared to our* kūpuna *(ancestors) and the other ethnic groups that reside in our ancestral homeland of Hawai'i.*

This essay is simply a reflection of my personal and professional experiences guided by a common ancestral knowledge inherited by all Hawaiians. However, any hewa *(mistakes or transgressions) in this essay are mine alone.*

Who Are Kānaka Maoli?

Ke ēwe hānau o ka 'āina
The lineage born of the land
(Pukui, 1983, p. 1691)

Geologists tell us that the Hawaiian archipelago was created by volcanic activity and natural erosion over the millennia. Anthropologists tell us that the Kānaka Maoli[1] (meaning true or real humans and used to refer to all Hawaiians today) are descendants of early Polynesians who migrated out of Southeast Asia and Malaysia and who eventually settled in Hawai'i about two thousand years ago. However, our *kūpuna* (ancestors) have a different account of our existence. They tell us that the islands of Hawai'i-nui-ākea (the great and vast Hawai'i) were born of the gods—Papa-hānau-moku (mother earth) and Wākea (sky father)[2]—and that all Kānaka Maoli share a common genealogical lineage to Hāloa—the first human. And because of this, our kūpuna were part and parcel of the 'āina (land) that nurtured them, of the *kai moana* (ocean) that surrounded them, and of the *lewa* (space) that embraced them.

We contemporary Kānaka Maoli are direct descendants of ancient Kānaka Maoli who inhabited the islands of Hawai'i for nearly two thousand years. Although we are no longer biologically and socioculturally[3] homogeneous as were our kūpuna, we still maintain the traditional values and beliefs that connect us to our 'āina and our *mo'okū'auhau* (ancestral lineage). We continue to hold fast to our unique identity and way of life as a distinct ethnocultural group amid a multiethnic society that now comprises Hawai'i. And like our kūpuna, we continue to believe that our physical, emotional, and spiritual wellbeing are directly tied to our 'āina, kai moana, and lewa. As were our kūpuna, we are the younger siblings of Hawai'i. We are Kānaka Maoli.

Huli Aku, Huli Mai: *Change Was Not for the Better*

Lawe li'ili'i ka make a ka Hawai'i, lawe nui ka make a ka haole
Death by Hawaiians takes a few at a time;
death by foreigners takes many.
(Pukui, 1983, p. 211)

The Kānaka Maoli world, as our kūpuna understood it to be, was forever altered in the year 1778—the year Kānaka Maoli were fortuitously introduced to the Western world. This was the year Captain James Cook haphazardly came across the Hawaiian archipelago. The writings of Cook and his crew shed some light on the health[4] and social status of our kūpuna at the beginning of contact between these two worlds. They observed that the inhabitants of the islands of Hawai'i were "above middle size, strong, well made and of a dark copper colour, and . . . a fine handsome set of people" (Beaglehole, 1967, p. 1178). On a socio-psychological note, these fair-skinned strangers also observed that Kānaka Maoli were "truly good natured, social, friendly, and humane, possessing much liveliness and . . . good humour" (Beaglehole, 1967, p. 1181). By these firsthand accounts, it is clear that our kūpuna at the dawn of Western contact were physically and emotionally healthy. By healthy, I mean the absence or very low prevalence of chronic medical (e.g., obesity and diabetes), psychological (e.g., depression), and social (e.g., poverty and marginalization) diseases. (For a review of the pre-Western contact health status of Kānaka Maoli, see Blaisdell, 1993.) This is in sharp contrast to the poor health status of contemporary Kānaka Maoli.

Current U.S. and state of Hawai'i health data indicate that we Kānaka Maoli, as an ethnic group, have the worst health and social status compared to all other ethnic groups in Hawai'i and most other ethnic groups in the United States. (For a review of the health status of contemporary Kānaka Maoli, see Johnson, Oyama, LeMarchand, & Wilkens, 2004.) We are among the most impoverished, undereducated, and socially disadvantaged people in our own homeland (Marsella, Oliveira, Plummer, & Crabbe, 1995). We have the highest rates of chronic medical diseases such as diabetes, heart disease, and certain types of cancers of most ethnic groups in the continental United States and Hawai'i. We have the poorest health behaviors, as reflected in the high prevalence of cigarette smoking, drug and alcohol use, and obesity (State of Hawai'i Behavioral Risk Factor Surveillance System [BRFSS], 2003). It is suspected that we Kānaka Maoli also suffer from high rates of emotional distress (Crabbe, 1999; Marsella et al., 1995). Consequently, our overall mortality and morbidity rates far exceed those of most other U.S. ethnic groups. Indeed, the poor health condition of contemporary Kānaka Maoli is a far cry from the excellent health condition our kūpuna enjoyed before the arrival of foreigners to Hawai'i. What happened to us Kānaka Maoli to create such an ominous circumstances?

Effects of U.S. Colonialism and Acculturation on Kānaka Maoli

'Ai nō ke kōlea a momona ho'i i Kahiki
The plover eats until fat, then returns to the land from which it came.
(Pukui, 1983, p. 12)

Aside from the infectious diseases that decimated our kūpuna,[5] we Kānaka Maoli have been subjected to over 180 years of U.S. occupation and exploitation of our islands (Trask, 1999). We have undergone, and continue to undergo, insidious assimilation into the U.S. Euro-American dominant culture via the process of acculturation. At the same time, we are also undergoing acculturation with other ethnic groups (e.g., Filipinos and Vietnamese) in Hawai'i. The Social Science Research Council (1954) in the United States described acculturation as follows:

> Culture change that is initiated by the conjunction of two or more autonomous cultural systems. Acculturative change may be the consequence of direct cultural transmission; it may be derived from non-cultural causes, such as ecological or demographic modification induced by impinging culture; it

may be delayed, as with internal adjustments following upon the acceptance of alien traits or patterns; or it may be reactive adaptation of traditional modes of life. (p. 974)

Certainly, we Kānaka Maoli have experienced, and continue to experience, "culture change" due to the "direct cultural transmission" of U.S. Euro-American values, beliefs, and practices, the "demographic modifications" (e.g., influx of foreigners and urban development) to our ʻāina, and the "reactive adaptation of traditional modes of life." As a result, many Kānaka Maoli in the beginning of U.S. colonialism were forced to abandon their native language, religious and spiritual beliefs, and other cultural practices (e.g., traditional healing) that were deemed not marketable for tourism or not consistent with the American way of life (Trask, 1999).

The process of U.S. acculturation for Kānaka Maoli formally began with the arrival of the Calvinist missionaries from New England in Hawaiʻi in 1820. They converted the *aliʻi* (chiefs) and, thereby, most Kānaka Maoli, to Christianity, which altered our traditional religious and spiritual beliefs and our unique genealogical connection to the world around us.[6] It must have been emotionally devastating to our kūpuna, who were made to believe that the gods they had worshipped for generations did not exist and that the infectious diseases that plagued them were the wrath of this new God. While the Calvinist missionaries were introducing the dogmas of Christianity, they were also introducing Euro-American values, beliefs, and ideologies to Kānaka Maoli. This began a series of detrimental events that led to the alienation of Kānaka Maoli from their beliefs, customs, and sovereignty, which has had significant physical, psychological, and social ramifications for many Kānaka Maoli to this day. In regards to the psychological ramifications, Bushnell (1993) writes the following:

> Beyond all doubt, psychological traumata of almost intolerable intensity and variety afflicted most Hawaiians after foreigners with their strange artifacts and alien values disrupted the indigenous society. Those new psychological stresses, as well as the new kinds of microbes [diseases], most certainly played important parts in the long dying of the Hawaiian race. (pp. 55–56)

Other significant events in Hawaiʻi that are believed to have had detrimental effects on the physical, psychological, and social wellbeing of Kānaka Maoli are also worth noting here. In 1848, Kauikeaouli, also known as Kamehameha III, signed into effect the Great Māhele, which abolished traditional communal land use for the Western notion of land privatization (Kameʻeleihiwa, 1992). This ultimately led to many Kānaka Maoli being landless and impoverished, which remains a problem for Kānaka Maoli to this day. The Western concept of land ownership was an alien concept to our kūpuna, who believed that the ʻāina was an elder sibling and, therefore, could not be owned or sold. In 1893, Queen Liliʻuokalani, the sovereign ruler of Hawaiʻi, was illegally overthrown by white businessmen, some of whom were descendants of the Calvinist missionaries, with support from representatives of the United States (Osorio, 2002). Despite strong protest by Kānaka Maoli against the overthrow, Hawaiʻi was annexed to the United States in 1898 (Silva, 2004). About this time, Kānaka Maoli were forced to abandon their native language for the English language exclusively through legislative acts (e.g., Act 57; see Kahumoku, 2003) under the provisional government following the overthrow. As a result, Kānaka Maoli were effectively precluded from learning and using their native language in the public education system, which led to the near-extinction of the Hawaiian language. Despite continued attempts by Kānaka Maoli to regain their sovereignty, Hawaiʻi was proclaimed the fiftieth state of the United States in 1959. Many of us contemporary Kānaka Maoli actively continue to seek the return of our nation, language, and traditional beliefs and practices (Osorio, 2002).

Because of the destruction of our native identity, our way of life, and our nation, some people believe that many contemporary Kānaka Maoli suffer from feelings of demoralization, alienation, and marginalization (Marsella et al., 1995). In a reactive adaptation to the impinging U.S. dominant mainstream culture, many Kānaka Maoli have had to alter their traditional modes of life. Some Kānaka Maoli have chosen to abandon their Kānaka Maoli heritage for full assimilation into the U.S. mainstream culture. Other Kānaka Maoli have chosen not to adopt U.S. mainstream practices in favor of maintaining a more traditional Hawaiian lifestyle. A Canadian cross-cultural psychologist, John Berry (2003), has presented a model of individual adaptation to the acculturation process that accounts for the various ways an acculturating group or person can adapt. He notes that

> it is essential to make the distinction between orientations toward one's own group and toward other groups . . . This distinction is rendered as a relative preference for maintaining one's heritage culture and identity and a relative preference for having contact with and participating in the larger society along with other ethnocultural groups. (p. 22)

In his model of acculturation adaptation, Berry (2003) highlights how cultural changes at the group level (e.g., changes in political and religious institutions) lead to changes at the individual level (e.g., beliefs, attitudes, and behaviors). Regardless of the circumstances of contact (e.g., immigration or occupation by another nation) between two groups, the acculturating group, usually the minority or conquered ethnocultural group, must eventually develop an adaptive coping style to the situation. However, individuals within an acculturating group could adapt differently from other individuals of the same group. Berry identified four modes of adaptation an acculturating person could adopt: integration, assimilation, separation, and marginalization. The integration mode of adaptation reflects a person who maintains his or her traditional heritage and identity while also adopting the cultural practices and beliefs of the dominant culture. This adaptation mode is also called biculturalism. The assimilated mode of adaptation reflects a person who does not maintain or identify with his or her traditional heritage, but fully adopts the cultural practices and beliefs of the dominant culture. Inversely, a person could maintain his or her traditional heritage and identity and not affiliate with the dominant culture, as is the case with the separation mode of adaptation. Finally, a person could inadvertently adopt the marginalization mode of adaptation in which he or she neither identifies with his or her traditional heritage nor the dominant culture.

Berry (2003) further theorizes that the physical and mental health status of a person can vary across the four acculturation modes of adaptation. People in the integrated and assimilated modes are believed to have a better physical and mental health status, whereas people in the traditional and marginalized modes are believed to be at a higher risk for physical and mental health concerns (Berry & Kim, 1988). Such differences in health status across acculturation modes are believed to be due to differences in people's experiences of acculturative stressors (e.g., language barriers and perceptions of racism and prejudices) and attitude toward, and willingness to assimilate into, the dominant culture. However, the degree to which a person is affected by these acculturative stressors and his or her attitude toward the dominant mainstream culture are influenced by the reasons for acculturation (e.g., conquered by another group versus voluntary immigration) and the dominant mainstream culture's acceptance (e.g., multiculturalism versus assimilation policies) of a person's traditional ethnic heritage (Berry & Kim, 1988). These factors can have a stronger impact on people in the traditional and marginalized modes compared with people in the integrated and assimilated modes for apparent reasons. Certainly, a person who is forced to acculturate to the lifestyle of another ethnocultural group or nation is likely to have a more negative attitude toward that group than a person who voluntarily entered into the acculturation process (e.g., immigrants). In the case of Kānaka Maoli, who involuntarily entered into the U.S. acculturation process, it stands to reason that the degree of cultural discord experienced would be high and that many would be apprehensive about the idea of full assimilation into the U.S. mainstream culture.

Using Berry's model of acculturation adaptation, Kamana'opono M. Crabbe (also a Hawaiian psychologist) and I, along with other colleagues, have examined the acculturation modes of Kānaka Maoli. We found that a majority (roughly 74 percent) of Kānaka Maoli identify themselves as being integrated or bicultural; nearly a quarter (roughly 21 percent) identify themselves as separatist (which we re-termed as traditional); a small minority (about 4 percent) identify themselves as being marginalized; and only one percent identify themselves as being assimilated (Crabbe, Kaholokula, Kenui, & Grandinetti, 1996; Kaholokula, 2004). From this data, it is apparent that 95 percent of Kānaka Maoli strongly identify with their traditional heritage (i.e., integrated and traditional), while only 5 percent of Kānaka Maoli do not strongly identify with their traditional heritage (i.e., marginalized and assimilated). It is clear that a vast majority of us Kānaka Maoli still value and want to maintain our unique Hawaiian heritage despite attempts by U.S. colonialism to assimilate us. However, what has been the cost of this cultural discord on Kānaka Maoli wellbeing, given that we live in an American-influenced society?

ʻEhaʻeha Ka Naʻau: *A Collective State of Depression*

Pulu ʻelo i ka ua o ka hoʻoilo.
Filled with grief and despair.
(Pukui, 1983, p. 300)

Psychological data on Kānaka Maoli support the idea that we could be suffering from higher rates of emotional distress compared to other ethnic groups in Hawaiʻi and the continental United States. Although no cross-ethnic comparisons of depression rates have been published among adults in Hawaiʻi, two community-based studies have found the prevalence of depressive symptoms to be 15 to 20 percent among adult Kānaka Maoli (Kaholokula, Grandinetti, Crabbe, Chang, & Kenui, 1999; Nelson, Kaholokula, Grandinetti, & Chang, 2003), which is much higher than the estimated 10 percent prevalence of depressive symptoms in the general U.S. population (Judd, Akiskal, & Paulus, 1997). Kānaka Maoli (37.4 percent) are more likely to perceive themselves as having a poorer mental health status compared to Caucasians (33 percent), Japanese (26.8 percent), Filipinos (20.2 percent), and other ethnic groups (30.8 percent) in Hawaiʻi (State of Hawaiʻi BRFSS, 2003). A study comparing the suicide rates of youth in Hawaiʻi has found that Kānaka Maoli youth are considerably more likely to attempt suicide (13 percent) compared to youth from other ethnic groups (Yuen, Nahulu, Hishinuma, & Miyamoto, 2000). It is without question that we contemporary Kānaka Maoli are at a higher risk for depression and other associated emotional disturbances when compared to other ethnic groups in Hawaiʻi.

It is believed that many Kānaka Maoli are suffering from these high rates of emotional distress because of the adverse health and social effects of U.S. colonialism and its acculturation process (Marsella et al., 1995). The idea that we Kānaka Maoli could be suffering from emotional distress associated with the loss of our culture and nation was formally documented by the Native Hawaiian Educational Assessment Project (NHEAP) in 1983. Regarding emotional distress among Kānaka Maoli, they stated the following: "Modern Hawaiians seem to suffer from a new kind of depression, a being 'beaten down', but not by rain, rather, by a sense of enormous personal loss . . . caused by two centuries of rapid change away from Hawaiian culture" (NHEAP, 1983, p. 418).

Since the NHEAP (1983) report, other Kānaka Maoli mental health professionals have further elaborated on the relationship between emotional distress and acculturation among Kānaka Maoli. A Hawaiian psychologist, William C. Rezentes III (1996), postulates that some contemporary Kānaka Maoli might be suffering from what he terms the *kaumaha* (meaning sadness, heaviness, or burden) syndrome, described as

> a collective sadness and moral outrage felt by many Hawaiians stemming from events such as the 1848 Māhele (division of lands), the 1887 Bayonet Constitution, or the 1893 overthrow of the ruling monarch of the independent nation of Hawai'i which led directly to the 1898 annexation of Hawai'i by the United States and then to U.S. statehood in 1959. (p. 37)

In relation to the kaumaha syndrome, Rezentes (1996) further explains the following:

> Hawaiians were coerced into submitting to foreign institutions, laws, and cultures and forced to either give up or be punished for practicing their traditional culture. Some Hawaiians have internalized their oppressors' messages. They have become trapped in vicious cycles of poor health practices, abuse of *'ohana* [family] members, neglect or prostitution of traditional Hawaiian culture, and the abandonment of their spirituality. (p. 37)

Crabbe (1999) also believes that many contemporary Kānaka Maoli suffer from a collective form of depression that he refers to as *hō'ino'ino,* or "broken-spirit." He describes hō'ino'ino as follows: "Perhaps it is this subtype [hō'ino'ino] that best reflects the plight of the modern Hawaiian today. This type of depressed 'broken-spirit' may be the psychological repercussion from years of cultural conflict with Westerners, acculturative discord, and progressive cultural regress" (p. 125).

The kinds of depression in Kānaka Maoli that NHEAP, Rezentes, and Crabbe have described are similar to the kind of depression the American psychologist Martin Seligman (1974) termed *learned helplessness.* The theory of learned helplessness describes persons with this kind of depression as "passive people who have negative cognitive sets about the effects of their own actions, who become depressed upon the loss of an important source of gratification" (Miller, Rosellini, & Seligman, 1985, pp. 182–183). Seligman and colleagues believe it is a reactive depression caused not by internal events (e.g., negative thoughts about self-worth) but rather by environmental events (e.g., loss of control over gratification and relief of suffering). Therefore, this reactive depression in people develops because they have come to learn that their attempts to bring about desired changes in their lives are futile. They develop a negative cognitive set (e.g., "others are against me and my people and we have no power to change it") that leads them to believe that, no matter what they do, no positive outcome will be achieved and, eventually, abandon any attempts to remedy the problem.

Consistent with the theory of learned helplessness, some researchers contend that depression is an adaptive response to subjugation and exploitation among defeated peoples (Gilbert, 2000; Sloman, 2000). The lack of resources (e.g., failure to maintain highly valued goals and wealth), the experience of internal (e.g., negative cognitive sets about the self) and external (e.g., social comparisons that lead to feelings of inferiority) conflict, and social discrimination and humiliation by others are believed to contribute to a depressive state among people who have been conquered and exploited (Gilbert, 2000). In such a case, depression is conceptualized as a person's defeat response (e.g., learned helplessness) to an inescapable and unchangeable situation, which ultimately results in feelings of powerlessness and demoralization, and counter-productive behaviors (e.g., social withdrawal and health-compromising behaviors; Sloman, 2000).

Indeed, the overwhelming influences of Euro-American culture and the U.S. military's presence in Hawai'i, as well as the influx of other foreigners to Hawai'i, leave many of us Kānaka Maoli with a sense of having no control over our own lives and our own destiny in our own homeland. Many people of other ethnic groups in Hawai'i hold negative stereotypes of us Kānaka Maoli, which only serve to reinforce the belief among many Kānaka Maoli that they are powerless and socially disadvantaged. It is common to hear Kānaka Maoli being referred to as lazy, uneducated, irresponsible, aggressive, and wanting a free ride, to name a few. Benjamin B. C. Young (1980), a respected Hawaiian psychiatrist, commented that "these stereotypes . . . have hindered many young Hawaiians from seeking high goals" (p. 21). With such feelings of helplessness and overt prejudices, is it any wonder why Kānaka Maoli have a collective kaumaha and hō'ino'ino?

To address the question of whether or not the psychological wellbeing of Kānaka Maoli is associated with acculturation, Crabbe and I (Crabbe et al., 1996; Kaholokula, 2004) conducted two studies that examined the association between acculturation modes and depressive symptoms in 522 (study 1) and 429 (study 2) Kānaka Maoli. Using Berry's modes of acculturation described earlier in this essay, we found that depressive symptoms were related to the acculturation mode of Kānaka Maoli. In both our studies, Kānaka Maoli who reported being in the traditional mode of acculturation had considerably more symptoms of depression than Kānaka Maoli who reported being in the bicultural (integrated) mode, and slightly more than those in the marginalized mode.[7] Furthermore, these differences in depressive symptoms across acculturation modes could not be explained away by differences in sex, age, education level, and degree of social support or Hawaiian ancestry (i.e., Hawaiian blood quantum).

Among Kānaka Maoli, the fact that traditional individuals experience more depressive symptoms than bicultural or marginalized individuals could be due to increased acculturative stressors experienced by traditional individuals. Some examples of these acculturative stressors for Kānaka Maoli in the traditional mode of acculturation could be increased perceptions of racism and discrimination; conflict with Euro-American values, beliefs, and practices; and problems with U.S federal and Hawaiʻi state laws that restrict a person's ability to practice traditional Hawaiian culture and ways of life (e.g., gathering rights and access to beaches and shorelines). Although we did not specifically examine acculturative stress among Kānaka Maoli in our studies, a significant association between acculturative stress and depression has been empirically observed among other U.S ethnic groups.

Anecdotal evidence from my own clinical experience suggests that many Kānaka Maoli could be experiencing a high degree of acculturative stress. Many Kānaka Maoli I have worked with, particularly older individuals, have a strong mistrust of Western medicine and healing practices. Other health professionals have also found Kānaka Maoli to be mistrustful of Western medicine (Hughes, 2004), to the extent that many prefer to place their fate exclusively in *ke Akua* (God) and/or traditional Hawaiian healing practices (e.g., *lāʻau lapaʻau*) than in the hands of their Western-trained physicians and mental health professionals. We also experience racism and prejudices from other U.S. ethnic groups who challenge our status as indigenous people and who use the U.S. Constitution to limit our access to education, quality health care, and social services. Indeed, we Kānaka Maoli must constantly defend our identity and way of life in our own *kulāiwi* (ancestral land). Could these acculturative stressors mediate the relationship between modes of acculturation and depressive symptoms among Kānaka Maoli?

The relationship between chronic psychosocial stressors and depression has been well documented in the scientific literature. For example, it has been reported that stressful events (e.g., health, marital, occupational, and financial problems) in a person's life over a one-year period can lead to an increase in depressive symptoms and that an increase in depressive symptoms can exacerbate existing stressful events in a person's life (Pianta & Egeland, 1994).

Applying this to the case of Kānaka Maoli, it would be a logical proposition to assert that the years of acculturative stressors experienced by Kānaka Maoli, coupled with their daily life stressors, could account for the high levels of depressive symptoms observed in this population. Reciprocally, these high levels of depressive symptoms among many Kānaka Maoli could, thereby, be contributing to an increase in acculturative and other psychosocial stressors for them. Finally, the high degree of depressive symptoms and acculturative and psychosocial stressors among Kānaka Maoli could also be contributing to their high susceptibility to health-compromising behaviors (e.g., overeating and alcohol and tobacco use) and chronic medical diseases (e.g., diabetes and heart problems). Empirical studies have found a significant association between depression and health-compromising behaviors (e.g., Kaholokula et al., 1999) and between depression and chronic medical conditions (e.g., Scalco, Scalco, Azul, & Lotufo Neto, 2005). Therefore, both anecdotal and empirical evidence suggests that these relationships could hold among Kānaka Maoli.

To better understand the relationship between acculturative stress and the physical, mental, and social health of Kānaka Maoli, the NHEAP (1983) formulated the cultural loss/stress hypothesis. The hypothesis describes the relationship among cultural loss, acculturative stressors, and the physical and mental health status of Kānaka Maoli using Bronfenbrenner's (1979) ecological model as a framework. It states that Hawaiian cultural loss has led to negative social outcomes (e.g., weakening of Kānaka Maoli cultural institutions and their connection to the ʻāina) which, in turn, has adversely impacted the ʻohana (families; e.g., domestic violence, broken homes), resulting in physical (e.g., obesity) and psychological (e.g., depression) problems for the individual. Furthermore, those who are negatively affected only serve to perpetuate Hawaiian cultural loss, negative social outcomes, and problems in the ʻohana. Although the cultural loss/stress hypothesis has yet to be empirically examined, it is consistent with historical data, the observations of many Kānaka Maoli mental health professionals, and the few epidemiological data available on Kānaka Maoli such as those discussed previously.

The complex interplay among biological, psychological, and environmental factors in influencing a person's overall wellbeing is only beginning to be fully appreciated by the Western medical and behavioral sciences. However, this is something ancient Kānaka Maoli have long realized—that there needs to be a harmonious balance among the individual, his or her social and spiritual relationships, and the environment to achieve optimal health (Pukui et al., 1972). Our kūpuna understood that the physical, emotional, and spiritual realms were interconnected and that they shared a complex reciprocal relationship. Each realm had a direct influence on the other and vice versa. When any one of these realms was compromised, so were the others. The current condition of contemporary Kānaka Maoli exemplifies this belief. As a result of being disenfranchised from our elder sibling, the ʻĀina, and having experienced spiritual and cultural disintegration, we have become vulnerable to physical, psychological, and social diseases. For many Kānaka Maoli, the healing process can only truly begin by reconnecting to our ʻĀina and our holistic sense of spirituality.

Nānā i Ke Kumu: *Looking Back to Move Forward*

In summary, I have suggested in this essay that U.S. colonialism in Hawaiʻi and its acculturation process have led to adverse physical, psychological, and social consequences for many contemporary Kānaka Maoli. Several Kānaka Maoli mental health professionals (Crabbe, 1999; Marsella et al., 1995; Rezentes, 1996) have theorized that we could be suffering from a collective type of depression (e.g., the kaumaha syndrome and hōʻinoʻino) associated with the effects of U.S. colonialism and resulting acculturative stressors. I have presented historical, epidemiological, empirical, and anecdotal evidence to support the assertions made in this essay. However, no type of evidence is needed to convince us Kānaka Maoli that, as a group, we have not fared well under U.S. occupation of our islands. Every time I see a fellow Kānaka Maoli homeless, incarcerated, or debilitated by disease, I am reminded of what we have lost under U.S. rule. Despite all this, I remain hopeful of our future as Kānaka Maoli, for our kūpuna have left us a rich legacy. They have left us their *ʻike* (knowledge) through *moʻolelo* (history), *oli* (chants), and *mele* (songs) and our *ʻōlelo makuahine* (native language), and they have given us their *mana* through our *moʻokūʻauhau*. For many of us Kānaka Maoli, we believe that it is from our kūpuna that the answer to our survival resides. We must *nānā i ke kumu*—look to the source for guidance.[8]

Notes

1. The term *Kānaka Maoli* (or *Kanaka Maoli* in the singular) is used here to mean Hawaiian(s) and refers to any person(s) who resided and/or had ancestors residing in the Hawaiian archipelago prior to Captain Cook's arrival to Hawaiʻi in 1778. The term was first used in 1852 Kingdom of Hawaiʻi documents to distinguish between Hawaiians and non-Hawaiians at the time.

2. There are many *moʻolelo* (historical accounts) of how the islands of Hawaiʻi were created. This particular account is from the *koʻi honua* (creation chant) called Mele a Pākuʻi (Fornander, 1916, vol. IV, pp. 12–16).

3. The majority of contemporary Kānaka Maoli are of mixed-ethnic ancestry, for example, Hawaiian, Chinese, and German or Hawaiian, Filipino, and Portuguese. Today, Hawaiʻi is comprised of many different ethnic groups that have had a significant influence on the local culture (e.g., food preference, religion, language, and politics).

4. The word *health* in this essay is used in a holistic sense, recognizing the interplay between physical, psychological, spiritual, and social wellbeing. This is consistent with the traditional Hawaiian view of wellbeing.

5. The population of Kānaka Maoli at the time of Cook's arrival in 1778 was estimated to be about 800,000 but, by the time of the illegal overthrow of the Hawaiian Kingdom in 1893, the native population had declined to about 40,000 (Stannard, 1989). This decline was mostly due to infectious diseases, such as gonorrhea and syphilis, smallpox, and measles, introduced by European and American foreigners (Bushnell, 1993). In 1893, Kānaka Maoli were out numbered by non-Hawaiians (approximately 50,000). Today, the number of Kānaka Maoli in Hawai'i is estimated to be 239,655 (approximately 21 percent of the total population), and another 161,507 are estimated to live in the continental United States (State of Hawai'i Data Book, 2001).

6. Following the death of Kamehameha Nui in 1819, his wife, Ka'ahumanu, influenced the abolition of the ancient *Kapu* socio-religious system, which was the hierarchical form of religious, government, and social order in place since the arrival of Pa'ao to Hawai'i in the twelfth century. This set the stage for the conversion of Kānaka Maoli to Christianity.

7. In these studies, data from the assimilation mode could not be statistically analyzed because of the small number of people who identified themselves as assimilated.

8. The phrase, *nana i ke kumu*, figuratively means to look to our ancestors for guidance and wisdom, and it is also the title of a valuable two-volume resource book for health professionals working with Kānaka Maoli (see Pukui, Haertig, & Lee, 1972).

References

Beaglehole, J. C. (Ed.). (1967). *The journals of Captain James Cook on his voyage of discovery*, vol. III: *The voyage of the Resolution and the Discovery, 1776–80*. London: Cambridge University Press.

Berry, J. W. (2003). Conceptual approaches to acculturation. In K. M. Chun, P. B. Organista, & G. M. Marín (Eds.), *Acculturation: Advances in theory, measurement, and applied research* (pp. 17–37). Washington, DC: American Psychological Association.

Berry, J. W., & Kim, U. (1988). Acculturation and mental health. In P. Dasen, J. W. Berry, & N. Sartorius (Eds.), *Health and cross-cultural psychology: Towards applications* (pp. 207–236). Beverly Hills: Sage.

Blaisdell, K. (1993). Historical and cultural aspects of native Hawaiian health. *Social Process in Hawai'i, 31*, 37–57.

Bronfenbrenner, U. (1979). *The ecology of human development*. Cambridge, MA: Harvard University Press.

Bushnell, O. A. (1993). *Germs and genocide in Hawai'i*. Honolulu: University of Hawai'i Press.

Crabbe, K. M. (1999). Conceptions of depression: A Hawaiian perspective. *Pacific Health Dialog, 6*(1), 122–126.

Crabbe, K. M., Kaholokula, J. K., Kenui, C. K., & Grandinetti, A. (1996, January). *Prevalence of depression, degrees of Hawaiianess, and modes of acculturation among Native Hawaiians living in rural North Kōhala, Hawai'i.* Paper presented at the National Institute of Health–Asian and Pacific Islander American Health Research Conference, Honolulu, HI.

Finch, B. K., Kolody, B., & Vega, W. A. (2000). Perceived discrimination and depression among Mexican-origin adults in California. *Journal of Health and Social Behaviors, 41*(3), 295–313.

Fornander, A. (1916). *Hawaiian antiquities and folk-lore.* Vol. IV. Honolulu: Bishop Museum Press.

Gilbert, P. (2000). Varieties of submissive behavior as forms of social defense: Their evolution and role in depression. In L. Sloman & P. Gilbert (Eds.), *Subordination and defeat: An evolutionary approach to mood disorders and their therapy* (pp. 3–45). Englewood Cliffs, NJ: Lawrence Erlbaum.

Hughes, C. K. (2004). Factors associated with health-seeking behaviors of Native Hawaiian men. *Pacific Health Dialog, 11*(2), 176–182.

Johnson, D. B., Oyama, N., LeMarchand, L., & Wilkens, L. (2004). Native Hawaiian mortality, morbidity, and lifestyle: Comparing data from 1982, 1990, and 2000. *Pacific Health Dialog, 11*(2), 120–130.

Judd, L. L., Akiskal, H. S., & Paulus, M. P. (1997). The role and clinical significance of subsyndromal depressive symptoms (SSD) in unipolar major depressive disorder. *Journal of Affective Disorders, 45,* 5–17.

Kaholokula, J. K. (2004, July). The effects of colonization and acculturation on the well-being of Native Hawaiians. In K. Nickerson (Chair), *Mana Maoli: Connecting the past with the present to preserve the future for native Hawaiians.* Symposium conducted at the American Psychological Association Annual Convention, Honolulu, HI.

Kaholokula, J. K., Grandinetti, A., Crabbe, K. M., Chang, H. K., & Kenui, C. K. (1999). Depressive symptoms and cigarette smoking among Native Hawaiians. *Asia-Pacific Journal of Public Health, 11*(2), 60–64.

Kahumoku, W. (2003). A tragic indigenous mo'olelo: The decline of Kanaka Maoli linguistic identity. *'Ōiwi[3]: A Native Hawaiian Journal: Huli Au,* Pō 160–167.

Kame'eleihiwa, L. (1992). *Native land and foreign desires: Pehea La E Pono Ai? How shall we live in harmony?* Honolulu: Bishop Museum Press.

Marsella, A. J., Oliveira, J. M., Plummer, C. M., & Crabbe, K. M. (1995). Native Hawaiian (kanaka maoli) culture, mind, and well-being. In H. I. McCubbin, E. A. Thompson, & J. E. Fromer (Eds.), *Resiliency in ethnic minority families: Native immigrant American families* (pp. 93–113). Madison: University of Wisconsin, Center for Excellence in Family Studies.

Mbeki, T. M. (n.d.). Quote retrieved June 27, 2005, from BrainyQuote Web site: http://www.brainyquote.com/quotes/quotes/t/thabomvuye178908.html.

Miller, W. R., Rosellini, R. A., & Seligman, M. E. P. (1985). Learned helplessness and depression. In J. C. Coyne (Ed.), *Essential papers on depression* (pp. 181–219). New York: New York University Press.

Native Hawaiian Educational Assessment Project. (1983). *Native Hawaiian educational assessment project report*. Honolulu: Kamehameha Schools/Bernice Pauahi Bishop Estate.

Nelson, K., Kaholokula, J. K., Grandinetti, A., & Chang, H. K. (2003, November). *CES-D factor structure among four distinct ethnic groups of Hawai'i.* Poster session presented at the 37th Annual Association for the Advancement of Behavior Therapy Convention. Boston, MA.

Oh, Y., Koeske, G. F., & Sales, E. (2002). Acculturation, stress, and depressive symptoms among Korean immigrants in the United States. *Journal of Social Psychology, 142*(4), 511–526.

Osorio, J. K. (2002). *Dismembering Lāhui: A history of the Hawaiian nation to 1887*. Honolulu: University of Hawai'i Press.

Pianta, R. C., & Egeland, B. (1994). Relation between depressive symptoms and stressful life events in a sample of disadvantaged mothers. *Journal of Consulting & Clinical Psychology, 62*(8), 1229–1234.

Pukui, M. K. (1983). *'Ōlelo No'eau: Hawaiian proverbs and poetical sayings.* Bishop Museum Special Publication No. 71. Honolulu: Bishop Museum Press.

Pukui, M. K., Haertig, E. W., & Lee, C. A. (1972). *Nānā I Ke Kumu: Look to the source.* Vols. I and II. Honolulu: Queen Lili'uokalani Children's Center.

Rezentes, W. C. (1996). *Ka Lama Kukui: Hawaiian psychology: An introduction.* Honolulu: 'A'ali'i Books.

Scalco, A. Z., Scalco, M. Z., Azul, J. B., & Lotufo Neto, F. (2005). Hypertension and depression. *Clinics, 60*(3), 241–250.

Seligman, M. E. P. (1974). Depression and learned helplessness. In R. J. Friedman & M. M. Katz (Eds.), *The psychology of depression: Contemporary theory and research* (pp. 83–109). Oxford: John Wiley & Sons.

Silva, N. K. (2004). *Aloha betrayed: Native Hawaiian resistance to American colonialism.* Durham, NC: Duke University Press.

Sloman, L. (2000). How the involuntary defeat strategy relates to depression. In L. Sloman & P. Gilbert (Eds.), *Subordination and defeat: An evolutionary approach to mood disorders and their therapy* (pp. 47–67). Englewood Cliffs, NJ: Lawrence Erlbaum.

Social Science Research Council. (1954). Acculturation: An exploratory formulation. *American Anthropologist, 56*, 973–1002.

Stannard, D. (1989). *Before the horror: The population of Hawai'i at the eve of Western contact.* Honolulu: Social Science Research Institute, University of Hawai'i.

State of Hawai'i Behavioral Risk Factor Surveillance System. (2003). *Behavioral risk factor surveillance system.* Honolulu: Hawai'i State Department of Health.

State of Hawai'i Data Book. (2001). *State of Hawai'i data book: A statistical abstract*. Honolulu: Hawai'i State Department of Health.

Trask, H-K. (1999). *From a native daughter: Colonialism and sovereignty in Hawai'i*. Rev. ed. Honolulu: University of Hawai'i Press.

Young, B. B. C. (1980). The Hawaiians. In J. F. McDermott, W-S. Tseng, & T. W. Maretzki (Eds.), *People and cultures of Hawaii: A psychocultural profile* (pp. 5–24). Honolulu: University of Hawai'i Press.

Yuen, N. Y. C., Nahulu, L. B., Hishinuma, E. S., & Miyamoto, R. H. (2000). Cultural identification and attempted suicide in Native Hawaiian adolescents. *Journal of the American Academy of Child and Adolescent Psychiatry, 39*(3), 360–367.

Acknowledgments

I would like to *mahalo nui aku* (thank very much) my dear friends and colleagues who so graciously read initial drafts of this essay and who provided me with their *'ike* (knowledge) and *mana'o* (thoughts): Ty Kawika Tengan, PhD, assistant professor of ethnic studies and anthropology at the University of Hawai'i at Mānoa; Laiana Wong, PhD, assistant professor of Hawaiian languages at the University of Hawai'i at Mānoa; Jill Oliveira, PhD, clinical psychologist at Nā Pu'uwai Native Hawaiian Health Care Systems Clinic on Moloka'i, Hawai'i; and Jana Silva, MD, assistant professor of medicine in the Department of Native Hawaiian Health, John A. Burns School of Medicine at the University of Hawai'i at Mānoa. It is because of these people, and many like them, that we Kānaka Maoli and our heritage will never perish.

16

Crisis in Paradise
Family Violence in Samoan Communities

KARANINA SIAOSI SUMEO

I am a mother of three children with the stretch marks to prove it. I have spoken Samoan to my children since they were in my stomach so that they knew who they were and would never have to try to find themselves in non-Samoan environments. My childhood in my island home in the Pacific was a time of spiritual, physical, and emotional freedom—feelings I wish my own children to have throughout their lives. Childhood is therefore a very precious time, and I try to pack as many positives and challenges on my children, as they do to their parents and wider family, as we give each other love, strength, character, knowledge, skills, and aspirations as we journey through life.

It has taken some time to realize my passion in my professional and academic paths, migrating from a background in chemistry to social work and social policy. One of the significant landmarks in my learning was a research thesis on child abuse within Samoan families that I conducted for my social policy degree. That research is the basis for the following essay on child abuse, human rights, justice, and cultural identity. While the essay is concerned centrally with Samoan children and their families, I believe that there are parallels between Samoans and other minority groups, in particular, people whose political, economic, social, and cultural identities have been reshaped over time by foreign laws, religions, economies, philosophies, and governments that pursue goals without a necessarily shared vision with the people.

Violence of any kind within the home has a direct impact on the mental and spiritual health of children. This essay looks at child abuse and domestic violence within Samoan communities. The essay offers some perspectives and learning to those who work with Samoan families, in the hope it may assist intervention to support them.

Physical Abuse

The most dominant of all influences upon family life and child rearing within Samoan communities has been, and continues to be, religion (Meleisea, 1992; Ngan-woo, 1985). While there is an opinion that violent methods of child discipline have always been present in Samoan communities (Freeman, 1985), perpetrators of physical abuse have often manipulated biblical teachings to justify their actions (Cahill, 2000; Ngan-woo, 1985; Siaosi Sumeo, 2004).

The narrow interpretation of the word *rod* from the English Bible, translated as *lāʻau* (stick) in the Samoan Bible, a physical instrument, is perhaps one of the leading contributors to child abuse. In a recent study, Siaosi Sumeo (2004) found that the Bible was quoted readily by participants as justification for using physical discipline and extreme violence upon children by caregivers in families and by religious leaders themselves. Siaosi Sumeo found that wives of some pastors (*faletua*) were openly abusive to children, and indeed perceived it as their right and duty to use extreme disciplinary measures, to the degree that some children were seriously injured. What was more frightening was that witnesses to the abuse condoned it, as they perceived both *faletua* and *faifeʻau* (pastors) as servants of God Himself. In the Family Health and Safety Study (FHSS) (Ministry of Women's Affairs [MWA], 2003), women reported that pastors were some of the main perpetrators of physical abuse upon women in their lives (Siaosi Sumeo, 2004).

A broader interpretation of the rod concept (Proverbs 23:13–14) implies that it can be an instrument of protection and guardianship (Hille, 1985). Some Christian writers advocate that Jesus emphasized the importance of obedience and respect to parents, but he never advocated the physical punishment of children. Jesus instead warned people against the mistreatment of children, and elevated the position of children in society by promoting their care and protection as characteristics of greatness in people (Cahill, 2000; Capps, 1995; Fruean, 1991). As powerful agents of social engineering, religious institutions in Samoan communities have a responsibility to reverse the promotion of the use of violence toward children in their communities, and to model this reversal, in order to stop abuse (Siaosi Sumeo, 2004).

Siaosi Sumeo (2004) found that in Samoa, physical abuse of children occurred directly from generational modeling of the use of extreme violence in parenting, the inability to manage children's behavior, scapegoating, and resentment of the child. The last two factors featured predominantly in the study as a major contributing factor to abuse, according to participants in the study. It is significant that in the two cases over the past ten years where children have died from direct acts of caregiver abuse, both offenders were stepfathers who were known in their communities to be frequent abusers of their stepchildren.

Abuse also occurred as a consequence of low or no partner support in the home; an accumulation of financial, social, and emotional stressors; and current victimization of women caregivers by their partners or by members of the partner's family, as it is common for the nuclear unit to live with the father's family. It was significant to see that the abuse of women had a direct link to the abuse of children. The findings consistently suggested that violence has been perpetuated from one generation to the next through role modeling. The FHSS study had found that of the men who self-disclosed as being abusive to their partners, 93 percent had experienced physical abuse before they reached 15 years of age, and 42 percent had witnessed their own fathers abusing their mothers for answering back or disobedience (MWA, 2003).

Sexual Violence

Sexual abuse is no new phenomenon to Samoan society, as it has been documented in its history and legends (Kramer, 1994; Lafai-Sauoaiga, 2000; Mead, 1943; Stueble, 1976). Historical processes of justice against sexual crimes also indicate that such acts are not new, and have resulted in extreme consequences such as banishment and death (Sunia, 1997). In more recent times, Samoa and its local communities are finding it increasingly difficult to address sexual abuse and to prevent offending. Abuse of children in Samoan society has been found to be perpetrated largely by those in the immediate circles of the child—family members, acquaintances of family members, and other members of the community, with very few offenses being committed by total strangers (Siaosi Sumeo, 2004).

In Samoa, there are very few accessible therapeutic agencies for traumatized child victims, and no support through statutory agencies for counseling or rehabilitation. Religious leaders, most with no training in the area, are somehow expected to provide therapeutic support. For some families, acknowledgment of the crime by authorities, if not a successful prosecution, may be the only form of recognition of their suffering. The lack of expertise and resources to deal with the problem is compounded by attitudes and compromises within communities and professional organizations that make addressing sexual abuse difficult.

In the Samoan Supreme Court in September 2000, a Catholic catechist was convicted of sexual offenses toward a 12-year-old girl. The judge's statement disclosed that the offender had been convicted of a similar offense eight years earlier, while practicing in the same role. While the judge acknowledged possible embarrassment to the church from the conviction, he noted that the church knew of the man's history yet allowed him to continue practicing, implying that the church brought embarrassment upon itself and contributed to the crime (University of South Pacific, *Police v. Paulo*, September 29, 2000).

In New Zealand in 1991, a Samoan pastor was suspected of sexual abuse of a 12-year-old girl who lived in his home. State authorities removed the child from the home, but the alleged perpetrator denied the allegations, and there was no supporting evidence. The child concerned was later found dead under suspicious circumstances. A year later, in 1992, the alleged perpetrator was convicted on two charges of unlawful sexual intercourse with a 14-year-old girl from his church and sentenced to eleven months in jail. In 2001, it was reported in a local newspaper that the convicted perpetrator was once again practicing as a pastor in a local church (Coddington, 2004).

In Samoa, traditional processes of justice still operate, particularly in rural areas where the national police force is virtually invisible and the *matai* (chiefly) councils (*fono*) are the authority. Sexual crimes are dealt with to varying degrees, from material and monetary fines to banishment. In some villages, particularly in the urban areas, there is no intervention by the fono and the matters are referred to the police. People have a choice about which authority they take matters to, and there are villages that also strongly discourage people from taking such matters outside the village council (Siaosi Sumeo, 2004).

Processes vary from one village to another and the consequences are completely at the discretion of each council, according to established rules and protocols in that village. As with physical abuse, sexual crimes committed across different *'āiga* are easily addressed through the traditional processes of the *īfoga* (ritualized public apology instigated by the offender's family independent of any authority intervention) and the fono. The processes, however, are not as visible when crimes such as incest or rape are committed within the same *'āiga*. Crimes committed "in house" are not as readily addressed unless a formal approach to the council has occurred, as the fono is primarily there to govern the use of land and to manage relationships between 'āiga, leaving individual families their own autonomy. Processes for dealing with child sexual abuse are problematic because of local attitudes and beliefs around family autonomy, limitations on the powers of the fono to intervene, and the lack of objective justice, particularly where the offender may be a matai of the family who also sits in the fono (Siaosi Sumeo, 2004).

Sexual abuse in Samoa is largely seen as a problem inflicted by men on female children, with some indicators from the FHSS study that there is also abuse to males from females, namely, mother to son (MWA, 2003). The first study on domestic and sexual violence in Samoa found that convictions for sexual crimes against people under 16 years of age outnumbered those for adults (Mapusaga o Aiga [MOA], 1996). This finding was further confirmed by a later study, along with the fact that all victims except one were females (Siaosi Sumeo, 2004). The findings suggest that children are certainly targeted by perpetrators of sexual violence.

The invisibility of male victims is of concern, considering research from other societies that found that the rate of re-offending by men who victimized boys was estimated to be twice as high as men who offended against females (Finkelhor, 1986). These findings suggest that boys are victimized possibly at a much higher rate than police reports suggest or than societies would like to believe.

Social attitudes in Samoa about the *fa'afāfine* (a general term to describe males who are perceived to be effeminate, gay cross-dressers) do not protect boys who may be perceived as such from abuse, and who may be blamed for possibly inviting the abuse. One study found that offenders against boys were predominantly heterosexual men, with a smaller category of bisexual men, but rarely homosexual men (Dorais, 2002). In addition, some perpetrators abused because they believed it was their male right to use females as well as weaker males (boys and homosexual men) to achieve sexual gratification (Dominelli, 1991). Negative attitudes and beliefs in society around homosexuality, patriarchy, and expectations that real men are not victimized therefore continue to silence victims, shield perpetrators from accountability, and close society's eyes and ears to the abuse of male children.

Perceptions distorted by ignorance and denial—such as blaming sexual offending on youthful experimentation, foolishness, temptation (in the form of children), and lapses in judgment by men—contribute to minimizing the violation and trauma for children. Statements from perpetrators such as "the devil made me do it" or "I was overcome by Satan," as well as blaming teenage girls for having seduced or invited the perpetrators, reflected a rejection of responsibility, yet were readily accepted by personnel in both local and state authorities as acceptable reasons for committing offenses (Siaosi Sumeo, 2004).

A study of the prevalence of sexually transmitted infections, called "The Antenatal Clinical STI Survey" and sponsored jointly by the Samoan government and the World Health Organization (WHO), was recently conducted (Bourke, 2002). The research tested 427 women in Samoa, from the age of 15 upwards, for sexually transmitted infections (STIs), between October 1999 and April 2000. Of the 66 women aged 15–19 years, 39.4 percent had at least one STI. The rate of STIs peaked with the next group, 20–24 years, with 44.6 percent having at least one STI. These rates were comparable with those found in Asia and Africa. Assuming the majority were in heterosexual relationships, the findings suggest that there would be a significant number of men carrying STIs, which consequently has implications for victims of sexual abuse through transmission.

This raises questions about the protection of children from men who view them as opportunities for sex, the testing of victims for STIs, and follow-up treatment. Additional concerns include the absolute lack of accessible, appropriate therapeutic services for victims, the reliance of supportive nongovernmental organizations (NGOs) in Samoa on overseas funds in order to run, and an absence of rehabilitation programs for offenders.

Domestic Violence

Research on domestic violence conducted in Samoa in recent years (MOA, 1996; MWA, 2003) has alluded to links between family violence and child abuse, yet did not explore any connection in depth, as the main focus of the research was violence between adults. Nevertheless, the studies provide useful insights for initial analysis.

The Family Health and Safety Study (FHSS) conducted in Samoa in 2003 showed that of 1,646 women interviewed, 48 percent had experienced partner abuse (38 percent physical, 19 percent emotional, 20 percent sexual). Alarmingly, 24 percent of the physically abused victims in the FHSS study were pregnant at the time of the assault (MWA, 2003). Of the women who disclosed their victimization, 73 percent believed that domestic violence was "normal and not serious." Of the men surveyed, 57 percent believed that domestic violence was a private matter between husband and wife (MWA, 2003). Half of the women in the FHSS study who experienced abuse never sought help or spoke to anyone about it. The close proximity of houses and the lack of privacy between households, especially in rural villages, suggest that the so-called private incidents were often witnessed by many in the community, including children.

Due to the lack of exploration and, one may argue, recognition of the link between domestic violence and child abuse in Samoan studies, it is helpful to reflect on other materials from the Pacific region. A study conducted in Fiji by Adinkrah (2003) found a link between domestic violence and child abuse. In one case, a father became so enraged when his wife would not warm up his meal that he burned down the house while his wife and four children slept. Another father hacked his wife and five children to death because he suspected his wife was having an affair. A 2-year-old child, who ran to his mother who was being beaten, was thrown against a wall by his father. The child's head hit the wall and he consequently died as a result of the impact. The mother told authorities that the child accidentally fell, in order to cover up for her husband. Two months later, another incident of domestic violence occurred and this time the mother disclosed what truly happened to her son (Adinkrah, 2003).

A study by Kruger and Duddridge (1997) of child abuse cases in Queensland, Australia, also found links between family violence and child abuse. The study looked at cases of homicide between 1989 and 1992. It was found that 68.6 percent of the dead children were killed by a parent (mother, father, stepparent), and a further 19.8 percent were killed by another family member. Approximately 45.5 percent of the victims were under one year, and another 40 percent were between one and 5 years of age. Very young children were at highest risk of death due to abuse.

Similar to some of the findings of the Fijian study, the Queensland children died from varying reasons such as an unwanted child (infanticide); discipline killings, where parents did not intend to kill the child but through constant and brutal abuse caused the death; psychotic parents (those who suffered from some form of psychiatric illness at the time of the killing); and retaliation killings. The retaliation killings occurred when the offender killed the child as revenge against the other partner. In one case, a father got angry with his partner for telling him to leave and cut the 15-month-old baby's throat (Kruger & Duddridge, 1997). Another Australian study found that child abuse contributed to partnership breakdown, or occurred as a consequence (Brown, Sheehan, Frederico, & Hewitt, 2002).

Adinkrah (2003) found that police did not automatically assess the safety of children during domestic violence call-outs, and recommended that child assessment become a routine part of investigations. In light of his findings, Adinkrah raised the possibility that there may have been unrecognized cases of accidental deaths to children that were purposely inflicted during incidents of domestic violence.

Responses by the courts to accusations of child abuse in custody battles in which there were allegations of domestic violence between applicants were also found to be inadequate. Because of the acrimonious relationship between the parents, allegations of abuse were not always taken seriously by child protection agencies, or responded to as quickly through the court system (Brown, Sheehan, Frederico, & Hewitt, 2002).

Cribb (1997) conducted a study on domestic violence in New Zealand, with thirty Samoan women, mostly under 40 years of age. The study found that violence was accepted by one-third of the respondents. The younger women in the sample who were more educated and more accepting of assistance were found to be less tolerant of partner violence. The older women remained in violent households, even in a society where support services were available to them. Cribb suggested that the older women who came from Samoa had been accustomed to using the fono system in the village to counter the violence, but neither the fono nor the village support networks existed in the New Zealand context. The older women therefore felt trapped, compounded by their lack of skills to access and utilize Western support services (Cribb, 1997).

Cribb's suggestion that traditional structures in Samoa were relied upon to prevent domestic violence contradicted the MOA and FHSS studies, which found a significant rate of tolerance for, if not acceptance of, domestic violence within villages and general society. There was a strong belief (98 percent) by the male participants in the FHSS study that a good woman obeyed her husband (MWA, 2003). When women were asked in the MOA study (1996) about how they thought domestic violence could be stopped, the most frequent responses were to develop a better relationship with God, and for wives to be more patient and not answer back to their husbands, according to biblical principles. In the MOA study (1996), only 2 percent of the women sampled who had been abused by their partners reported incidents to police.

In addition to the beliefs and attitudinal barriers within local communities around domestic and patriarchal authority, the police were not trusted to take the complaints seriously. Some victims reported being turned away by individual officers and told (incorrectly) that there were no laws against abuse. Of the 12 percent of men in the FHSS study who admitted being abusive to their partners, 74 percent said they did so because their partners were disobedient or answered back; 26 percent hit their partners for disrespecting their in-laws and refusing to have sex.

In Samoan villages where the council of chiefs (fono) derive their power and authority from the collective of chiefs, the fono must recognize the right, duty, and authority of each chief (matai) to have responsibility for the care and maintenance of his own family relationships (Siaosi Sumeo, 2004). While there are existing rules within villages to address offenses between two separate families, prevailing attitudes about male dominance and the autonomy of the ʻāiga suggest that intervention by members of the local community in cases of family violence would not have been likely.

Changing Culture

Clearly, Samoan society, as it was, is changing, along with the values and attitudes of its people, depending on the various environmental influences upon them. One may wonder what the Samoan culture might look like twenty years from now and if there is a future for collective existence as the people have known it. While globalization is not the focus of this essay, it is clear that the Pacific nations have to engage in economic arrangements with bigger Western nations, which will have a lifelong impact on the culture (Kelsey, 2004). Globalization has had a direct effect on employment, income distribution, wealth, and poverty in the island nations.

Alongside globalization and free trade are the philosophical ideals promoted by the United Nations, such as the United Nations Convention on the Rights of the Child (UNCROC) and the United Nations Convention on the Elimination of All Forms of Discrimination Against Women (CEDAW). These have been regarded by many Samoans as pro-individualistic policies that degrade the interests of both the collective and the traditional chiefly authority, as they change fundamental social and political structures around gender and children. Even more disturbing to Samoans is that such policies are being ratified, with or without consultation with the people. Most matai who participated in one study on the processes of justice to address child abuse in Samoa stated that there was no public consultation prior to the ratification of the UNCROC by Samoa in 1994. Consequently, traditional authorities have felt increasingly sidelined by governments over these issues (Siaosi Sumeo, 2004). Many efforts in recent years by state agencies and NGOs to promote these conventions have therefore encountered significant public opposition.

As a people who were taken over by superpowers in the 1800s, and later won back their independence in 1962, Samoans take pride in self-ownership and the ability to determine their own future. Samoa has a multitude of constitutions—each village fono has its own, and the state has one as well—yet this is seen as acceptable. The simplistic view that Samoa will simply adopt UN conventions and move on with the rest of the world ignores the fact that, at least for now, the people of Samoa, not the government, own their lands and belong to collectives, which are physical and psychological assets. These factors instill identity, pride, and strength in all Samoans, even when they live in foreign societies.

Traditional values and beliefs that were internalized within the culture to counter acts such as rape, incest, and bloodshed are changing with the new realities. The valuing of the female child as the *taupou*, as a social and political asset to her family and community, meant that she was treasured and protected. Today this word is commonly used simply to refer to the physical state of female virginity. The traditional role and duty of the brother to protect and care for his sister, even after she is married, in a cultural covenant between male and female siblings called the *feagaiga*, exists today only in general and optional terms, as siblings do their own thing.

These elements of the culture were a significant form of social control, as the brother and sister definitions in Samoan culture extended beyond blood siblings to include cousins and relatives through marriage (Stuebel, 1976). Due to the shrinkage of the family unit and the necessities of survival for many families, especially in foreign countries, historical structures that guided social relationships are for some now irrelevant.

The more limited definitions of siblings and family members under existing legislation, and the way that Samoan society has changed today, have undermined these traditional lines of respect and accountability. The interdependence and collaborative nature of family relationships has weakened to the point where one unit does not consider connection with another unit necessary, and families become increasingly independent—and for some, isolated—a particularly dangerous situation for victims of abuse. While obtaining independence from the collective supports the idea of ʻāiga autonomy, for a family in which there is abuse, it benefits only the abuser, and distances the family from the eyes of the wider collective.

Traditional laws focus on the protection and preservation of the collective and its relationships with other collectives, not on individuals. Traditional methods of justice are weakening in their ability to enforce local laws and prevent re-offending, as society changes through urbanization, through exposure to alternative philosophies in foreign societies directly and indirectly through foreign goods and services, and through state laws that overrule traditional authorities in support of individual human rights. On the other hand, while statutory bodies are legally established and government-funded, resources are by no means adequate for authorities to fulfill the requirements of ensuring the protection and enforcement of basic rights of citizens, especially children (Siaosi Sumeo, 2004).

The problem of child abuse and domestic violence within Samoan communities requires appropriate and sensitive address. This is about protecting thc future, the healing of our men and women who abuse, and reclaiming the cultural buffers that existed prior to our alleged development. Without address, physical and sexual violence to women and children will continue to stifle the achievement of the social, economic, and spiritual aspirations of our people.

References

Adinkrah, M. (2003). Men who kill their own children: Paternal filicide incidents in contemporary Fiji. *Child Abuse & Neglect, 27*, 557–568.

Bourke, T. (2002, April 23–29). Sexually transmitted infections in Samoa. Sourced from World Health Organization research on "The Antenatal Clinical STI Survey." *Le Samoa*, 8.

Brown, T., Sheehan, R., Frederico, M., & Hewitt, L. (2002). Child abuse in the context of parental separation and divorce. *Children Australia, 27*(2), 35–40.

Cahill, L. S. (2000). *Family: A Christian social perspective*. Minneapolis: Fortress Press.

Capps, D. (1995). *The child's song: The religious abuse of children*. Louisville: Westminster/John Knox Press.

Coddington, D. (2003). *The New Zealand paedophile & sex offender index 2004*. Auckland: Alister Taylor.

Cribb, J. (1997, November). "Being bashed is just something I have to accept": Western Samoan women's attitudes towards domestic violence in Christchurch. *Social Policy Journal of New Zealand, 9*, 164–170.

Dominelli, L. (1991). *Gender, sex offenders and probation practice*. Norwich: Novata Press.

Dorais, M. (2002). *Don't tell: The sexual abuse of boys*. Trans. I. Denholm Meyer. Montreal: McGill-Queens University Press.

Finkelhor, D. (1986). *A sourcebook on child sexual abuse*. Beverley Hills: Sage.

Freeman, D. (1985). *Margaret Mead and Samoa: The making and unmaking of an anthropological myth*. Ringwood, Victoria: Penguin Books.

Fruean, M. (1997). *The moral status of children: Essays on the rights of the child.* The Hague, Netherlands: Martinus Nijhoff.

Hille, S. (1985). *The rod of guidance.* FaithTrust Institute (Reprinted from *SCAN Advocate*, Spring 1985). Retrieved July 3, 2003, from http://www.faithtrust-institute.org/Articles/rod-of-guidance.htm.

Kelsey, J. (2004, April). *Big brothers behaving badly: The implications for the Pacific Islands of the Pacific Agreement on Closer Relations (PACER).* Suva, Fiji: Pacific Network on Globalisation.

Kramer, A. (1994). *The Samoa Islands: An outline of a monograph with particular consideration of German Samoa.* Vol. 1. Trans. T. Verhaaren. Auckland: Polynesian Press.

Kruger, M., & Duddridge, D. *The sentencing of parents who kill their children: A Queensland study 1979–1997.* Unpublished manuscript.

Lafai-Sauoaiga, F. S. A. (2000). *O le vamaega i le tai: The will by the sea.* Salelologa, Samoa: Methodist Printing Press.

Mapusaga O Aiga [MOA]. (1996). *A study of domestic and sexual violence against women in Western Samoa research report.* Unpublished manuscript.

Mead, M. (1943). *Coming of age in Samoa: A study of adolescence and sex in primitive societies.* Harmondsworth, England: Penguin. (Original work published in 1928).

Meleisea, M. (1992). *Change and adaptation in Western Samoa.* Christchurch: Macmillan Brown Centre.

Ministry of Women's Affairs, Samoa. (2003, February 17–19). *Family health and safety study in Samoa.* Presentation at the Regional Workshop on Strengthening Partnerships to Eliminate Violence Against Women, Suva, Fiji.

Ngan-woo, F. (1985). *Faasamoa: The world of Samoans.* Wellington: The Office of the Race Relations Conciliator.

Siaosi Sumeo, K. (2004). *An exploratory study on the physical and sexual abuse of children in Samoa.* Unpublished master's thesis, Massey University, New Zealand.

Stuebel, C. (1976). *Tala o le vavau: Myths and legends of Samoa.* Trans. Brother Herman. Wellington: A. H & A. W. Reed.

Sunia, F. I. F. (1997). *Lupe o le foaga (Vaega Muamua).* Apia: Malua Printing Press.

The Bible Society in South Pacific. (1979). *O le Tusi Paia: The Holy Bible.* Reprinted from the edition of 1884. Suva, Fiji: United Bible Societies.

University of the South Pacific. *Police v Paulo, 29 September 2000.* Retrieved January 26, 2003, from http://www.vanuatu.usp.ac.fj/paclawmat/Samoa_cases/N-Z/Police_v_Paulo_(Sentence).html.

17

Doing Good Work and Finding a Sense of Purpose

The Nature and Treatment of Substance Abuse among Native Hawaiians

A. AUKAHI AUSTIN

My name is Ayda Aukahi Austin. I am a Native Hawaiian woman with a PhD in clinical psychology, which puts me in a relatively uncommon position. I understand the world both as a trained scholar and from my na'au, *my internal way of knowing that comes from being Kānaka Maoli and a proud member of my* 'ohana. *In my field, I am both a researcher and a clinician: one who respects the value of science and at the same time is driven primarily by a desire to serve my people. This essay combines my research on Native Hawaiian substance use with my experiences doing clinical work with Native Hawaiians in our communities. The causes I suggest are by no means exhaustive, nor are the clinically relevant aspects of Hawaiian culture that I have described. They are the factors that I chose to highlight because of their relevance to the people I have worked with. My work is offered with gratitude and the hope that it will be useful to my people and throughout the Pacific.*

According to most estimates, substance abuse among Native Hawaiians is increasing to an all-time high, with rates that are significantly higher than those for non-Hawaiians (Allan, 1998; Gartrell, Wood, & Ovenden, 2000; Hammond, 1988; Marsella, Oliveira, Plummer, & Crabbe, 1995; Office of Hawaiian Affairs, 2002). This increase is believed to be due in large part to the crystal methamphetamine (ice) epidemic that has taken hold in Hawai'i. Alcohol and other drug abuse rates are also increasing rapidly, with serious negative health consequences for our people. The higher prevalence rates for these problem behaviors among Native Hawaiians, and their apparent resistance to typical interventions (Gartrell et al., 2000; Hammond, 1988), suggest that something about Native Hawaiians and the conditions they live under is different from other groups.

A fundamental question to ask about Native Hawaiian substance use is: Why? Native Hawaiians are disproportionately represented among Hawai'i residents for substance dependence and abuse. What explains this difference? Do the same factors that contribute to this behavior among other ethnic and cultural groups hold for Native Hawaiians? Are there other factors? For example, an important factor that predicts substance abuse in adulthood is the age at which a person first tries alcohol. This relationship seems to be consistent across a variety of ethnic groups in the United States, and is true for Native Hawaiians as well (Austin, 2004a & b). At the same time, what is not understood is whether factors other than age at first use matter more for Native Hawaiians, and what predicts age at first use among Native Hawaiians.

The next critical question to ask is: What can we do to address this problem? Once we understand the factors that predict substance abuse, how do we use this understanding to improve the quality of the services that Native Hawaiians receive? This essay opens with a discussion of the nature of substance abuse among Native Hawaiians and the factors that predict its occurrence. Two factors are emphasized: the substance use and violent behavior of members of an individual's social network, and the impact that working and having a sense of purpose has on Native Hawaiian identity and health, as illustrated by the examples of three clients: Isaiah, Nohea, and Kaleo. The chapter then moves into a discussion of therapy and intervention for substance abuse within a Native Hawaiian context.

CASE EXAMPLE: ISAIAH

Isaiah is a 59-year-old Native Hawaiian man with Type II diabetes, major depression, and liver failure resulting from decades of drug and alcohol abuse. Isaiah began behavioral health treatment to support his recovery from drug and alcohol abuse and to assist him in coping with depression. Isaiah has a wife and two adult sons, although he did not live with any of them when he started treatment. Isaiah had been clean and sober for six months at the start of treatment and regularly attended self-help support group meetings to maintain his sobriety. He attended all scheduled appointments and maintained regular contact with his parole officer to update him on his treatment progress and take regular drug tests. Isaiah had relapsed back into drug use four or five times during his recovery process, which spanned over three years.

At the start of treatment, we focused our efforts on addressing Isaiah's depressed mood and health concerns, because his abstinence seemed rather well controlled. Isaiah's personal goals for treatment were to remain clean and sober, improve his health, and get a job. Frequent conflict with his wife and exposure to his drug-using social network were identified early on as triggers for relapse. Since Isaiah's first treatment goal was to remain clean and sober, we focused initially on using problem-solving strategies to help him avoid these triggers and keep his focus on recovery. In addition,

Isaiah successfully initiated a weight-loss program and showed improvement in his daily mood as a result of the exercise regimen he maintained. These improvements moved Isaiah much closer to his second goal, of improving his health overall.

Substance Use in Social Networks

There are many known individual factors that predict substance use, including early exposure to substance use, age at first use, initial tolerance, alcohol and drug expectancies, stress, education, and gender (Austin, 2004b; DeWit, Adlaf, Offord, & Ogborne, 2000; Paschall, Flewelling, & Faulkner, 2000; Petraitis, Flay, Miller, Torpy, & Greiner, 1998; Ritter, Stewart, Bernet, Coe, & Brown, 2002; Werner & Smith, 2001). Another important factor that explains alcohol use among Native Hawaiians is an individual's social network. The greater the number of substance users present in one's environment, within either the community or immediate family, the more likely a person is to have substance-use-related problems (Howard, Walker, Walker, Cottler, & Compton, 1999; Kumpfer & Hopkins, 1993). Individuals are influenced by the behavior around them. For Native Hawaiians, this connection is particularly strong, given the collectivist nature of the culture and the powerful influence of social norms within this group. Native Hawaiians who live and socialize with people who drink alcohol will themselves drink more alcohol. Johnson, Nagoshi, Ahern, Wilson, and Yuen (1987) found that Native Hawaiian cultural norms for alcohol use were important predictors of the level of alcohol use and risk of alcohol abuse among adults. Focus group data about mimicking what is around us also support this notion: "I'm doing exactly what I was bred to do, drink beer, cuz that's what my uncles did, and I thought that was cool" (Austin, 2004b, p. 54).

Native Hawaiians tend to drink socially, in garages, at family parties, and with relatives. Drinking occurs in a variety of settings and without need for a special occasion, as was historically the case. "Dad and I think nothing of driving to [the store] and buying a cold pack. Before, they only drink when there was a party, now, we drink cuz it's hot!! It's hot! Get me a cold beer! We had a good day, have a beer, we had a bad day, have a beer. It's not just to celebrate anymore" (Austin, 2001, Appendix D).

What this means for an individual Native Hawaiian is that there are numerous opportunities during the course of any week when drinking alcohol would be a completely normal and appropriate behavior. This makes detecting excessive or problematic drinking more difficult because one of the traditional identifiers of excessive use—drinking alone—may never be necessary in order to drink to abuse. The other issue here is that the amount of alcohol that individuals consume may increase as norms for consumption increase. Families where everyone has just one glass of wine with dinner may promote very different drinking behavior from a family that plans to consume one six-pack of beer per person.

ʻOhana

The family unit has been the fundamental component of Native Hawaiian social structure. It organized labor and dictated family leadership. The family unit was also primarily responsible for intervening in problem situations (Pukui, Haertig, & Lee, 1972). Today, Native Hawaiian families are cohesive units that include both immediate and extended family members across multiple generations (Austin & Marsella, 2005). An examination of Native Hawaiian adolescents suggests that family connectedness is higher among Native Hawaiians than non-Hawaiians (Nahulu et al., 1996). In addition, having a supportive family appears to be a more powerful protector against anxiety and depression for Native Hawaiians than non-Hawaiians (Goebert et al., 2000).

Much of what we understand about how substance abuse affects our communities comes from identifying what changes in a family system as a result of these behaviors. In Native Hawaiian families, greater substance use among family members was related to less family cohesion, greater family conflict, and less organization within the family (Kameoka, 1998).

ISAIAH ON *ʻOHANA*

Isaiah and I talked often about family and what it means to be a man. Despite his own challenges, Isaiah took care of his elderly father, who had significant health problems. His proudest achievements resulting from his hard work in rebuilding his life were repairing the relationship he had with his oldest son and being allowed to take care of his 2-year-old granddaughter during the day. His sense of family was so strong that when his estranged wife became ill, he reunited with her, despite knowing that she had often been a trigger for substance use in the past. Knowing how important it was for him to be able to take care of his family, I focused my efforts on strengthening his ability to cope with the inevitable frustrations she would bring, rather than trying to convince him not to bring her back into his life. Trying to convince him that taking care of her was the wrong thing to do, while logical from some perspectives, would have been contrary to his most fundamental assumptions about himself and the world.

Although it is well documented that having high family conflict increases a person's risk for relapse following treatment (Finney & Moos 1991; Kelly, Halford, & Young, 2000; Moos & Moos 1984; Schutte, Brennan,

& Moos, 1994), supporting Isaiah's efforts to care for his family was more important clinically than trying to reduce the overall level of conflict in his household.

CASE EXAMPLE: NOHEA

Nohea is a 35-year-old Native Hawaiian woman who first presented for treatment at the Health Center to assist in her recovery from drug and alcohol abuse. Nohea had successfully remained clean and sober for the better part of one year when we began treatment together, but continued to struggle with both depression and anger.

Nohea is married and has three children. Her children have lived with her mother since she lost custody of them almost a year prior to the start of treatment. Missing her children appeared to be the primary source of Nohea's depression. Nohea made numerous attempts to convince her mother to allow her to see her children, but these efforts were typically unsuccessful outside of the occasional one- to two-hour visit. Nohea often resorted to sitting outside of her children's school to see them as they came out. Nohea's husband continued to use drugs even after Nohea had stopped.

In addition to alcohol, crystal methamphetamine (ice) also has devastating effects on Native Hawaiian families and communities. A focus group of Native Hawaiians living in the continental United States identified the growing ice problem as a primary reason for moving away from Hawai'i (see Austin, 2004b). One of the most damaging aspects of ice on Native Hawaiian families is that it is so addictive that it compels the individual taking it to ignore core values and connections to other people. Individuals who are addicted to ice undergo complete shifts in personality and seem nearly unrecognizable to other members of their family.

CASE EXAMPLE: KALEO

Kaleo was a patient at a substance-abuse day-treatment program. Kaleo had been addicted to ice for over five years when he was mandated by the court to attend day treatment following a relatively minor offense at the age of 21. Kaleo had completed one week of detoxification at the time that he first presented to group treatment. After days of self-reported irritability and explosive anger, Kaleo was quiet and somewhat dazed for most of the group session. Finally, near the end of the session, he said, "Wow . . . this is heavy." He went on to tell us about how he could feel his mind clearing, which was a good feeling except that now he was totally awake to remember all of the bad things he had done, such as lying to everyone he knew, stealing money from his parents and relatives, and failing to show up for visits he'd arranged with his 4-year-old son. The full weight of his actions over the past several years appeared to hit him all at once and he was stunned by how little he had cared about his family's feelings and well-being while he was high. He viewed himself as fortunate for having been arrested and forced to participate in a treatment program, believing that he would have been unable to quit on his own.

Kaleo's experience is not novel, except that he was able to recover enough to realize what he had done to his family. Unfortunately, the pain of this realization actually put him at greater risk of relapse. Therefore, a primary therapeutic goal in working with Kaleo was to use his desire to make things right with his family in order to motivate him to participate in treatment and avoid ice use. Connecting Kaleo's love of his family to treatment made each step forward for him more meaningful. He could stay focused on a single path with clear expectations rather than trying to negotiate whether or not to use ice at every opportunity.

Doing Good Work and Having a Sense of Purpose

Again and again in my work treating Native Hawaiians with alcohol and drug abuse problems, I hear the recurring theme of losing purpose. Inevitably, alcohol and drug abuse problems co-occur with disruptions in every aspect of life. By the time most of my clients enter treatment, they have lost both their families and their jobs. In recounting their paths to substance abuse, clients talk about how they had initially sought relief from work and family pressures through substance use. This was typically followed by a period during which heavy substance use put a strain on their families and made them likely to miss work. Inevitably, this period resulted in family disruption and job loss, which, ironically, often led to greater substance use and depression. Native Hawaiians without a family or work to provide a sense of purpose can feel an overwhelming sense of hopelessness that makes it difficult for them to seek help.

NOHEA ON DOING GOOD WORK

Although Nohea had successfully remained clean and sober for a year at the time we started treatment, a key factor in her successful recovery was whether or not she'd be able to get a job. Nohea spent large blocks of time each day sitting inactive or arguing with her husband. Though by increasing her physical activity, we were able to reduce the amount of time she spent each day doing nothing, we struggled to find ways to keep her mind occupied. After a number of weeks of searching for a good solution to this problem, we decided that she would work toward getting a job. Almost immediately upon coming up with this plan, her mood lifted. She became excited about planning her future and completed each assignment with renewed energy. From then on, we organized her treatment plan around the steps required to attain her goal. We made timelines for how long it would take to complete each step toward getting a job, and talked a great deal about what working would mean for her life.

Nohea was ambivalent about working because she was worried about the inevitable stress associated with reentering the workforce and resuming her parenting responsibilities. At the same time, we had identified how important it was for her to feel productive again. She needed to occupy her time somehow and knew that the more useful the activity, the better she would feel.

This case study illustrates some of the particular issues faced by Native Hawaiian women involved in substance use. Prior to their fall into alcohol and drug abuse, most had busy, productive lives, where they worked and cared for their families. They saw themselves as the glue of their families and proudly recounted how they endured most of the burden and heartache for their families as well. The path into excessive use began differently for each of them, with some being casual alcohol users throughout their lives, while others joined in with their husband's drug use to be closer to him, and still others had endured horrific tragedies and deliberately sought escape in alcohol and drugs. What is shared by these women is that whatever the path, their fall into substance abuse inevitably led to unemployment, loss of home, and loss of children. What they mourn most as they come through recovery, and face the consequences of their substance abuse as sober women for the first time, is their identity. "I used to be able to work twelve hours and then come home and take care of the kids and my husband, and now look at me. I got nothing. I cannot handle nothing." The shame and guilt associated with not being able to parent their children or hold down a job is nearly crippling.

The importance of being able to do good work and to be productive is central to a Native Hawaiian's sense of self. Of all the consequences of colonization and the dispossession of land in Hawai'i, losing the socioeconomic structure that clearly defined a person's work and familial roles has been among the most destructive to Native Hawaiian individuals' identity. Families were organized in such a way that adults worked in close proximity to the families they were supporting. This organization was lost when families moved into cities to work for cash wages. Urban employment required a completely different skill set than had been cultivated in the traditional family system. The legacy of this disrupted socioeconomic structure continues to affect Native Hawaiians today. Native Hawaiians as a group are poorer than non-Hawaiians living in Hawai'i, make up the greatest portion of prison inmates, and have unemployment rates that are 3 percent higher than the state's rate of 4.3 percent (Office of Hawaiian Affairs, 2002).

A key therapeutic goal when working with Native Hawaiians who have lost their jobs and families to substance abuse is to restore their sense of purpose. Working steadily to accomplish a goal has a positive influence on an individual's self-esteem that cannot be achieved any other way.

ISAIAH ON DOING GOOD WORK

It appeared, after over eight months of sobriety and slow but steady improvements in weight, blood sugar levels, and mood, that we would be able to move toward addressing Isaiah's final goal of getting a job. We had used a workday format throughout treatment to help Isaiah remain physically active, complete assigned practices, and attend his almost-daily doctor's appointments and substance abuse meetings. Each week we reviewed his prior week's work and planned the coming week. He exuded pride in retelling his successful completion of all of his obligations, and each week we checked in on the progress he had made toward each of his treatment goals. His mood was much improved from the start of treatment and stable across weeks. Discussing the steps required to get a job was the logical next focus of treatment. The key question was how quickly to move toward that goal, given his history of relapse.

Therapy and Intervention in a Native Hawaiian Context

Although a number of substance abuse treatment models exist, including both group and individual formats, there are some consistencies across therapeutic models that appear to be relevant in working with Native Hawaiian clients. The nature and boundaries of the therapeutic relationship, self-disclosure practices, gift giving, the sense of time, and a process-versus-outcome orientation are all elements of the client-therapist relationship that need to be considered when working with Native Hawaiians.

Therapeutic Boundaries and Self-Disclosure

An individual's culture and worldview can impact upon every aspect of a therapeutic relationship, from the way in which information is shared to the outcome expected. The traditional therapeutic relationship in a Western sense involves establishing appropriate boundaries such as minimal therapist self-disclosure, maintaining a narrow focus on the specific problem at hand, and emphasizing a one-directional relationship where the therapist delivers help to the client, and not the other way around. In working with Native Hawaiian adults and children, many of these boundaries must be altered because they are so incongruent with Native Hawaiian values. For example, it is a convention of social interaction among Native Hawaiians to exchange information about where you are from and what your family name is. This information helps the other person place you in a context and possibly allows additional connections to be made between relatives and shared acquaintances. An individual may be viewed as more trustworthy if she or he is connected to a good family or to an area that is familiar to the listener. Further, in traditional times, individuals were thought to take on the traits associated with particular regions in Hawaiʻi. To some extent, this practice persists, as Native Hawaiian adults will often ask what school a person attended to get an idea of his or her characteristics such as wealth or athleticism, as well as similarity of experiences.

When extending this practice into a therapeutic setting, these same types of information are shared at the start of a therapeutic relationship as part of rapport building. At times, in addition to asking about what region I'm from and what high school I went to, Native Hawaiian clients will ask about my family names to see if there are any that they recognize. This type of information can be exchanged between client and therapist to establish a common ground, a mutual investment in the therapeutic process. In the context of substance abuse treatment, exchanging this information becomes even more important, as it allows clients to express pride in their background rather than beginning with an assessment of problems, which can evoke guilt and shame.

Gift Giving

Other Native Hawaiian beliefs and values can also appear in the therapeutic process, such as gift giving. In traditional Western therapeutic contexts, taking gifts from clients is considered problematic because the therapist may feel a sense of indebtedness to the client that could complicate client-therapist dynamics. The therapeutic exchange in this context is inherently not mutual, with obvious power differences between help-seeker and help-provider. In contrast, gift giving in a Native Hawaiian context has a different significance, one that is more generally grounded in culturally appropriate social interaction. It is customary when visiting others to bring a small gift. We make offerings to our ancestors and *akua* (gods/spirits) to honor them and express gratitude as a customary part of social and ceremonial protocols.

With this as a cultural backdrop, accepting gifts within a therapeutic context has a different meaning, which makes it more necessary and appropriate. In fact, there are times when not accepting a gift would be insulting to a Native Hawaiian family in a way that would be damaging to the therapist's work. Gift giving in a Native Hawaiian sense is less a form of payment and more an expression of gratitude and honor. Receiving a gift that someone has given allows that person to honor you. There is no explicit expectation of reciprocity, other than the receiver's responsibility to accept what has been given. Refusing a person's attempt to honor you dishonors him or her and suggests that you felt the gift was not good enough. Obviously, there must be some measure of caution applied to gift giving so that the client is not burdened financially by giving the gift or given any cue that such gifts are expected. In my experience with Native Hawaiian families, gifts that are offered at the end of treatment tend to be either food or something that is more thoughtful than it is expensive. These gifts tend to demonstrate that the person or family knows something about you and chose something that reflects that. Accepting a gift in the spirit it was given is the most appropriate choice for a therapist.

Sense of Time

The Hawaiian sense of time is also relevant to the therapeutic process. Time from a Native Hawaiian perspective is more relative and less linear than the Western perspective assumes. Events happen when they are meant to happen; they cannot be rushed or delayed. This has significant implications for short-term psychological interventions, which are about addressing problems through step-by-step problem solving. Having this view of time does not necessarily rule out short-term interventions, but it does require that these activities be reframed, and an effort be put into helping the client evaluate which indicators might suggest when the appropriate time to work toward change would be.

Process Orientation

The Native Hawaiian belief system also places greater emphasis on process rather than outcome. The effort put into an act, and the lessons learned from successes and failures, matter much more than the end product. This belief is particularly helpful in substance abuse treatment, where relapse rates are extremely high, making failure, even with good effort, more likely. This belief also has implications for the value of the therapeutic relationship. Native Hawaiian clients may attempt changes they otherwise wouldn't because they feel connected to their therapist and believe that making this effort is their contribution to the relationship.

Managing Termination

For this same reason, termination of treatment must proceed more carefully when working within a Native Hawaiian context, in order to avoid offending the client and undoing the positive steps that have been made therapeutically. If clients make an effort to change in large part because they value the *pilina* (relationship, connection) they have with you, then the same clients may undo the good work they have achieved if they feel that you are ending the interaction prematurely. One of the strategies that I have used when coming to the end of treatment with a Native Hawaiian family was to talk about the importance of their family unit being strong on its own. I wanted them to think of me as still being connected to them, just not through regular contact. I had them practice facing the problems and concerns of their daily life and thinking about what I would tell them to do to address them, what questions I would ask, what tools I would remind them to use. In some ways, preparing for termination happens throughout the course of treatment. By setting goals, we acknowledge that when those goals are met, it is a natural time to move on.

Another strategy that I have used in helping families deal with termination is to draw a parallel between myself and a family member who lives on another island. Although I may not see my relative very often or be able to share daily ups and downs with her or him, the connection is still there, what they shared with me is still there, and I can reach them whenever I need to. This is a particularly useful metaphor for substance abuse treatment because of the high relapse rates. It is likely that individuals with substance abuse problems will need to seek treatment more than once before they are successful in sustained recovery.

ISAIAH ON TREATMENT: DEFINING SUCCESS

After experiencing initial gains from treatment, Isaiah had a series of relapses that began when his wife moved back into their home. We had discussed relapse prevention on several occasions during the time that we had been working together, so that when the first of his most recent relapses occurred, we had a foundation for talking about what had happened. As predicted, marital conflict, paired with a chance encounter with a drug-using friend, triggered the initial relapse episode. We redefined success so that Isaiah's recovery from the relapse was our primary goal again. Interestingly, the same strategies that had proven to be successful for Isaiah in the past—daily exercise, following a schedule, relaxation techniques for tension and anger management, and problem solving—were the strategies that Isaiah selected to support his recovery. We talked about how his recovery was absolutely a success because he resumed sobriety within a few days this time, rather than after a period of months, as had been his pattern to this point.

Rather than blaming or being disappointed by relapse, I worked with him in treatment to view the relapse as useful information—perhaps an indicator that his life had gotten more complicated with increased demands and uncertainty too quickly for him to adjust to. We talked about how it was actually a good thing that he had relapsed while still in treatment with me, rather than having to go through the relapse and recovery process without support once treatment had ended.

Conclusions

For Isaiah, Nohea, and Kaleo, the journey through recovery never really ends. I concluded my work with each of them at very different points in their recovery. I knew Kaleo for less than one week, while my work with Isaiah and Nohea extended over a year. Isaiah continued to battle against relapse after we stopped working together, while at last report, Nohea was maintaining full-time employment and had permission to visit with her children regularly. The learning in each instance was mutual. I learned from them as they learned from me. Hawaiian identity, and the role of culture in therapy, was never really discussed explicitly in the context of treatment, but I feel certain that our work could not have proceeded without my attention to it. It affected the easy rapport that was established. It affected the tone and pace of our conversations. It affected the goals we set and how we chose to work toward them.

Substance abuse in the Native Hawaiian community presents a difficult set of challenges to our health and wellbeing as a people. Treatment and prevention efforts aimed at reducing substance abuse in our communities must proceed with sensitivity and understanding of the complex nature of this problem for our people, and the individual, social, and cultural factors that influence its expression.

References

Allan, A. T. (1988). No-shows at a community mental health clinic: A pilot study. *The International Journal of Social Psychiatry, 34*, 40–46.

Ary, D. V., Duncan, T. E., Biglan, A., Metzler, C. W., Noell, J. W., & Smolkowki, K. (1999). Development of adolescent problem behavior. *Journal of Abnormal Child Psychology, 27*, 141–150.

Austin, A. A. (2001). *Alcohol, tobacco, and other drug use, and violent behavior in a Native Hawaiian community*. Unpublished master's thesis, University of Hawai'i at Mānoa.

Austin, A. A. (2004a). Alcohol, tobacco, other drug use, and violent behavior among Native Hawaiians: Ethnic pride and resilience. *Substance Use & Misuse, 39*, 771–796.

Austin, A. A. (2004b). *Native Hawaiian risky behavior: The role of individual, social, and cultural factors in predicting substance use and violence*. Unpublished doctoral dissertation, University of Hawai'i at Mānoa.

Austin, A. A., & Marsella, A. J. (2005). Understanding substance abuse and violent behavior in a Native Hawaiian community. In A. J. Marsella, A. A. Austin, & B. A. Grant (Eds.), *Social change and psychosocial adaptation in the Pacific Islands: Cultures in transition* (pp. 171–186). New York: Springer.

Damphousse, K., & Kaplan, H. B. (1998). Intervening processes between adolescent drug use and psychological distress: An examination of the self-medication hypothesis. *Social Behavior and Personality, 26*, 115–130.

DeWit, D. J., Adlaf, E. M., Offord, D. R., & Ogborne, A. C. (2000). Age at first alcohol use: A risk factor for the development of alcohol disorders. *American Journal of Psychiatry, 157*, 745–750.

Downs, W. R. (1987). A panel study of normative structure, adolescent alcohol use and peer alcohol use. *Journal of Studies on Alcohol, 48*, 167–175.

Finney, J. W., & Moos, R. H. (1991). The long-term course of treated alcoholism: I. Mortality, relapse, and remission rates and comparisons with community controls. *Journal of Studies on Alcohol, 52*, 44–54.

Gartrell, J., Wood, D. W., & Ovenden, A. (2000). *Substance abuse in Hawai'i: Adult population household telephone survey (1998)*. Technical Report. Honolulu: Department of Health.

Goebert, D., Nahulu, L., Hishinuma, E., Bell, C., Yuen, N., Carlton, B., Andrade, N. N., Miyamoto, R., & Johnson, R. (2000). Cumulative effects of family environment on psychiatric symptomatology among multiethnic adolescents. *Journal of Adolescent Health, 27*, 1–9.

Hammond, O. W. (1988). Needs assessment and policy development: Native Hawaiians as Native Americans. *American Psychologist, 43*, 383–387.

Howard, M. O., Walker, R. D., Walker, P. S., Cottler, L. B., & Compton, W. M. (1999). Inhalant use among urban American Indian youth. *Addiction, 94*, 83–95.

Jenkins, J. E. (1996). The influence of peer affiliation and student activities on adolescent drug involvement. *Adolescence, 31*, 297–306.

Johnson, R. C., Nagoshi, C. T., Ahern, F. M., Wilson, J. R., & Yuen, S. H. L. (1987). Cultural factors as explanations for ethnic group differences in alcohol use in Hawaii. *Journal of Psychoactive Drugs, 19*, 67–75.

Kameoka, V. A. (1998). Psychometric evaluation of measures for assessing the effectiveness of a family-focused substance abuse prevention intervention among Pacific Island families and children. In N. Mokuau (Ed.), *Responding to Pacific Islanders: Culturally competent perspectives for substance abuse prevention, CSAP Cultural Competence Series 8*, (pp. 25–47). Rockville, MD: Department of Health and Human Services.

Kelly, A. B., Halford, W. K., & Young, R. M. (2000). Maritally distressed women with alcohol problems: The impact of short-term alcohol-focused intervention on drinking behavior and marital satisfaction. *Addiction, 95*, 1537–1549.

Kumpfer, K. L., & Hopkins, R. (1993). Prevention: Current research and trends. *Psychiatric Clinics of North America, 16*, 11–20.

Marsella, A. J., Oliveira, J. M., Plummer, C. M., & Crabbe, K. M. (1995). Native Hawaiian (Kanaka Maoli) culture, mind, and well-being. In H. I. McCubbin, A. I. Thompson, & J. E. Fromer (Eds.), *Resiliency in ethnic minority families,* vol. 1: *Native and immigrant American families,* (pp. 93–112). Madison: University of Wisconsin Press.

Moos, R. H., & Moos, B. S. (1984). The process of recovery from alcoholism III. Comparing functioning of families of alcoholics and matched control families. *Journal of Studies on Alcohol, 45,* 111–118.

Nahulu, L. B., Andrade, N. N., Makini, G. K., Yuen, N. Y. C., McDermott, J. F., Danko, G. P., Johnson, R. C., & Waldron, J. A. (1996). Psychosocial risk and protective influences in Hawaiian adolescent psychopathology. *Cultural Diversity and Mental Health, 2,* 107–114.

Office of Hawaiian Affairs (2002). *Native Hawaiian data book.* Honolulu: Author.

Paschall, M. J., Flewelling, L., & Faulkner, D. L. (2000). Alcohol misuse in young adulthood: Effects of race, educational attainment, and social context. *Substance Use & Misuse, 35,* 1485–1506.

Petraitis, J., Flay, B. R., Miller, T. Q., Torpy, E. J., & Greiner, B. (1998). Illicit substance use among adolescents: A matrix of prospective predictors. *Substance Use & Misuse, 33,* 2561–2604.

Pukui, M. K., Haertig, E. W., & Lee, C. A. (1972). *Nānā i ke kumu (Look to the source),* Vol. 2. Honolulu: Hui Hānai.

Ritter, J., Stewart, M., Bernet, C., Coe, M., & Brown, S. A. (2002). Effects of childhood exposure to familial alcoholism and family violence on adolescent substance use, conduct problems, and self-esteem. *Journal of Traumatic Stress, 15,* 113–122.

Schutte, K. K., Brennan, P. L., & Moos, R. H. (1994). Remission of late-life drinking problems: A 4-year follow-up. *Alcoholism: Clinical and Experimental Research, 18,* 835–844.

Werner, E. E., & Smith, R. S. (2001). *Journeys from childhood to midlife: Risk, resilience, and recovery.* Ithaca, NY: Cornell University Press.

18

Pregnancy, Adoption, FASD, and Mental Illness

SUIAMAI SIMI

I was born in the village of Fasito'otai in Samoa. A few hours after I arrived, my grandmother Sa'ese'ese Afamasaga Aukuso held me close to her frail body, looked me eye to eye (hers dimmed; mine, unaccustomed to light, were closed tight), and said that she was ready to go. She named me Suia-mai (a changeover) to signify the generational link that she and I were about to effect. She explained that she was ready to go and that I had come to take her place. She blessed me, then died two days later. Two years went by and her son Simi Savai'inaea Sekai followed her, leaving his creative and resourceful wife Lualua'i (nee Tamaseu) widowed, with their ten children. I am number nine.

Weeding was a task my mother and I often did together and during those times, she repeatedly and unconsciously (when she told me to pull out the roots) planted deep within me a principle that has left a lasting influence on how I should deal with problems, that is, to find and remove the roots and the problems will go. I have learned though that some problem roots are permanent, and others difficult to remove because, to start with, we don't know what to look for. Problems often need to be observed over time within and without their dynamic milieu of associated problems woven tightly together in subtle patterns that defy any attempt to find the roots. Losses associated with adoption, abandonment, poor parenting, and being born prematurely have received, I believe, far more than their just share as being the roots of antisocial behaviors and learning and mental problems that afflict many. Many books, research reports, and articles have been written on these issues. In this essay fetal alcohol spectrum disorder (FASD) is added to the matrix, and is presented as being a significant root of many of the problems mentioned.

Permanent roots cannot be removed and we just have to learn to dance with the resulting problems to the tune of the roots. FASD belongs to this type—it is for life. Correct diagnosis attracts right treatment. When we can identify and understand FASD, we can make a big difference in the lives of those affected. Often, through a lack of understanding problems, we can end up hurting the very people we try to help. This essay challenges us all to protect our future generations from FASD.

Through the twentieth century, research produced mounting evidence that in vitro exposure to alcohol can have devastating effects on the development of the unborn child. At a molecular level, "alcohol itself acts as a teratogen (an agent causing deformities) and specifically, as a neurotoxin (an agent that is toxic to brain cells and other nerve cells in the body)" (Kitson & Parackal, 2005). Throughout the lifespan, the consequent developmental impairment can result in complex psychological, learning, and behavioral problems. In a study of more than four hundred participants with a history of prenatal exposure to alcohol, Streissguth and O'Malley (1997) found that almost all had experienced mental health difficulties for which they had been referred to psychiatrists, psychologists, or social workers. This essay is therefore a conch shell, calling Pacific Island professionals and communities around the world to rise up and protect our unborn babies from FASD and to provide support and protection to those in our communities affected by it.

Fetal Alcohol Spectrum Disorder (FASD)

Although pregnant women have been warned against drinking alcohol in writings as ancient as the Bible and the works of Aristotle, and poor birth outcomes and patterns of birth defects were noted in studies by Sullivan (1899) in Britain and Lemoine (1968) in France, respectively, it was not until the later years of the twentieth century that fetal alcohol syndrome (FAS) was identified by Smith and Jones (Alberta Learning, Special Programmes Branch, 2004). These researchers noted a characteristic set of facial features and neurological changes in infants and children of mothers who were alcoholics while pregnant. Currently, a full diagnosis of FAS is based on a history of maternal drinking during pregnancy, as well as the presence of: (1) growth deficiencies; (2) a specific cluster of facial anomalies; and (3) central nervous system disorder.

The term *fetal alcohol effects* (FAE) was coined by Clarren in 1978 to describe a set of characteristics now known as alcohol-related neuro-developmental disorder (ARND), which he observed in a large group of physically healthy children and adults who seemed to be of relatively normal intelligence, but who experienced difficulties coping with the long-term effects of maternal alcohol abuse during pregnancy. Although these people were minimally affected by the facial characteristics of FAS, which had often disappeared by their mid-teens, they struggled with learning and behavioral problems that indicated dysfunctional central nervous systems (Buxton, 2004).

It is helpful to be familiar with other terms that have developed out of further research in the field, including partial fetal alcohol syndrome (PFAS) and alcohol-related birth defects (ARBD). As FAS was found to denote only the tip of the iceberg, and these other, hidden aspects related to FAS became more apparent, the need was evident for a term to describe the broad range of effects of prenatal alcohol exposure that do not apparently qualify for a FAS diagnosis. "By the end of the twentieth century," as Buxton (2004) reports, "fetal alcohol spectrum disorder (FASD) began to be used as an umbrella term denoting several kinds of diagnosis, just as the word *cancer* can refer to a number of debilitating conditions" (p. 45). In April 2004, the following definition was constructed by leaders in the field:

> Fetal Alcohol Spectrum Disorder (FASD) is an umbrella term describing the range of effects that can occur in an individual whose mother drank alcohol during pregnancy. These effects may include physical, mental, behavioral, and/or learning disabilities with possible lifelong implications. The term FASD is not intended for use as a clinical diagnosis. (NOFAS, 2004)

In the context of FASD, the term *primary disabilities* refers to the effect of alcohol on the fetus, including brain damage, facial characteristics, and small head or body. *Secondary disabilities* are those that develop after a person is born, particularly in the absence of appropriate care and protection to meet the special needs created by FASD.

In a study of secondary disabilities associated with FAS and FAE involving 473 participants, Streissguth and O'Malley (1997) found that of the six main secondary disabilities studied, mental health problems were by far the most prevalent, experienced by over 90 percent of the sample. Additionally, in participants age 12 and over, disrupted school experience (suspension, expulsion, or dropping out) and trouble with the law (defined as ever having been in trouble with authorities, charged, or convicted of a crime) characterized 60 percent of the sample. Approximately 50 percent experienced confinement (including inpatient treatment for mental health problems or alcohol/drug problems, or having been incarcerated for a crime), and a similar percentage had engaged in inappropriate sexual behavior. Approximately 30 percent of the participants were noted as having had alcohol and/or drug problems.

A list in the Royal Canadian Mounted Police FASD Guidebook (2003) identifies a range of problems that provide an indication of the scope of potential secondary disabilities: fear, anxiety, avoidance, withdrawal; victimization of and by others; shutting down, lying, running away, dropping out of school, joblessness, homelessness; willingness to please and comply; mental illness, depression, self-injury; violent or threatening behavior, impulsivity, trouble with the law; addiction issues; suicide. Malbin (2002) has also identified a number of these characteristics, including the broader categories of trouble at home and/ or school and mental health problems, and has added to the list fatigue, tantrums, irritability, frustration, anger, and aggression. Kellerman (2002), herself an adoptive mother of an FASD child, has also noted the psychological manifestations of brain damage: emotional lability; inability to learn from consequences; attention deficits (not always hyperactive, but easily distracted by external stimuli); short-term memory deficits; inappropriate social interactions; difficulty managing money; poor judgment; vulnerability and naiveté.

Streissguth headed a team of researchers who studied 415 clients who had been diagnosed with FAS. The study identified a series of protective factors in the environment that might mitigate the long-term effects of FASD. The two most significant factors were obtaining an early diagnosis (before the age of 6) and living in a stable, nurturing environment (University of Washington, 2004). What this and many parallel studies emphasize is that while the negative effects of a mother's alcohol consumption during pregnancy cannot be reversed, the long-term damage can be contained through environmental stability, non-exposure to violence in the home, and particular attention during the formative years of late childhood and early adolescence.

Adoption, Premature Birth, and the Case of Fala

My own curiosity to understand what I now recognize as FASD started in the 1990s while I was working as an adoption social worker. I read everything on adoption that came my way. The lack of literature on Pacific Island adoption meant that most of my reading was from pālagi resources. It did not matter, because what I observed was that while the reasons for adoptions and the processes for effecting them varied with each case, culture, and country, the issues for those who were party to adoption relationships were basically the same.

People can be deeply affected by the losses and grief associated with adoption. For birth mothers/parents, it is the grief of having to give up children. For the adoptive parents with infertility issues, it is grief over the loss of the children that they could not have. For adopted people, it is loss associated with not growing up in their biological families, and not knowing who they are in the case of closed adoptions. Older children placed for adoption may also have suffered from multiple placements and often, from abuse. I came across all these issues among many of the Pacific Island adoption cases that were allocated to me.

I also became aware of the existing concern over the behavioral and/or learning problems known to be common among adopted people and of their disproportionate representation in psychotherapy in the United States, as well as in residential treatment centers, juvenile halls (correction centers), and special schools (Verrier, 1993). Consistent patterns of psychological and behavioral problems had been reported, and the individuals were characterized as impulsive, provocative, aggressive, and antisocial.

While still doing adoption work, however, I discovered through my reading that the antisocial behavior and other issues common among adopted children are also common among children who are born prematurely. I left the adoption work wondering whether there could be a common causal root to the behavior manifesting in these two groups of children—adopted/fostered and premature. The case of Fala illustrates the issues in question.

Fala is a Pacific Island teenager fostered by his aunt Lina (not their real names). Lina said that she was privileged to be foster mother to Fala. He was full of life, playful, and cheerful, and had a great sense of humor, a pleasure to have, but raising him had been a challenge. She said that knowing that Fala was born prematurely—at 29 weeks with a gestation weight of 1,460 grams (3.21 pounds)—forearmed her to deal with the problems that she had since learned were typical FASD characteristics. As a toddler, Fala had a number of seizures. When he was able to stand and hold on to things, rocking his new wooden cot became his favorite pastime, and the cot was a complete wreck before he was 3. As he grew older, he had become oppositional and reacted explosively to changes. He fought off both sleep and work. He had a short concentration span and had difficulty keeping on task.

Toward the end of intermediate school (junior high school), the teacher had written to Lina, concerned that Fala was not completing his homework, and that he had not developed the study skills required to succeed in high school. Getting him to do his homework was a struggle and Lina said that often she just gave up trying and instead directed her energy to ensuring that they had a happy relationship.

Fala had been suspended from school, and interviewed twice by police for his involvement in fights. Doing detention after school or during recess time was normal for him. (Detentions disappeared after Lina visited the school with FASD literature and explained that Fala was a potential FASD victim.) His high school reports were dominated by comments such as, "far too easily distracted and does not always behave in a positive manner . . . has more ability than his marks indicate, major problem has been that he has found it hard to settle into a pattern of work . . . seldom does his homework, although is capable of producing work of good quality . . . lacks concentration . . . needs to discipline himself to remain on task . . . tends to be talkative at inappropriate times . . . he finds it difficult to follow instructions," and so on.

Those who know Lina and the way she deals with others would say that she was extremely patient and lenient, but Lina admitted that she had smacked Fala a few times. Here are some examples of their experiences: Fala was about 12. He usually dressed the way he wished. On one cold wet winter morning, however, he was asked to wear his jersey (sweater). He resisted aggressively but finally put it on after Lina persisted. At the door, Lina noted that it was beginning to rain so she asked Fala to wear his cap; again the instruction was met with intense opposition. As the tension built, Fala, with big tears rolling down from glassy eyes red with anger and determination, looked up straight into Lina's eyes and politely screamed, "Please, aunty, don't make me do it." Shocked and puzzled by the defiance, Lina, who was struggling to remain calm, came near to slapping Fala on the face. She was sure, however, that Fala would be sick by the evening if he did not wear his cap, and she decided that that would be the time to say, "I told you so." So, controlling her anger, she bent down, kissed Fala and said, "Go." (Fala did not get sick in the evening or at all during that winter.)

When Fala was 16, a similar scenario occurred and again it was winter. This incident, however, provided Lina with a profound insight. Fala had missed school for a day due to a cold. He normally wet his hair in the morning and left it soaking wet. Because he had been sick, Lina asked him to dry his hair properly. He resisted, giving as his reasons that "people won't know that I have had a shower in the morning" and "my hair looks untidy when it is dry." As usual, he was articulate. Tension started to build. As in the first incident, Fala was asked to wear his jersey and he resisted, not accepting any reasoning. He was then told not to bus home after school, but that he would be picked up. He became more oppositional and did not want to comply with any of the three instructions given.

At that time Lina had learned that Fala's mother had drunk alcohol during her pregnancy and that much of Fala's learning problems and antisocial behavior, including his dislike of change and his oppositional behavior were common characteristics of children affected by fetal alcohol brain damage. So Lina bottled up all the pressure calmly, but firmly insisted that Fala obey all three instructions given.

In the kitchen, uncooperative Fala was having breakfast and had just put down an empty glass. Lina walked in and picked up the glass, thinking she would rinse it and put it aside to be washed later. Instead, she hurled the glass across the kitchen into the sink, shattering it to pieces. She was shocked and immediately regretted her impulsive action, thinking that if the inflamed situation had caused her (an adult, a social worker, a counselor to families with parenting problems, and an ex-teacher) to behave in this way, how would Fala's 16-year-old alcohol-affected brain be coping? How much longer could he cope? Fala, for his part, sat stunned and silent

It is well documented that people with FASD generally find it hard to handle changes in their routine. Evensen and Lutke (1997), in their brochure *8 Magic Keys,* advise caregivers to be consistent: "Because of the difficulty students with FAS experience trying to generalize learning from one situation to another, they do best in an environment with few changes. This includes language. Teachers and parents can coordinate with each other to use the same words for key phrases and oral direction" (n.p.). In her *Ain't Misbehavin'* brochure, Evensen reminds parents that FAS children "don't have moveable parts in the thinking process; so, when you change a piece of the routine for the child, you have created an entirely new routine" (n.p.).

Fala's case illustrates the importance of effective change management in the routine of someone affected by FASD, and that understanding this can make a big difference in the day-to-day interactions with them. Lina understood Fala's situation, but it took her a while to realize that it was not just a matter of Fala's not wanting to do what he was asked to do. For Fala, it was also a case of experiencing three unexpected changes to his routine and he was struggling to cope. Realizing this, Lina withdrew one of her instructions, and said he could bus home, but he must dry his hair (which he did to his standard) and wear his jersey (which he put on without a word). On their way to school, Lina was able to explain a few more things and they parted happily. Understanding Fala's condition did not save one of the few glasses they own, but it certainly saved their relationship for the rest of the day.

Connecting with the FASD family

In 2003 I read stories of Native American children affected by FASD who had been fostered and who were subjects of legal battles over whether they should be adopted by their foster families or returned to their native tribes who were demanding them. I thought of Fala. He was born prematurely, had been fostered, and had behavioral and learning problems similar to those I had seen in the adoption context, and more recently read about in the FASD literature, but I did not think his birthmother, Kana (not her real name), had drunk alcohol while pregnant. I shared my thoughts with Lina, who agreed to ask Kana. The answer was yes. A pediatrician later wrote that Kana "was working during the pregnancy; she took no drugs but she was a social drinker, particularly at parties on the weekends, and at times she thinks she probably got reasonably high but never totally intoxicated and this was a relatively infrequent occurrence."

When Lina told me that Kana drank while pregnant with Fala, my thoughts raced through the facts: Fala was fostered (in-family); he was born prematurely; he had a confirmed history of prenatal alcohol exposure; his behavior and learning problems were typical of those of children affected by FASD as well as a number of adopted children. Some children with prenatal alcohol exposure are born prematurely and remain with their birth families. Others are adopted or fostered. Some are born full-term and remain in their families while others are fostered or adopted, with the possibility of the recipient family's having no knowledge of FASD and that the mother drank during pregnancy. Whether a child is premature or not, or remains with the birth parents, or is adopted/fostered, the brain damage caused by alcohol in the uterus is permanent.

With respect to adopted children, Verrier (1994) had sought to find an explanation for the "high incidence of sociological, academic, and psychological disturbance among this population" and their predisposition to this vulnerability (p. xvi). The title of her own book on adoption includes the metaphor "the primal wound" and in the title of their book, Keck and Kupecky (1995) have used the metaphor "the hurt child" in addressing adoption issues for families in which the child has special needs. This led me to wonder whether Verrier's primal wound and Keck and Kupecky's hurt child, and their associated problems, may not stem solely from adoption or fostering issues, but that FASD may be a significant root of the problems in many adoption cases. Even ten years ago, at the time when these and many other books and articles on adoption were being published, FASD was not mentioned, or mentioned but not recognized as well as it is today. Intrigued, my curiosity led me to investigate further. In research by Streissguth et al. (2004), for example, 80 percent of their sample of 415 participants with FAS or FAE were not raised by their biological mothers. If they were not with their biological mothers, then it is possible that many may have been either adopted or fostered.

Speaking of the importance of identifying the influence of FAS on children's development and wellbeing, Ferry (1997) has urged:

> As adoption and FAS are often found together, every effort must be made to get these records and locate the birth mother or substantiate the cause of death if she is deceased. It is possible that her death may have been caused by an alcohol-related disease or accident. Follow her fate as far as possible because, even if she simply dropped out of sight, her trail up to her disappearance may indicate a life shattered by alcohol. Try to establish how many children she had (along with spontaneous abortions, if any) and whether any children were put up for adoption or removed from her care and whether or not their fate is indicative of FAS impairment. (p. 46)

The high incidence of children in foster care and available for adoption was underscored by Buxton (2004), who reported statistics from southern Alberta, Canada, an area with a total population of 146,000. "All children in care of child protection services were assessed for fetal alcohol damage, and 50 percent were found to have FASD. Among children in permanent care and thus available for adoption, 70 percent had FASD" (p. 50). In the absence of comparable statistics for our Pacific population here, there is no reason to believe the situation would be any different.

The Challenge

The mental health of our communities starts in the womb. As a child, I asked my mother where I came from. She said that I grew inside a beautiful bag situated close to her heart. The bag, I later learned, is the womb, including the *fanua* (in Samoan, meaning both land and afterbirth). Rooted in this fanua, the new life draws nutrients from whatever the *palapala* or *'ele'ele* (soil or earth, but metaphorically, blood) yields. The fetus grows, unfolds, and takes shape according to its unique complex blueprint inherited from its parents. As a community we are vigilant in protecting our lands—mother earth—from pollution, including environmentally persistent neurotoxins like mercury and lead. Wisdom and morality dictate that we should be equally vigilant in keeping the fanua/uterus, home to our unborn babies, including their developing brains, absolutely free from all such pollution, including alcohol.

This humble conch shell's final note is that it is time we all imitated the biblical angel who told a young woman that she was about to become pregnant and have a baby, and that she was therefore not to drink wine or any fermented drink (Judges 13). Our communities need leaders who will blow the conch shells, beat the *lali*, the *pātē*, the empty cabin-bread tin, the empty gas cylinder, sing, preach, teach, and by example, sound out the message that as a community we need to support our women in making the decision not to drink when pregnant, breast feeding, or likely to be pregnant. This is a community problem that needs community action. We must pass the message on and educate the whole community, including our children, relatives, friends, church members, club mates, and work mates, as a personal as well as a professional responsibility. We must also develop cultures and rituals that support our women in avoiding drinking alcohol while pregnant—cultures and rituals that can transcend this generation into the next, with the message that pregnancy and alcohol do not mix, because one child with FASD is one child too many.

A ritual that is now observed by many around the world is International FASD Awareness Day, held on the ninth day of the ninth month every year (http://www.fasday.com). As the first country to see in the dawn of each new day, New Zealand has proudly marked FASD Awareness Day since its inception in 1999. The challenge now is to build a broader awareness of this problem on the part of our professions and the wider Pasifika community, to develop our local knowledge of its consequences for individuals and their families, and to commit ourselves to action to address the damage alcohol has caused our babies, and prevent further devastation.

References

Alberta Learning, Special Programmes Branch. (2004). *Teaching students with Fetal Alcohol Spectrum Disorder: Building strengths, creating hope*. Edmonton, Alberta: Author.

Buxton, B. (2004). *Damaged angels: A mother discovers the terrible cost of alcohol in pregnancy*. Toronto: Alfred A. Knopf.

Evensen, D. (n.d.) *'Ain't Misbehavin': Understanding the behaviors of children and adolescents with Fetal Alcohol Syndrome*. Retrieved May 4, 2005, from www.fasstar.com.

Evensen, D., & Lutke, J. (1997). *8 magic keys: Developing successful interventions for students with FAS*. Fetal Alcohol Consultation and Training Services. Retrieved May 5, 2005, from http://www.fasalaska.com/8keys.html.

Ferry, D. (1997). Fetal Alcohol Syndrome: An effective capital defense. *California Attorneys for Criminal Justice Forum, 24*(2), 42–50.

Keck, G. C., & Kupecky, R. M. (1995). *Adopting the hurt child: Hope for families with special-needs kids*. Colorado Springs: Pinon Press.

Kellerman, T. (2002). *Fetal Alcohol Spectrum Disorders: Soft signs*. Tucson, AZ: FAS Community Resource Center.

Kitson, K. E., & Parackal, S. M. (2005). Alcohol in pregnancy—limiting the potential of our future sports people? *Proceedings of the Sport and Alcohol Conference, Massey University, Palmerston North, New Zealand,* February 8–10, 2005.

Malbin, D. (2002). *Understanding Fetal Alcohol Syndrome/Alcohol-Related Neurodevelopmental Disorder (FAS/ARND)*. Retrieved October 3, 2004, from www.fascets.org/info.html.

National Organization on Fetal Alcohol Syndrome (NOFAS). (2004, April 15). *Historical agreement heralds new era for prevention and treatment of Fetal Alcohol Spectrum Disorders*. Press release, retrieved April 26, 2005, from http://www.nofas.org/news/04152004.aspx.

Royal Canadian Mounted Police. (2003). *Fetal Alcohol Spectrum Disorder, FASD guidebook for police officers*. Ottawa: Royal Canadian Mounted Police.

Streissguth, A. P., Bookstein, F. L., Barr, H. M., Sampson, P. D., O'Malley, K. D, & Young, J. K. (2004). Risk factors for adverse life outcomes in Fetal Alcohol Syndrome and Fetal Alcohol Effects. *Developmental and Behavioral Pediatrics 25*(4), 228–238.

Streissguth, A. P. (1997). *Fetal Alcohol Syndrome: A guide for families and communities*. Baltimore: Brookes Publishing Company.

Streissguth, A. P., & O'Malley, K. D. (1997). Fetal Alcohol Syndrome/Fetal Alcohol Effects: Secondary disabilities and mental health approaches. *Treatment Today,* 9(2), 16–17.

University of Washington. (2004, August 10). *New hope for fetal alcohol syndrome shown in study.* Press release, retrieved October 10, 2004, from http://depts.washington.edu/fadu/.

Verrier, N. N. (1994). *The primal wound: Understanding the adopted child.* Baltimore: Gateway Press.

19

Misplaced Dreams
Tongan Gambling in Auckland

YVETTE GUTTENBEIL-POʻUHILA
AND SIONE TUʻITAHI

Yvette: *Many things and many people have contributed to* me *today. I hail from the "Fatafata Māfana" Moʻunga Talau/Fungamisi Vavaʻu, and the stormy waters of Hūfangalupe, Tongatapu.*

My family migrated from Tonga to Ponsonby, Aotearoa, when I was 3 and then to Avondale when I was 7—where like the market my life has been vibrant and mixed with many peoples, languages, music, and food! And like many other children from the Pacific, I have survived changes, socialization, and alienation to become me *today—daughter, mother, wife, sister, aunty, friend. In my other life I am a sociologist, researcher, consultant, project manager, and network coordinator. But in this context I am co-author.*

Gambling for Tongan people in Auckland is a complex issue. Understanding its nature involves addressing a mixture of sociocultural concepts, the effects of migration, intergenerational relationships, the power of money, and its links to dreams and perceptions. Central is surviving in the world with what you know and what you have.

This essay is by no means an exhaustive discussion but it is a start. At its heart are the Tongan people, families, and communities, which gambling, the industry, and its supporters entice, deprive, and eventually destroy.

Fakaʻapaʻapa Atu.

Sione: *My studies, work, and travel enrich the islander in me to operate as a world citizen, embracing cultural diversity while observing certain global phenomena such as migration and materialism that are transforming societies around the world, in particular, indigenous minorities. Although gambling is as old as humanity, repackaging it in the context of a more secular society (and with the aid of modern technology) makes it very enticing to low socioeconomic groups who are not fully aware of its adverse socioeconomic costs. Gambling was partly chosen for the research upon which this essay is based, largely because it was seen as an emerging health issue for Tongans in Auckland. It is one of many social and economic fac-*

tors that need to be researched for the benefit of Pacific peoples and other groups.

From teaching I recently moved to policy and strategic planning at Massey University, while managing the Pacific team, Vaka Ola, at the Auckland Regional Public Health Service, a branch of the Auckland District Health Board. Working simultaneously in health and education provides a greater opportunity to be more holistic and effective in serving Pacific peoples, since they have the highest needs for better health and education among all ethnic groups in New Zealand.

Anecdotal evidence that some Tongan families were suffering socially and economically as a result of gambling led to an investigation into why Tongan people in Auckland gamble. Tongans have been migrating from their group of 170 islands to Aotearoa/New Zealand since the 1960s in search of a better socioeconomic life. Discovering that problem gambling was already a major health and social issue within the Tongan community in Auckland, rather than an emerging one, was a rude awakening to the authors. In this essay we reflect on some of the findings from a study of gambling issues in the Auckland Tongan community (Guttenbeil-Poʻuhila & Tuʻitahi, 2004), and discuss specific sociocultural factors in Tongan culture that may contribute to problem gambling.

Research Methods

When embarking on this project, the team sought to find Tongan research frameworks to guide the data collection, analysis, and the dissemination of the results. This reflected the team's commitment to cultural integrity, and a desire to realize the various possibilities and understandings of "our own things" rather than trying to fit into Western research processes. Tongan values and principles were incorporated through the adoption of Helu-Thaman's (1999) *kakala* model that was chosen to guide the recruitment and interviewing of participants as data were collected, the analysis of the data, and the presentation and dissemination of the findings. In addition, to assist with the analysis and interpretation of the data, we included *pō talanoa*. Each of these is explained below.

The Kakala *Model: A Cultural Framework*

Helu-Thaman's (1999) model was developed out of a critique of Western educational constructs that reflect Western values, aims, and methods, and the way in which they have replaced the Tongan worldview, values, and processes. Based on Tongan values and principles such as reciprocity, sharing, respect, collectivism, and context-specific skills and knowledge, it describes the processes of gathering knowledge and information, analyzing and arranging it, and applying it through gift giving.

The kakala (flowers/fragrant flora used for adornment) model is based on the traditional process of fragrant garland making and is divided into three distinct stages. The first is the time of *toli kakala,* when experts are sent out to gather special flowers and flora to make the garland. These people are familiar with the natural materials, locations, scents, shades, sizes, textures, and the preservation of the raw materials so that they remain pristine. This is likened to the fieldwork stage, when information is gathered from appropriate people and communities by experts in recruitment and interviewing.

The next stage is the *tui kakala*, which Helu-Thaman (1999) likens to the time of data input, analysis, and authorship. This process involves taking the raw materials to the *kau tui kakala*, experts in traditional and contemporary design, to determine the best method of weaving the flowers and flora together. These experts hold knowledge about which designs are appropriate for certain occasions and for certain ranks in royalty, nobility, ministers, villagers, and so forth. They comment on the method and correctness of the weave, material, and design, and discuss symbolic meanings of the importance and rank of raw materials, and the intrinsic meanings of the kakala.

The final process is the time of *luva e kakala*, which follows the completion of the garland. This involves the dissemination and ownership of information from the research project. In the luva process, when the garland is completed, it is offered and/or presented as a gift to the person being honored at the special occasion—the festival, dance, birthday, or wedding. A kakala is not made to be kept by those who have created it. Even in death, a special kakala is made for the departed. Our participation in this publication is part of the dissemination of the information gathered in this research project, as it belongs to all the Tongan community as well as to those who contributed to this research.

Pō talanoa: *An Analysis of Findings*

In order to enhance our understandings of why Tongan people in Auckland gamble, *pō talanoa* (a conversational process) was included during the time of the kau tui kakala, when raw data from fieldwork and the thoughts and commentaries of leaders, professionals, ministers, academics, and community people were brought together for analysis and pō talanoa (Helu-Thaman, 1999). This reflected the spirit of Helu's (1999) advice about putting aside referencing from others and turning to our own internal and personal knowledge to develop further understandings.

Phases of the Research Process

This research was planned in two phases. Throughout the process, the researchers were assisted by advisory teams representing relevant perspectives including the gambling industry, gambling experts, Tongan sociocultural experts, as well as academics and research experts.

Information gathered for phase one was obtained through a series of individual and focus group interviews. The purpose was to ascertain whether Tongan people were indeed experiencing problem gambling, as anecdotal evidence suggested, and further, to identify factors that may contribute to the development of problem gambling. Participants in this phase included twenty ministers of different churches and denominations, fifteen health and social service providers, and fifteen community leaders who had been invited to take part. They were interviewed by the researchers during the time of toli kakala.

During the second phase, tui kakala, the analysis and interpretation of the data was extended and enriched by the inclusion of pō talanoa. Taking part were members of the research and advisory teams. Many of the emergent themes from the fieldwork, pointing to reasons why Tongan people in Auckland were gambling, needed more in-depth pō talanoa in order to unwrap and understand the underlying significance of some of the reasons that had been identified by participants. It was evident that these were manifestations or indicators of issues affecting the community at a deeper level. The contributions of those who took part included informed judgments, observations, and assessments from their professional perspectives, as well as others' personal observations from the perspective of their cultural expertise, leadership roles, and social awareness of New Zealand society.

Participation in Gambling by the Tongan Community

It is evident that Tongan people in Auckland take extensive advantage of an array of gambling opportunities available, including the casino, "pokies" (poker machines), TAB (state-sponsored sports gambling), and Lotto. The major source of problems identified was the pokies, which are located in neighborhoods near concentrations of the Tongan population. While Tongans do frequent the casino in the central business district, it is the increase in local venues with poker machines that can be seen as a major problem. At the community level, the increased availability of gambling activities and venues in local communities is contributing to a changing landscape in many of the most deprived areas throughout Auckland.

Prominent members of the community, leaders, and church groups, as well as groups of women, frequent gambling venues. This contributes to its normalization so that people feel gambling is a socially acceptable activity. Sociocultural sanctions, particularly regarding the participation of older women as well as young people, especially young women, in public places such as casinos, pubs, and bars, have shifted as a result of this normalization of gambling. In addition, youth from otherwise strict families drive older family members to the casino and are then left unsupervised for hours in town, sometimes at night. They may have been told to go home, but in some cases they hang around or gamble themselves while waiting for their mothers and the older groups.

Research participants reported that gambling had become a major health and social issue within the Tongan community, adversely affecting Tongan people and culture. The consequences of problem gambling and addictive gambling were seen in the financial difficulties that led to homes and vehicles being repossessed, marriage breakdown, an increasing number of people in debt, neglect of children, lack of supervision of young people, and leaving old people at home or at the casino alone.

Households were also suffering where the mother, expected to be the backbone of Tongan families' keeping everything together, and her partner became involved in gambling. Ironically, for a woman in an abusive relationship, gambling could be experienced as an escape from her personal problems. It could provide her with a sense of freedom outside the home, interacting with a machine she may think she can control, while pinning her hopes and dreams on a possible win.

Problem Gambling

Gambling can be defined on a continuum, with non-gamblers at one end and pathological gamblers at the other. Levels of gambling progress along the continuum, depending on the extent and effect of the gambling activity. Problem gambling would be located along the middle to upper end of the continuum, and it is important to note that it is socially defined. Although pathological gambling was acknowledged and given some consideration, an assessment of its prevalence was beyond the scope of this investigation. Rather, the current study specifically focused on identifying issues for the Tongan community associated with problem gambling.

Within the Tongan community, gambling and problem gambling are not clearly defined or well understood. Unlike alcohol, drugs, and tobacco, where the community has some understanding of the effects, gambling is an "unknown evil." Tongans generally have very poor knowledge about the way gambling venues operate and the technology that controls winning. Thus there is a misconception that gambling is not only socially sanctioned entertainment, but also that it is fair. The belief is widespread that there is generosity involved and that all money that is put into the machine is returned. Formulas circulate around the community regarding the best time to gamble and ways of locating the fullest machines, such as after midnight on a Sunday night. These contribute to the widespread notion that the machines are controllable, fair, reciprocal, and generous.

Understanding Gambling in the Tongan Context

Our cultural analysis uncovered a number of influences promoting gambling other than the most commonly stated reasons: entertainment, relaxation, and socializing. Tongans, like other groups, say they gamble in hope of winning, achieving financial freedom, and success. Winning is a blessing, a sign *of tāpuaki/monūʻia,* or being blessed/lucky. This suggests that they perceive their participation in gambling as rewarded, and therefore endorsed, by God.

The Tongan belief in dreams and signs contributes to the presumption that the activity of gambling is basically benign. Gambling is therefore seen as a logical and realistic option for improving one's status and upward class movement for Tongans in New Zealand. The hope of hitting a big win and being able to fulfill one's obligations and distribute winnings among family, friends, and church—in both New Zealand and Tonga—is a powerful motivation. Additional reasons given for gambling include the excitement of an urban venue; hope of financial gain; the sense of freedom and, for women especially, the chance of financial freedom; loneliness and lack of alternatives for recreation; the lack of opportunity for accumulating finances in low-waged work; addiction; and vulnerability to advertising and the gambling culture of New Zealand.

Tongan Concepts That Support Gambling

Analysis of Tongan concepts—such as *fua fatongiá* (carrying out one's rightful duties), *fua kavenga* (shouldering social and financial burdens), *feingá* (trying one's very best), and *tāpuaki/faingamālie* (taking advantage of opportunities one is blessed with)—has revealed that some cultural elements also support gambling.

Fua fatongiá/fua kavenga

This relates to the need to fulfill one's obligations to the family, church, community, and/or state. These obligations are often a combination of financial contributions; cultural, familial, and church knowledge; time; and the willingness to participate in the event or occasion associated with the obligation.

Communal living has involved maintaining interdependent relationships within and between the extended family unit, and the church community or village community, which in turn means that being a part of the group entails the fulfillment of responsibilities and obligations. Not being able to fulfill these obligations can ultimately mean that members are marginalized, and left to feel *ma* (shamed), which then affects the immediate family and, to a lesser extent, the extended family. Fua fatongiá/fua kavenga is a major part of Tongan life, and is also shared by Samoans in their practice of *fa'aaloalo* (cultural obligations and responsibilities).

Gambling can therefore be seen as a means to an end. Winning the jackpot or striking it lucky at the TAB or Lotto means that the obligations and any financial responsibilities to the family, church, community, and state could be fulfilled and completed. It means that one could thereby win favor from family, peers, and leaders.

Laukau

Another concept emerging from the discussion of fua fatongiá and fua kavenga is *laukau* (pride). Fulfilling obligations can contribute to building up Tongans' self-esteem, through enhancing one's importance as a family, church, or community member. Related principles are *ngali tangata/fefine e fua fatongiá* (fulfilling one's obligations dictated by gender role) and *ke lava lelei e fua fatongiá* (fulfilling one's obligations in an exemplary manner). These cultural understandings underpin the need to fulfill obligations well, the superior achievement of which builds oneself and one's family up to a higher level of status, desired by many Tongans.

Feingá

All of the people interviewed named feingá as a reason Tongans were gambling. Feingá means that you have essentially tried your best, have covered all alternatives, and have given it your all to either solve a financial problem or fulfill an obligation. It invokes feelings, attitudes, and philosophies of effort, courage, persistence, perseverance, and determination. Hence, feingá was cited many times by participants as a reason for gambling and a way of trying to meet obligations: fua fatongiá, fua kavenga.

The act of gambling was perceived as incorporating all the values and qualities associated with feingá, including trying another path and exhausting all avenues to get money. Understanding that the majority of Tongan people in New Zealand have low socioeconomic status, and that the options for generating alternative funds and finances are limited, gambling becomes a logical and rational pathway for feingá. For a people with limited options, gambling activities and venues offer ways of increasing feingá, demonstrating persistence and determination; it is often justified as *ko e lava ia e feingá/ko e 'osi ia e feingá* (I've exhausted all my options, that was my final effort). Health professionals observed that it has therefore become a viable and common option in order to make ends meet, fulfill obligations, and provide for families, the community, or church.

The research team tried to identify and understand why a people who have had little or no history of gambling in their homeland turn to gambling as a logical and sensible option in New Zealand. We also attempted to understand why gambling for some must be considered before they can say they have done their best or tried their hardest.

It seems that the legal regulation of gambling has served as a de facto endorsement of it as a legitimate and proper activity. Beset by limited options, Tongans now see regulated and legal gambling as a legitimate way of making some money and therefore an acceptable and favorable avenue to explore for feingá. Furthermore, the attraction of gambling is that wagering is a type of play that regulates chance, thereby imparting a sense of control in the players.

Feingá is therefore also associated with beliefs about chance and luck. It was mentioned throughout the interviews that people participating in gambling opportunities as viable options believed that they had a chance of winning, or that it could be their lucky day—like the Lotto slogan, "Be in to Win." In addition, research participants described people who dreamed of being lucky and winning, and who would get up in the middle of the night and go to the casino because they believed it was a sign. They feared that if they didn't go, they would miss out on their fortune. Gaming venues have therefore become perceived as places where dreams can come true, enabling all your problems to disappear once you hit that jackpot. According to participants, these beliefs are strongly held within the Tongan community.

The Transfer of Dreams: From New Zealand to Gambling Venues

An underlying phenomenon identified to explain the use of gambling as another area for feingá was the transfer of dreams. Before immigration, New Zealand was perceived by Tongans as the land of milk and honey. It was seen as a place where all dreams come true and, for many, the dream was to provide for the family, fulfill obligations, and enjoy some form of material comfort.

On their arriving in New Zealand, however, the dream has proven elusive; the reality is that it is not so easily attained. Factors such as loss of support and new demands associated with migration, ethnic prejudice, membership in a minority community, language and communication problems, limited work skills, and low socioeconomic status have made the dream of a better life for the family appear almost impossible to achieve.

It seems that these dreams are being physically transferred to gambling venues such as casinos, local bars, mini-casinos, TABs, and such. Though the dreams have remained the same, the site has now changed, from New Zealand as the land of opportunity, to gambling venues and machines as the new site for achieving promised opportunities. Gambling venues are now perceived as the places where anything is possible, where dreams can be realized, and, for people with limited resources and limited alternatives, these sites provide a logical and sensible avenue for feingá, for achieving those dreams.

Gambling thereby becomes perceived as a rational approach to coping and problem solving, given the lack of other opportunities for poorly paid individuals to amass a large sum of money. When this motivation is coupled with the belief that there is an even chance of winning, gambling seems a realistic hope. Furthermore, many Tongans maintain connections with spiritual and symbolic worlds and meanings. These then become interrelated with their beliefs and practices around luck and chance.

Many Tongan people attribute particular meanings to signs from nature and other symbolisms that appear in their dream. They look to both the physical and spiritual environment for answers to questions, or explanations of their environment and events that may or may not occur. For some, there is often no real distinction between the physical and spiritual: the two worlds coexist simultaneously. Common Tongan expressions that capture the coexistence of these worlds are *naʻe pau pē ke hoko* (it was predestined, it was meant to be), *tamasiʻi monūʻia* (that person is blessed with luck; good things will always happen to that person), and *naʻe ʻosi ʻi ai pē ʻae ngaahi fakaʻilonga* (there were signs to warn/tell/inform us this was going to happen).

Therefore, *misi* (dreams), and belief in symbols, signs, and messages that come from dreams and their interpretation, provide another explanation for Tongan gambling. It was reported many times that people would experience dreams about numbers, then would buy a Lotto ticket the next day; if they did not, there would be a feeling of missing out on luck or losing a chance. This could result in depression or obvious stress.

Another significant factor identified was the belief that a win was a blessing. It is not uncommon for Tongan people to pray before using machines or another means of gambling, asking for God's intervention or blessing. An individual may also pray while engaging in a gambling activity, possibly making a pact with God in the case of a significant win. Thus another cultural change highlighted is that blessings can now be bestowed by way of a machine.

The practice itself is not exceptional, in that praying is common practice for many Tongans. Prayer is offered at the opening and closing of formal meetings, state, religious, or familial events like birthdays, weddings, and anniversaries, and at informal occasions such as sports events, fundraisers, and social events. This reflects Tongan beliefs that God is omnipotent, and that all things are predestined according to the will of God. The irony is that, as dreams and blessings are received by way of machines, Tongan people's perceptions of relationships may change: they may be increasingly regarded or experienced as commodities, and gamblers may also be vulnerable to developing distorted perceptions of their relationships with machines, as if they were human.

The combination of factors such as low socioeconomic status, limited options, targeted marketing, and stressors associated with migration have increased the vulnerability of Tongans to participating in gambling activities. Gambling for some Tongans possesses the elusive mystical power that can answer their prayers and help them realize their dreams through bringing good fortune and blessing. Casinos have become the physical place to which the dreams and hopes of a people have been transferred and where prayers are being offered. The social context in which this is taking place, however, also requires examination in order to understand this phenomenon.

Migration and the Breakdown of Traditional Kāinga *Support Networks*

The *kāinga* system (extended or communal family) serves as both the Tongan social network and a welfare system (Helu, 1999). Traditionally it dictated the distribution of resources, maintained peaceful relations, mediated conflicts, ensured appropriate caregiving, and managed the correct fulfillment of responsibilities and obligations. Many researchers, however, have commented on the breakdown of the kāinga system due to the various effects of migration and to Western influences such as capitalist business enterprise and individualism.

It has been noted that Tongan people gamble because they want to fua kavenga, fua fatongiá. However, it became apparent in this study that gambling to fulfill obligations was essentially filling a gap that had been created by breakdowns within the kāinga system. The capacity of the kāinga system to discharge its responsibility for fulfilling obligations within the familial context, and for distributing familial wealth and resources, depends upon the effectiveness of its processes and procedures. Even if the kāinga system has collapsed, it is probable that familial responsibilities and obligations remain the same, or have even increased due to the demands of changing social environments. With increased obligations outside the kāinga system, individuals and nuclear families are therefore left to fulfill these obligations either on their own or with one or two other relatives.

Furthermore, if these families/individuals are typical of Tongan migrants to New Zealand, they will be living on or below the poverty line and have few, if any, alternatives or options for making extra money. The themes of *fusimo'omo e mo'ui, fe'amokaki e mo'ui, taufā 'a e mo'ui* come into play. Feelings of hopelessness, severe financial hardship, and poverty become central to understanding the far-reaching effects of the kāinga system's breakdown and the difficulty of achieving fua kavenga, fua fatongiá on an individual and nuclear family basis.

The fundamental importance of fulfilling one's obligations is part of the Tongan definition of good health. For a Tongan person to achieve good health and wellbeing, areas of *mo'ui fakasino* (physical health), *mo'ui faka'atamai* (mental health), and *mo'ui fakalaumālie* (spiritual health) must be addressed, and one's obligations must be fulfilled in each of these areas. By meeting one's obligations to family, country, church, and God, one helps to maintain harmonious and mutually beneficial relationships, and therefore contributes to one's own relational wellbeing with those key institutions in life (Finau, 1996).

According to 'Okusitino Mahina (personal communication, 2004), in failing to fua fatongiá, fua kavenga, a family commits the "worst social sin of fakamā." *Fakamā* (shame, loss of face) harms the health of Tongan people in deep and meaningful ways. For a people that operate at a communal level, fakamā adversely affects all aspects of health for people who are touched by it—physically, mentally, and spiritually.

Isolation from the kāinga and/or breakdown of the kāinga system means that there is no longer adequate support for Tongan families as they struggle to build a life in their new homeland. Furthermore, the new societies often do not understand communal lifestyles and all the responsibilities and obligations that come with operating as a larger group.

Gambling in this sociocultural context has appeared as a beacon of hope, albeit false, to combat poverty and to fulfill all financial obligations facing the family so as to avoid fakamā. As already indicated, however, obligations remain consistent and still require fulfillment. Continued availability and accessibility of gambling facilities proffer an easy solution to the situation, offering false support for a people whose traditional networks have at some levels disintegrated. Families cannot depend on the kāinga distribution of resources and wealth, but gambling venues entice people to participate, enjoy, and "be in to win," so that resources from gambling such as hitting the jackpot, accumulation of credits, blackjack, betting, scratchies, and Lotto can be shared with them.

Laukau *and Class Mobility*

Prior to having easy access to material goods and resources, movement between the highly stratified hierarchies within Tongan society was possible through education, intermarriage, ordination, and business. Even these means, however, were only available to an elite few. The majority had to remain content with commoner status, although even here the stratification of rank and power was evident. So if by birth, placement, social environment, and relational consequences, one could not move easily through the hierarchy, access to material resources was a sure way to improve one's own and one's family's status. In order to demonstrate this improvement of status and wealth, more generous contributions would be made when meeting obligations to church, family, and the village, whether in terms of money, crafts, livestock, and/or harvest goods.

In addition to laukau (pride), the expressions *fakavahavaha'a* (rivalry), and *fesiosiofaki* ("keeping up with the Joneses") are also salient here, associated with the concept of competition through and by material gain, in order to achieve upward social mobility. These notions are not new to many people who participate in gambling, and definitely not unique to Tongans. However, understanding the communal nature of Tongan lifestyles and the close interrelationships of people, it is fair to claim that for Tongans, "everything is defined by the environment and the people around us" (Mahina, personal communication, 2004). Everything and everyone is interconnected in some way or another, and both private and public life must be understood from a holistic perspective, including people and the environment.

Once it is understood that everything in Tongan society and the kāinga system is stratified, that mobility is difficult to achieve, and that status is predetermined by birth and genealogy, then the emphasis on materialistic gain/competition, increased donations, "bigger means better," and the desire to "keep up with the Joneses" can also be understood in relation to *laukau, ngali tangata—ngali fefine,* and *kuo lava lelei e fatongiá* (the duty has been accomplished well). For many Tongans, this equates with attaining wellbeing and health, as obligations have been fulfilled well and family status and social ranking have improved.

The reality, however, for the majority of Tongans in Auckland is one of a young population of low socioeconomic status, dealing with recent migration, coping with English as a second language, and living in extended family situations, with affiliation to some form of organized religion. High numbers of Tongans reside in the more materially deprived areas of Auckland. In this situation, gambling again presents itself as a logical and realistic option for improving one's status and upward social mobility. If they hit a big win, the *tāpuaki*/blessings, *monū'ia*/luck, and winnings will be shared with their community, in both New Zealand and Tonga, reflecting their loyalty to the kāinga system. We have discussed the effects of its breakdown, but it seems that if resources are available, a priority for Tongan people is providing support for members of their kāinga network, thereby strengthening the kāinga welfare system.

Fakapotopoto: *Working against Gambling*

In contrast to these interrelated factors that influence Tongan gambling, the attributes associated with *fakapotopoto* (maturely capable), a quality that is admired, were frequently mentioned as a reason for *not* gambling or for the ability to control gambling habits. People who are fakapotopoto are sensible with resources, proficient in their distribution, wise, practical, smart, and consistent. Success and leadership in any field, fulfillment of obligations, leadership qualities, and attainment of wealth, are linked to this quality, and people who are not fakapotopoto are believed unlikely to succeed. Instead, they are likely to experience sadness and financial hardship.

Tongans understand and value people-centered relationships—*tauhi vā* (building harmonious relations)—as an essential part of Tongan culture and kāinga systems. Fakapotopoto in this context is concerned with the development of these relationships, systems, and networks, by fulfilling obligations well and contributing to the overall wellbeing of the kāinga, church, village, or community. Within the New Zealand context, fakapotopoto includes skills related to budgeting, planning, and forward thinking to meet basic needs and obligations. This reflects the adjustment Tongan people have had to make, from not knowing the value of money or not valuing money, to viewing money as a means to an end, and using it for tauhi vā, developing, maintaining and nurturing relationships, kāinga, acquaintances, or friendships.

Closing Comments

This study has led to the identification of a number of interrelated concepts and themes that provide explanations for gambling within the Tongan community. Further investigation is needed to uncover additional, significant sociocultural concepts that may support, encourage, and contribute to the development of problem gambling within the Tongan community.

Tongan people in Auckland face the challenges of migration and the uncertainty of settling into a new homeland. Like many other migrant peoples, they do the best they can with what they have and what they know. Recurring stories of lost and/or repossessed goods and property, disconnected utilities, neglected children and elders, false hopes, and misplaced dreams were a stark awakening to how quickly gambling hurts the individual, family, community, and society as a whole. When gambling becomes a problem, one of the most dangerous consequences is the speed with which it affects almost every area of life.

Given the targeting of poorer and under-resourced communities by the gambling industry, possible cultural congruence (as explained by the overlap between gambling myths and cultural values), lack of opportunities for social and financial progress, a lack of education about the odds of winning and the hazards of gambling, and existing addiction, it would be surprising if the rate of gambling did not continue to increase within the Auckland Tongan community. With it will come inevitable increases in the socio-cultural problems identified. In order to prevent this escalation, further research needs to be undertaken to extend the analysis developed in this investigation. The knowledge we are developing must be shared within the community in this luve e kakala phase of the research process, and creative means must be found to apply it in developing effective ways to address this challenge that threatens the wellbeing of our community.

References

Finau, S. 'A. (1996). Health, environment and development: Towards a Pacific paradigm. *Pacific Health Dialog: Journal of Community Health and Clinical Medicine for the Pacific, 3*(2), 266–278.

Guttenbeil-Po'uhila, Y., & Tu'itahi, S. (2004). *Gambling issues in the Auckland Tongan community: Palopalema 'oe Va'inga Pa'oanga 'ihe Kainga Tonga 'i Aokalani.* A research project hosted by Auckland Regional Public Health and funded by the Health Research Council of New Zealand. Retrieved May 15, 2005, from http://www.camh.net/egambling/archive/pdf/JGI-issue12/JGI-Issue12-tuitahi.pdf.

Helu, I. F. (1999). *Critical essays: Cultural perspectives from the South Seas.* Canberra: ANU Printing Service.

Helu-Thaman, K. (1999). *A matter of life and death: Schooling and culture in Oceania.* Keynote address presented at Innovations for Effective Schooling Conference, Auckland.

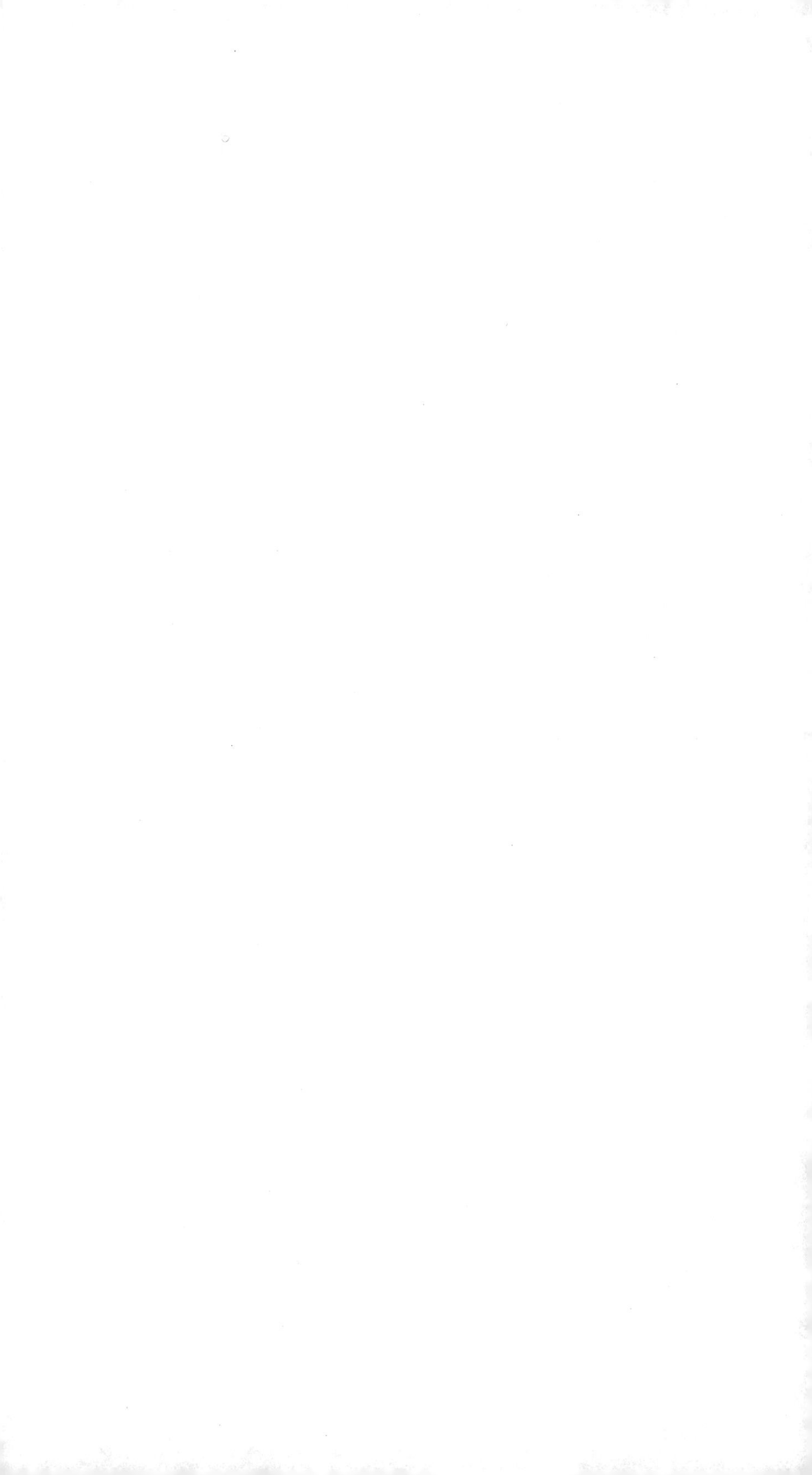

A Bibliography of Pasifika Mental Health Resources

TO'OA JEMAIMA TIATIA, WITH MARGARET AGEE AND PHILIP CULBERTSON

This final section of this book is provided to enable readers to access additional resource material in areas related to Pasifika mental health. In searching for literature to construct the bibliography, sources used included Google searches, using the following key words and phrases: Pacific health; Pacific mental health; Pacific arts; Pacific myths and legends; Pacific research methodology; alcohol and drugs; and identity. Items were also identified from a search of current student theses, from library searches, and from the bibliographies found in recent relevant Pacific works.

We believe the material included in this bibliography will be helpful for students, researchers, and practitioners, providing further information to enrich our understandings as we engage in an ongoing *talanoa* (conversation) about the issues raised in this book. The contents have been organized into categories that reflect major pertinent themes of both professional and academic interest. These are listed below, in alphabetical order.

As the *fale* is open, so too is the range and potential of the resources that may be identified and created in order to contribute to this talanoa. This bibliography, originally prepared by Jemaima Tiatia (tiatia@hibiscusresearch.co.nz) is by no means exhaustive. The editors welcome annotations, additions, and corrections, including either print- or web-based resources. Additions and corrections can be sent to p.culbertson@auckland.ac.nz or m.agee@auckland.ac.nz.

Contents

Medicine and Traditional Healing
Mental Health
Pastoral Care and Spirituality
Psychology, Psychiatry, and Psychotherapy
Research Methodology
Sexuality and Gender
Substance Abuse and Addictions
Suicidal Behaviors
The Arts
Violence
Youth

Counseling

Afoa, I. (1997). Marriage and divorce among Samoan couples. In P. Culbertson (Ed.), *Counselling issues and South Pacific communities* (pp. 189–213). Auckland: Snedden & Cervin.

Autagavaia, M. (2001). A Tagata Pasifika supervision process: Authenticating difference. In L. Beddoe & J. Worrell (Eds.), *Supervision: From rhetoric to reality: Conference proceedings*. Auckland: Auckland College of Education.

Christensen, C. (1989). Cross-cultural awareness development: A conceptual model. *Counselor Education and Supervision, 28*, 270–287.

Culbertson, P. (Ed.). (1997). *Counselling issues and South Pacific communities*. Auckland: Snedden & Cervin.

Di Nicola, V. (1997). *A stranger in the family: Culture, families, and therapy*. New York: W. W. Norton.

Foliaki, L. (1981). Pacific Island counselling. In F. Donnelly (Ed.), *A time to talk: Counsellor and counselled*. Auckland: George Allen & Unwin.

Gherardi, P., & E. Tanoi. (2000). Working with Pacific Island people. In H. Love & W. Wittaker (Eds.), *Practice issues for clinical and applied psychologists in New Zealand* (pp. 158–163). Wellington: The New Zealand Psychological Society.

Hesslegrave, D. (1984). *Counseling cross-culturally*. Grand Rapids: Baker Book House.

Lee, C. L. (1997). *Multicultural issues in counseling*. Alexandria: American Counseling Association.

Metge, J., & Kinloch, P. (1978). *Talking past each other: Problems of cross cultural communication*. Wellington: Victoria University Press.

Pedersen, P. B. (2002). Ethics, competence and other professional issues in culture-centered counseling. In P. B. Pedersen & J. G. Draguns (Eds.), *Counseling across cultures*. Thousand Oaks: Sage Publications.

Pedersen, P. B., & Ivey, A. (1993). *Culture-centered counseling and interviewing skills: A practical guide*. Westport: Praeger.

Schuster, F. S. (2001). Counselling against all the odds: The Samoan way.

Pacific Health Dialog: Journal of Community Health and Clinical Medicine for the Pacific, 8(1), 193–199.

Seiuli, B. (2004). *Mea'alofa, a gift handed over: Making accessible and visible Samoan counselling in New Zealand*. Unpublished master's thesis, University of Waikato, Hamilton, New Zealand.

Su'a-Hawkins, A., & Mafile'o, T. (2004, December). What is cultural supervision? *Social Work Now, 29*, 10–16.

Sue, D. W., & Sue, D. (2003). *Counseling the culturally diverse: Theory and practice* (4th ed.). New York: John Wiley & Sons.

Webber-Dreadon, E. (1999). He taonga mo o matou tipuna (A gift handed down by our ancestors): An indigenous approach to supervision. *Te Komako: Social Work Review, 11*, 7–11.

Culture and Customs

Bargatzky, T. (2002). "To be like God": Reflections on the nature of the Samoan matai. In *5th Conference of the European Society for Oceanists (ESfO): Recovering the past: Resources, representations and ethics of research in Oceania*. Vienna: ESfO.

Barnhill, D. L. (Ed.). (1999). *At home on the earth: Becoming native to our place, a multicultural anthropology*. Berkeley: University of California Press.

Benguigui, G. (1989). The middle classes in Tonga. *Journal of Pacific Studies, 98*, 451–463.

Biersack, A. (1982). Tongan exchange structures: Beyond descent and alliance. *Journal of the Polynesian Society, 91*, 181–212.

Biersack, A. (1990). Under the toa tree: The genealogy of the Tongan chiefs. In J. Siikala (Ed.), *Culture and history in the Pacific*. Helsinki: Transactions of the Finnish Anthropological Society.

Craig, R. D. (1989). *Dictionary of Polynesian mythology*. New York: Greenwood.

Donald, J., & Rattansi, A. (1992). *Race, culture and difference*. London: Open University.

Drozdow-St. Christian, D. (1004). *Body/work: Aspects of embodiment and culture in Samoa*. Unpublished doctoral dissertation, McMaster University, Hamilton, Canada.

Duranti, A. (1985). Famous theories and local theories: The Samoans and Wittgenstein. *The Quarterly Newsletter of the Laboratory of Comparative Human Cognition, 7*(2), 46–51.

Eves, R. (1996). Colonialism, corporeality and character: Methodist missions and the refashioning of bodies in the Pacific. *History and Anthropology, 10*(1), 85–138.

Finnegan, R., & Orbell, M. (Eds.). (1995). *South Pacific oral traditions*. Bloomington: Indiana University Press.

Formander, A. (1916). *Hawaiian antiquities and folk-lore*. Cambridge: Bishop Museum Press.

Gardner, L. (1965). *Gautavai: A study of Samoan values*. Unpublished master's thesis, University of Hawai'i.

Garsee, J. W. (1965). *A study of Samoan interpersonal values*. Unpublished master's thesis, University of Oklahoma, Norman, Oklahoma.

Gell, A. (1993). *Wrapping in images: Tattooing in Polynesia*. Oxford: Clarendon Press.

Gifford, E. (1971). *Tongan myths and tales*. Milwood: Kraus Reprint Co.

Gifford, E. (1985). *Tongan society*. Milwood: Kraus Reprint Co.

Grattan, F. J. H. (1948). *An introduction to Samoan custom*. Auckland: R. McMillan.

Graves, T. D., & Graves, N. B. (Eds.). (1985). *Kinship ties and preferred strategies of urban migrants: Patterns of social behavior*. Hamilton: New Zealand and the South Pacific Academic Press.

Hart, J. H. (1996). *Samoan culture*. Apia: Ati's Samoan Print Shop.

Hirsh, S. (1958). The social organization of an urban village in Samoa. *Journal of the Polynesian Society, 67*, 266–301.

Holmes, L. D. (1958). *Ta'u: Stability and change in a Samoan village*. Wellington: The Polynesian Society.

Holmes, L. D. (1974). *Samoan village*. New York: Holt, Rinehart and Winston.

Horst, C. (1971). The sacred child and the origins of spirits in Samoa. *Anthropos, 66*, 173–181.

James, K. (1991). The female presence in heavenly places: Myth and sovereignty in Tonga. *Oceania, 61*(4), 237–308.

Ka'ili, T. O. (2005). Tauhi vā: Nurturing sociospatial ties in Maui and beyond. *The Contemporary Pacific, 17*(1), 83–114.

Keene, D. (1978). *Houses without walls: Samoan social control*. Unpublished doctoral dissertation, University of Hawai'i.

Keesing, F., & Keesing, M. (1956). *Elite communication in Samoa: A study in leadership*. New York: Farrar, Strauss & Giroux.

Linnekin, J. (1990). The politics of culture in the Pacific. In J. Linnekin & L. Poyer (Eds.), *Cultural identity and ethnicity in the Pacific*. Honolulu: University of Hawai'i Press.

Love, J. W. (1983). Review of Sala'ilua: A Samoan mystery by Bradd Shore. *Pacific Studies, 7*(1), 122–145.

Macpherson, C., & Macpherson, L. (2005). The ifoga: The exchange value of social honour in contemporary Samoa. *Journal of the Polynesian Society, 114*(2), 109–133.

Moore, S. E., Leslie, H. Y., & Lavis, C. A. (2004). *Subjective well-being and life satisfaction in the Kingdom of Tonga*. Dordrecht: Kluwer.

Morton, H. (1996). *Becoming Tongan: An ethnography of childhood*. Honolulu: University of Hawai'i Press.

Morton, H. (1998). How Tongan is a Tongan? Cultural authenticity revisited. In D. Scarr, N. Gunson, & J. Terrell (Eds.), *Echoes of Pacific war*. Canberra: Target Oceania.

Moyle, R. (1981). *Fagogo: Fables from Samoa in Samoan and English*. Auckland: Auckland University Press.

O'Meara, T. J. (1990). *Samoan planters: Tradition and economic development in Polynesia*. Fort Worth: Holt, Rinehart, Winston.

Pau'u, T. H. (2002). My life in four cultures. In J. Spickard, J. Rondilla, & H. Wright (Eds.), *Pacific diaspora: Island peoples in the United States and across the Pacific*. Honolulu: University of Hawai'i Press.

Perelini, O. (1973). *Christian marriage: A critical study of Christian marriage with specific reference to Samoa society*. Unpublished master's thesis, St. John's Theological College, Auckland.

Perminow, A. A. (1993). *The long way home: Dilemmas of everyday life in a Tongan village*. Oslo: Scandinavian University Press (available through Oxford University Press).

Polu, L. (2000). Cultural rights and the individual in the Samoan context. In M. Wilson & P. Hunt (Eds.), *Culture, rights, and cultural rights: Perspectives from the South Pacific*. Wellington: Huia.

Pukui, M. K. (1983). *'Olelo No'eau: Hawaiian proverbs and poetical sayings*. Honolulu: Bishop Museum Press.

Shore, B. (1977). *A Samoan theory of action*. Unpublished doctoral dissertation, University of Chicago.

Shore, B. (1982). *Sala'ilua: A Samoan mystery*. New York: Columbia University Press.

Spickard, J., Rondilla, J., & Wright, H. (Eds.). (2002). *Pacific diaspora: Island peoples in the United States and across the Pacific*. Honolulu: University of Hawai'i Press.

Stuebel, C. (1976). *Myths and legends of Samoa: Ala o le vavau*. Wellington & Apia: A. H. and A. W. Reed and Wesley Productions.

Sutter, F. (1980). *Communal versus individual socialization at home and in school in rural and urban Western Samoa*. Unpublished doctoral dissertation, University of Hawai'i.

Toafa, I. (1976). *The myths, legends and customs of old Samoa*. Auckland: Polynesian Press.

Tu'itahi-Tahaafe, S. (2003). *Introducing disability concepts with integrity into Tongan cultural context*. Unpublished master's thesis, Massey University, New Zealand.

Education

Bishop, R., & Glynn, T. (1999). *Culture counts: Changing power relations in education*. Palmerston North: Dunmore Press.

Bray, D., & Hill, C. (Eds.). (1973, 1974). *Polynesian and Pakeha in New Zealand education*. 2 vols. Auckland: Heinemann.

Carpenter, V., Dixon, H., Rata, E., & Rawlinson, C. (2001). Pacific Nations people in Aotearoa/New Zealand. In *Diversity: Theory in practice for educators*. Palmerston North: Dunmore Press.

Helu-Thaman, K. (1995). Concepts of learning, knowledge and wisdom in Tonga, and their relevance to modern education. *Prospects, 25*(4), 723–733.

Lloyd, M. (1995). Bridging the cultural gap: A literature review of factors influencing Samoan students' acculturation to Western education. *Many Voices, 8*, 11–13.

Mafi, M. (1998). *Factors affecting educational achievement of Tongans in Auckland*. Unpublished master's thesis, The University of Auckland.

Manu'atu, L., & Kepa, M. (2005). Unending curiosity and empowering Tongan people: Indigenous Tongan & Maori perspectives on partnership & practice in secondary schooling. In *Ministry of Education Northern Region Conference—Partnership and Practice in the 21st Century*. Auckland: Ministry of Education.

Tofi, T., Flett, R., & Timutimu-Thorpe, H. (1996). Problems faced by Pacific Islands students at university in New Zealand: Some effects on academic performance and psychological wellbeing. *New Zealand Journal of Educational Studies, 31*(1), 51–59.

Tupuola, A. M. (2000). Making sense of human development: Beyond western concepts and universal assumptions. In K. Helu-Thaman & C. Benson (Eds.), *Pacific cultures in the teacher education curriculum*. Suva: The University of the South Pacific.

Utumapu, T. (1992). *Finau i mea sili: Attitudes of Samoan families in New Zealand to education*. Unpublished master's thesis, The University of Auckland.

Williams, B. T. (2005). *The gift of dreams: Effective mentoring for Pacific secondary school students*. Unpublished master's thesis, The University of Auckland.

Emotions

Aune, R. K., & Waters, L. L. (1994). Cultural differences in deception: Motivations to deceive in Samoans and North Americans. *International Journal of Intercultural Relations, 18*(2), 159–172.

Beaglehole, E. (1940). Psychic stress in a Tongan village. In *Proceedings of the Sixth Pacific Science Congress of the Pacific Science Association, IV*, 43–52. Berkeley: University of California Press.

Gerber, E. (1975). *The cultural patterning of emotions in Samoa*. Unpublished doctoral dissertation, University of California.

Gerber, E. (1985). Rage and obligation: Samoan emotion in conflict. In G. White & J. Kirkpatrick (Eds.), *Person, self and experience: Exploring Pacific ethnopsychologies*. Berkeley: University of California Press.

Goodman, R. A. (1990). Laughter and anger: On Samoan aggression. In H. Caton (Ed.), *The Samoan reader: Anthropologists take stock*. Lanham: University Press of America.

Hassed, C. S. (2000). Depression: Dispirited or spiritually deprived? *eMJA*, Retrieved June 18, 2005, from http://www.mja.com.au/public/issues/173_10_201100/hassed/hassed.html.

Kanahele, G. H. S. (2002). The dynamics of aloha. In J. Spickard, J. Rondilla, & H. Wright (Eds.), *Pacific diaspora: Island peoples in the United States and across the Pacific*. Honolulu: University of Hawai'i Press.

Kitayama, S., & Markus, H. R. (Eds.). (1994). *Emotion and culture: Empirical studies of mutual influence*. Washington, DC: American Psychological Association.

Mageo, J. M. (1988). Malosi: A psychological exploration of Mead's and Freeman's work and of Samoan aggression. *Pacific Studies, 112*(2), 25–65.

Mageo, J. M. (1989). Amio/aga and loto: Perspectives on the structure of the self in Samoa. *Oceania, 59*, 181–199.

Mageo, J. M. (1991). Samoan moral discourse and the loto. *American Anthropologist, 93*(2), 405–420.

Mageo, J. M. (1998). *Theorizing self in Samoa: Emotions, genders and sexualities*. Ann Arbor: University of Michigan Press.

Olson, E. (1994). Female voices of aggression in Tonga. *Sex Roles, 30*(3 & 4), 237–249.

Government Agencies and Policy

Afeaki, E. (2001). A practical Pacific way of social work: Embrace collectivity. *Social Work Review/Tu Mau, 13*(3), 35–37.

Afeaki, E. (2004). *The effects of social policy upon the Tongan kainga*. Unpublished master's thesis, Massey University, New Zealand.

Coxon, E. (1997). *The politics of modernisation in Western Samoa*. Unpublished doctoral dissertation, The University of Auckland.

Hanlon, D. L., & White, G. M. (2000). *Voyaging through the contemporary Pacific*. London: Rowman & Littlefield.

Helu-Thaman, K. (2002). Shifting sights: The cultural challenge of sustainability. *Higher Education Policy, 15*, 133–142.

Ivison, D., Patton, P., & Sanders, W. (Eds.). (2000). *Political theory and the rights of indigenous peoples*. Cambridge: Cambridge University Press.

Latukefu, S. (1974). *Church and state in Tonga: The Wesleyan Methodist missionaries and political development*. Canberra: Australia National University.

Melesia, M. (1987). *The making of modern Samoa: Traditional authority and colonial administration in the modern history of Western Samoa*. Suva: Institute of Pacific Studies.

Meleisea, M. (1992). *Change and adaptations in Western Samoa*. Christchurch: Macmillan Brown Centre for Pacific Studies.

Ministry of Health. (1997). *Making a Pacific difference: Strategic initiatives for the health of Pacific people*. Wellington: Author.

Ministry of Social Development. (2002). *Briefing to the incoming Minister: Improving wellbeing for all New Zealanders*. Wellington: Author.

Mulitalo-Lauta, P. T. (2000). *Fa'a Samoa and social work within the New Zealand context*. Palmerston North: Dunmore Press.

Ongley, P. (1991). Pacific Islands migration and the New Zealand labour market. In P. Spoonley, D. Pearson, & C. Macpherson (Eds.), *Nga take: Ethnic relations and racism in Aotearoa/New Zealand*. Palmerston North: Dunmore Press.

Schoeffel, P., & Meleisea, M. (1996). Pacific Islands Polynesian attitudes to child training and discipline in New Zealand: Some policy implications for social welfare and education. *Social Policy Journal of New Zealand, 6*, 134–146.

Shore, B. (1978). Ghosts and government: A structural analysis of alternative institutions for conflict management in Samoa. *Man (N.S), 13*, 175–199.

Statistics New Zealand. (2002). *Pacific progress: A report on the economic status of Pacific peoples in New Zealand*. Wellington: Ministry of Pacific Island Affairs.

Tamasese, E. T. (2004). *Resident, residence, residency in Samoan custom*. University of Waikato, Retrieved May 5, 2005, from http://lianz.waikato.ac.nz/PAPERS/symposium/Customary%20Law%20conference%20paper%20Oct%2004.pdf.

History

Chapman, T. M., et al. (1982). *Niue: A history of the Island*. Suva: University of the South Pacific.

Hanlon, D. L. (2003). Beyond the English method of tattooing: Decentering the practice of history in Oceania. *The Contemporary Pacific, 15*(1), 19–40.

Kirch, P. V., & Green, R. C. (2001). *Hawaiki, ancestral Polynesia: An essay in historical anthropology*. Cambridge: Cambridge University Press.

Kramer, A. (1994). *The Samoan Islands*. Auckland: Polynesian Press.

Ledyard, P. (1982). *The Tongan past*. Vava'u: Matheson.

Marcus, G. H. (1980). *The nobility and the chiefly tradition in the modern Kingdom of Tonga*. Auckland: Auckland University Press.

Marcus, G. H. (1989). Chieftainship. In A. Howard & R. Borofsky (Eds.), *Developments in Polynesian ethnology*. Honolulu: University of Hawai'i Press.

Mead, M. (1969). *Social organization of Manu'a*. Honolulu: Bishop Museum Press.

Meleisea, M. (1987). *Lagaga: A short history of Western Samoa*. Suva: Institute of Pacific Studies.

Munro, D. (1995). Pacific Islands history in the vernacular. *New Zealand Journal of History, 29*(1), 83–96.

Osorio, J. K. (2002). *Dismembering lahui: A history of the Hawaiian nation to 1887*. Honolulu: University of Hawai'i Press.

Paongo, K. (1990). The nature of education in pre-European to modern Tonga. In P. Herda, J. Terrell, & N. Gunsen (Eds.), *Tongan culture and history: Papers from the 1st Tongan history conference held in Canberra 14–17 January 1987*. Canberra: Australia National University.

Poyer, L. (1992). Defining history across cultures: Islander and outsider contrasts. *A Journal of Micronesian Studies, 1*(1), 73-89.
Sahlins, M. (1995). *How 'natives' think: About Captain Cook, for example.* Chicago: Chicago University Press.
Silva, N. K. (2004). *Aloha betrayed: Native Hawaiian resistance to American colonialism.* Durham: Duke University Press.
Stair, J. B. (1897). *Old Samoa or, flotsam and jetsam from the Pacific Ocean.* London: Religious Tract Society.
Stannard, D. (1989). *Before the horror: The population of Hawai'i at the eve of Western contact.* Honolulu: Social Science Research Institute, University of Hawai'i.
Tiffany, S. (1975). Giving and receiving: Participation in chiefly redistribution activities in Samoa. *Ethnology, 14,* 267–286.
Turner, G. (1989). *Samoa: A hundred years ago and long before.* Suva: University of the South Pacific.
White, G. M., & Lindstrom, L. (Eds.). (1997). *Chiefs today: Traditional Pacific leadership and the postcolonial state.* Stanford: Stanford University Press.

Identity

Anae, M. (1995). *Papalagi redefined: Towards a NZ-born identity.* Paper presented at Ethnicity and Multiethnicity Conference, Brigham Young University, Hawai'i.
Anae, M. (1997). Towards a New Zealand-born Samoan identity: Some reflections on labels. *Pacific Health Dialog: Journal of Community Health and Clinical Medicine for the Pacific, 4*(2), 128–137.
Anae, M. (1998). *Fofoa-i-vao-'ese: The identity journeys of NZ-Born Samoans.* Unpublished doctoral dissertation, The University of Auckland.
Anae, M. (2001). The new vikings of the sunrise: New Zealand-borns in the information age. In C. Macpherson, P. Spoonley, & M. Anae (Eds.), *Tangata o te moana nui: The evolving identities of Pacific peoples in Aotearoa/New Zealand.* Palmerston North: Dunmore Press.
Anae, M. (2003). O A'u/I: My identity journey. In P. Fairbairn-Dunlop & G. Makisi (Eds.), *Making our place: Growing up PI in New Zealand* (pp. 89–101). Palmerston North: Dunmore Press Ltd.
Anae, M. (2005). Samoans. In *Te Ara: The Encyclopedia of New Zealand.* Retrieved September 9, 2005, from http://www.TeAra.govt.nz/NewZealanders/NewZealandPeoples/Samoans/en.
Blakely, T., & Drew, K. (2004). Ethnicity, acculturation and health: Who's to judge? *The New Zealand Medical Journal, 117,* 11–18.
Challis, R. L. (1973). Immigrant Polynesians in New Zealand: Aspects of stability in adjusting to change. In D. H. Bray & C. G. N. Hill (Eds.), *Polynesian and Pakeha in New Zealand education:* vol. 1: *The sharing of cultures.* Auckland: Heinemann.
Chun, M. K. (2000). *One person, two worlds?: Two persons, one world?: Cultural*

identity through the eyes of New Zealand born Samoans. Unpublished master's thesis, University of Hawai'i, Honolulu.

Cowling, W. E. (1990). Motivation for contemporary migration. In P. Herda, J. Terrell, & N. Gunsen (Eds.), *Tongan culture and history: Papers from the 1st Tongan history conference held in Canberra, 14–17 January, 1987*. Canberra: Australia National University.

Crocombe, R. (1975). *The Pacific way: An emerging identity*. Suva: Lotu Pasifika Productions.

Crosbie, S. (1993). Americanization: American popular culture's influence on Maori and Pacific Island identity. *Midwest, 3*, 22–29.

Filoiali'i, L. A., & Knowles, L. (1983). Attitudes of Southern California Samoans toward maintaining the Samoan way of life. *Sociology & Social Research, 67*(3), 301–311.

Finau, C. (2000). *The teaching of Tongan knowledge and culture in a Tongan early childhood centre: A case study of Akoteu 'o Tuigapapai-'O-Uesile*. Unpublished master's thesis, The University of Auckland.

Franklin, M. (2003). I define my own identity: Pacific articulations of 'race' and 'culture' on the internet. *Ethnicities, 3*(4), 465–490.

Fusitu'a, L. M. (1992). *Ko e poto mo hono tauhi 'o e 'ulungaanga fakatonga/knowledge and the maintenance of Tongan culture*. Unpublished master's thesis, The University of Auckland.

Hanna, J. M. (1998). Migration and acculturation among Samoans: Some sources of stress and support. *Social Science & Medicine, 46*(10), 1325–1336.

Helu, I. F. (1999). *Critical essays: Cultural perspectives from the South seas*. Canberra: Australia National University.

Holt, A. J. (1999). *Culture, ethnicity & identity: A look at first generation children from immigrant Samoan families*. Unpublished master's thesis, The University of Auckland.

Kavapalu, H. (1995). Power and personhood in Tonga. *Social Analysis, 37*, 14–28.

Keddell, E. (2006). Pavlova and pineapple pie: Selected identity influences on Samoan-Pakeha people in Aotearoa/New Zealand. *Kotuitui: New Zealand Journal of Social Sciences Online, 1*, 45–63.

Koloto, A. H. (2000). A Tongan perspective on development. In I. Bird & W. Drewery (Eds.), *Aotearoa: A journey through life* (pp. 34–39). Sydney: McGraw-Hill.

Krishnan, V., Schoeffel, P., & Warren, J. (1994). *The challenge of change: Pacific Island communities in New Zealand, 1986–1993*. Wellington: NZ Institute for Social Research Development.

Lealaiauloto, R. S. (1995, Winter). I am Samoan, but can Samoans accept me? The cultural identity crisis of a New Zealand reared Samoan. *Mental Health News*. Auckland: Mental Health Foundation.

Lee, H. M. (2003). *Tongans overseas: Between two shores*. Honolulu: University of Hawai'i Press.

Liu, D. M. (1991). *A politics of identity in Western Samoa*. Unpublished doctoral dissertation, University of Hawai'i.

Loomis, T. (1991). The politics of ethnicity and Pacific migrants. In P. Spoonley, D. Pearson, & C. Macpherson (Eds.), *Nga take: Ethnic relations and racism in Aotearoa/New Zealand*. Palmerston North: Dunmore Press.

Macpherson, C. (1991). The changing contours of Samoans. In P. Spoonley, D. Pearson, & C. Macpherson (Eds.). *Nga take: Ethnic relations and racism in Aotearoa/New Zealand*. Palmerston North: Dunmore Press.

Macpherson, C. (1997). The Polynesian diaspora: New communities and new questions. In K. Sudo & S. Yoshida (Eds.), *Contemporary migration in Oceania: Diaspora and network*. Osaka: The Japan Center for Area Studies, National Museum of Osaka.

Macpherson, C. (1999). Will the 'real' Samoans please stand up? Issues in diasporic Samoan identity. *New Zealand Geographer, 55*(2), 50–59.

Macpherson, C. (2001). One trunk sends out many branches: Pacific cultures and cultural identities. In C. Macpherson, P. Spoonley, & M. Anae (Eds.), *Tangata o te moana nui: The evolving identities of Pacific peoples in Aotearoa/New Zealand*. Palmerston North: Dunmore Press.

Macpherson, C. (2005). From Pacific Islanders to Pacific People and beyond. In P. Spoonley, C. Macpherson, & D. Pearson (Eds.), *Tangata Tangata: The changing ethnic contours of New Zealand*. South Bank: Thomson.

Macpherson, C., Spoonley, P., & Anae, M. (Eds.). (2001). *Tangata o te moana nui: The evolving identities of Pacific peoples in Aotearoa/New Zealand*. Palmerston North: Dunmore Press.

Mageo, J. M. (1995). The reconfiguring self. *American Anthropologist*, 97(2), 282–296.

Mageo, J. M. (2002). Toward a multidimensional model of the self. *Journal of Anthropological Research, 58*, 339–365.

Meleisea, M., & Schoeffel, P. (1998). Samoan families in New Zealand: The cultural context of change. In V. Adair & R. Dixon (Eds.), *The family in Aotearoa New Zealand*. Auckland: Longman.

Mulitalo, T. (2001). *My own shade of brown*. Christchurch: University of Canterbury School of Fine Arts in association with Shoal Bay Press.

Ngan-Woo, F. E. (1985). *Fa'asamoa: The world of the Samoans*. Wellington: New Zealand Office of the Race Relations Conciliator.

Niulevaea, M. (2001). *To code-switch or not to code-switch: Language use patterns of Samoan adolescents as a measure of attitude and perception on identity, culture, and social behaviour*. Unpublished master's thesis, The University of Auckland.

Phinney, J. (1990). Ethnic identity in adolescents and adults. *Review of Research Bulletin, 108*, 499–514.

Phinney, J., & Rosenthal, D. (1992). Ethnic identity in adolescence: Process, context, and outcome. In G. R. Adams, T. P. Gullotta, & R. Montemayer (Eds.), *Adolescent identity formation*. New York: Sage Publications.

Pilato, T., Su'a, T., & Crichton-Hill, Y. (1998). A Pacific Islands perspective: Colonialism affects Pacific Island families. In C. O'Brien (Ed.), *Social work now*. Wellington: Children, Young Persons and their Families Service.

Pitt, D., & Macpherson, C. (1974). *Emerging pluralism: The Samoan community in New Zealand*. Auckland: Longman Paul Ltd.

Stewart, P., & Strathern, A. (Eds.) (2000). *Identity work: Constructing Pacific lives*. Pittsburgh: University of Pittsburgh Press.

Strathern, A., Stewart, P., Carucci, L., Poyer, L. Feinberg, R., & Macpherson, C. (2002). *Oceania: An introduction to the cultures and identities of Pacific Islanders*. Durham: Carolina Academic Press.

Taumoefolau, M. (2005). Tongans. In *Te Ara: the Encyclopedia of New Zealand*. Retrieved September 10, 2005, from http://www.TeAra.govt.nz/NewZealanders/NewZealandPeoples/Tongans/en

Tawake, S. (2000). Transforming the insider-outsider perspective: Postcolonial fiction from the Pacific. *The Contemporary Pacific, 12*(1), 155–175.

Tiatia, J. (1998). *Caught between cultures*. Auckland: Christian Research Association.

Trimble, J. E., & Dickson, R. (2005). Ethnic identity. In C. B. Fisher & R. M. Lerner (Eds.), *Encyclopedia of applied developmental science*. Vol. I. Thousand Oaks: Sage Publications.

Tu'inukuafe, E. (1990). Tongans in New Zealand: A brief study. In P. Herda, J. Terrell, & N. Gunsen (Eds.), *Tongan culture and history: Paper from the 1st Tongan history conference held in Canberra, 14–17 January, 1987*. Canberra: Australia National University.

Tupuola, A. (1993). Raising research consciousness the Fa'aSamoa way. *New Zealand Annual Review of Education, 3*, 175–189.

Tupuola, A. (1998). *Adolescence: Myth or reality for Samoan women. Beyond the stage-like toward shifting boundaries and identities*. Unpublished doctoral dissertation, Victoria University, Wellington.

Tuwere, I. S. (1994). Mana and the Fijian sense of place. *South Pacific Journal of Missionary Studies, 11*, 3–15.

Vea, S. (1997). Migration from the Kingdom of Tonga. *The Pacific Journal of Theology, 2*(18), 55–63.

Wassman, J. (Ed.). (1998). *Pacific answers to Western hegemony: Cultural practices of identity construction*. New York: Berg.

Language

Duranti, A. (1981). *The Samoan fono: A sociolinguistic study*. Canberra: Australian National University Press.

Duranti, A. (1992). Language and bodies in social space: Samoan ceremonial greetings. *American Anthropologist, 94*(3), 657–691.

Duranti, A. (1998). *From grammar to politics: Linguistic anthropology in a Samoan village*. Berkeley: University of California Press.

Giovanni, B. (2000). Language and space in Tonga: "The front of the house is where the chief sits!" *Anthropological Linguistics*, *42*(4), 499–545.

Johri, R. (1998). *Stuck in the middle or clued up on both? Language and identity among Korean, Dutch and Samoan immigrants in Dunedin*. Unpublished doctoral dissertation, University of Otago, Dunedin.

Mageo, J. M. (1989). "Ferocious is the centipede": A study of the significance of eating and speaking in Samoa. *Ethos*, *17*, 387–427.

Milner, G. B. (1961). The Samoan vocabulary of respect. *Journal of the Royal Anthropological Institute*, *91*, 296–317.

Ochs, E. (1982). Talking to children in Western Samoa. *Language in Society*, *11*, 77–104.

Ochs, E. (1988). *Culture and language development: Language acquisition and language socialization in a Samoan village*. New York: Cambridge University Press.

Ochs, E. (1992). Indexing gender. In A. Duranti & C. Goodwin (Eds.), *Rethinking context: Language as an interactive phenomenon*. Cambridge: Cambridge University Press.

Tent, J., & Geraghty, P. (2001). Exploding sky or exploded myth?: The origin of 'papalagi.' *Journal of the Polynesian Society*, *110*(2), 171–214.

Medicine and Traditional Healing

Barnes, L., Moss, R., & Kaufusi, M. (2003). Illness beliefs and adherence in diabetes mellitus: A comparison between Tongan and European patients. *New Zealand Medical Journal*, Retrieved April 26, 2005, from http://www.nzma.org.nz/journal/117-1188/744/.

Blaisdell, K. (1993). Historical and cultural aspects of native Hawaiian health. *Social Process in Hawaii*, *31*, 37–57.

Bloomfield, S. F. (2002). *Illness and cure in Tonga*. Nuku'alofa: Vava'u Press.

Cox, P. A. (1991). Polynesian herbal medicine. In P. A. Cox & S. A. Banack (Eds.), *Islands, plants, and Polynesians: An introduction to Polynesian ethnobotany*. Portland, OR: Timber Press.

Drozdow-St. Christian, D. (2002). *Elusive fragments: Making power, propriety & health in Samoa*. Durham: Carolina Academic Press.

Finau, S. A. (1982). The Tongan family: Relevance to health. *New Zealand Medical Journal*, *95*, 880–883.

Finau, S. A. (1996). Health, environment and development: Towards a Pacific paradigm. *Pacific Health Dialog: Journal of Community Health and Clinical Medicine for the Pacific*, *3*(2), 266–278.

Finau, S. A., & Tukuitonga, C. (1999). Pacific peoples in New Zealand. In P. Davis & K. Dew (Eds.), *Health and Society in Aotearoa/New Zealand*. Auckland: Oxford University Press.

Howard, A. (1986). Samoan coping behavior. In P. T. Baker, J. M. Hanna, & T. S. Baker (Eds.), *The changing Samoans: Behavior and health in transition*. New York: Oxford University Press.

Johnson, D. B., Oyama, N., LeMarchand, L., & Wilkens, L. (2004). Native Hawaiian mortality, morbidity, and lifestyle: Comparing data from 1982, 1990, and 2000. *Pacific Health Dialog: Journal of Community Health and Clinical Medicine for the Pacific*, *11*(2), 120–130.

Laing, P., & Miteara, J. (1994). Samoan and Cook Islanders' perspectives on health. In J. Spicer et al. (Eds.), *Social dimensions of health and disease: New Zealand perspectives*. Palmerston North: Dunmore Press.

Macpherson, C., & Macpherson, L. (1990). *Samoan medical belief and practice*. Auckland: Auckland University Press.

Mavoa, H. (1999). Pacific children in the statistical record: The need for ethnic-specific data in New Zealand. *Pacific Health Dialog: Journal of Community Health and Clinical Medicine for the Pacific*, *6*(2), 213–215.

Mavoa, H., Park, J., Tupouina, P., & Pryce, C. (2003). Tongan and European children's home interactions with adults and older siblings in New Zealand. *Ethos*, *31*(4), 1–24.

McGregor, D., Minerbi, L., & Matsuoka, J. (1998). A holistic assessment method of health and well-being for native Hawaiʻian communities. *Pacific Health Dialog: Journal of Community Health and Clinical Medicine for the Pacific*, *5*(2), 361–369.

Tukuitonga, C., & Finau, S. (1997). The health of Pacific peoples in New Zealand up to the early 1990's. *Pacific Health Dialog: Journal of Community Health and Clinical Medicine for the Pacific*, *4*(2), 59–67.

Mental Health and Illness

Bathgate, M., & Pulotu-Endemann, F. K. (1997). Pacific people in New Zealand. In P. Ellis & S. Collings (Eds.), *Mental health in New Zealand from a public health perspective*. Wellington: Ministry of Health.

Bellringer, M. E., Cowley-Malcolm, E., Abbott, M., & Maynard, W. (2004). *Pacific Islands families: The first two years of life studies*. Auckland: National Institute for Public Health and Mental Health Research, Auckland University of Technology.

Berry, J., & Kim, U. (1987). Comparative studies of acculturative stress. *International Migration Review*, *21*, 491–511.

Berry, J. W., & Kim, U. (1988). Acculturation and mental health. In P. Dasen, J. W. Berry, & N. Satorius (Eds.), *Health and cross-cultural psychology: Towards applications*. Beverly Hills: Sage Publications.

Bridgman, G. (1993, Spring). The Pakeha ambulance at the bottom of the cliff: Trends in Maori mental health. *Mental Health News*, 7–11.

Bridgman, G. (1996, December). Different paradigms, different services. *Mental Health Quarterly*, 6–8.

Bridgman, G. (1997). Mental health awareness in 1997: Mental illness and Pacific people in New Zealand. *Te Maori: Nga hui hui nga korero o Aotearoa*, *2*(32), 10–11.

Bridgman, G. (1997). Mental illness and Pacific people in New Zealand. *Pacific Health Dialog: Journal of Community Health and Clinical Medicine for the Pacific*, 4(2), 95–104.

Calvert, A. (1997). Health of Pacific peoples: Problems and solutions into the new millennium. *Pacific Health Dialog: Journal of Community Health and Clinical Medicine for the Pacific*, 4(2), 45–49.

Crabbe, K. M. (1999). Conceptions of depression: A Hawaiian perspective. *Pacific Health Dialog: Journal of Community Health and Clinical Medicine for the Pacific*, 6(1), 122–126.

Crabbe, K. M., Kaholokula, J. K., Kenui, C. K., & Grandinetti, A. (1996). Prevalence of depression, degrees of Hawaiianess, and modes of acculturation among Native Hawaiians living in rural North Kohala, Hawaii. In *The National Institute of Health—Asian and Pacific Islander American Health Research Conference*. Honolulu: The National Institute of Health.

Cueller, I., & Paniagua, F. (Eds.). (2000). *Handbook of multicultural mental health*. San Diego: Academic Press.

Disley, B. (1997). An overview of mental health in New Zealand. In P. M. Ellis & S. C. D. Collings (Eds.), *Mental health in New Zealand from a public health perspective*. Wellington: Ministry of Health.

Foliaki, S. (2001). *Pacific mental health services and workforce: Moving on the blueprint*. Wellington: New Zealand Mental Health Commission.

Jilek, W. (1988). Mental health, ethnopsychiatry, and traditional medicine in the Kingdom of Tonga. *Curare, 11*(13), 161–176.

Kaholokula, J. K., Grandinetti, A., Crabbe, K. M., Chang, H. K., & Kenui, C. K. (1999). Depressive symptoms and cigarette smoking among Native Hawaiians. *Asia-Pacific Journal of Public Health, 11*(2), 60–64.

Mafi, G. (1999). Mental dis-ease in a Tongan general practice. *Pacific Health Dialog: Journal of Community Health and Clinical Medicine for the Pacific*, 6(2), 196ff.

Mageo, J. M. (1991). Ma'i aitu: The cultural logic of possession in Samoa. *Ethnos, 19*(3), 352–383.

Makasiale, C., & Culbertson, P. (2003). Mental health and Polynesian clients. *The GM Resource and Referral Directory, 2003*, 121–122.

Malo, V. (2000). *Pacific people in New Zealand talk about their experiences with mental illness*. Wellington: New Zealand Mental Health Commission.

Marsella, A. J., Oliveira, J. M., Plummer, C. M., & Crabbe, K. M. (1995). Native Hawaiian (kanaka maoli) culture, mind and well-being. In H. I. McCubbin, E. A. Thompson, & J. E. Fromer (Eds.), *Resiliency in ethnic minority families: Native immigrant American families*. Madison: University of Wisconsin Press.

Nonu-Reid, E. (1996). *Guidelines for the treatment and management of depression by primary health care professionals*. Wellington: National Health Committee.

Puloka, M. H. (1999). 'Avanga: Tongan concepts of mental illness. *Pacific*

Health Dialog: Journal of Community Health and Clinical Medicine for the Pacific, 6(2), 268ff.

Pulotu-Endemann, F. K., Crawley, L., & Stanley-Findlay, R. (1995). *Strategic directions for mental health services for Pacific Islands people*. Wellington: Ministry of Health.

Tamasese, K., Peteru, C., Waldegrave, C., & Bush, C. (1997). Ole taeao afua, the new morning: A qualitative investigation into Samoan perspectives on mental health and culturally appropriate services. *Australian and New Zealand Journal of Psychiatry 39*(4), 300–309.

Tu'itahi, S., Guttenbeil-Po'uhila, Y., Htay, T., & Hand, J. (2004, December). Gambling issues for Tongan people in Auckland, Aotearoa-New Zealand. *Journal of Gambling Issues, 12*. Retrieved July 4, 2005, from http://www.camh.net/egambling/issue12/jgi_12_tuitahi.html.

Valle, R. (1998). *Caregiving across cultures: Working with dementing illness and ethnically diverse populations*. Washington: Taylor & Francis.

Pastoral Care and Spirituality

Afutiti, L. (1996). Samoan church and church diaspora. *Pacific Journal of Theology, II, 16*, 14–35.

Augsburger, D. (1986). *Pastoral counseling across cultures*. Philadelphia: Westminster.

Augsburger, D. (1992). *Conflict resolution across cultures*. Louisville: Westminster/John Knox.

Besnier, N. (1994). Christianity, authority and personhood: Sermonic discourse on Nukulaelae Atoll. *Journal of the Polynesian Society, 103*, 339–378.

Bohn, C. (Ed.). (1995). *Therapeutic practice in a cross-cultural world: Theological, psychological, and ethical issues*. Decatur: Journal of Pastoral Care Publications.

Clark, P. Y. (2004). Exploring the pastoral dynamics of mixed-race persons. *Pastoral Psychology, 52*(4), 315–328.

Duncan, B. K. (1994). *A hierarchy of symbols: Samoan symbolism in New Zealand*. Unpublished doctoral dissertation, University of Otago, Dunedin, New Zealand.

Elder, D. (1993). *Cross-cultural conflict: Building relationships for effective ministry*. Downers Grove: InterVarsity Press.

Halapua, W. (1997). An approach to pastoral care with a difference: The case of forgotten people. In P. Culbertson (Ed.), *Counselling issues and South Pacific communities* (pp. 241–255). Auckland: Snedden & Cervin.

Havea, J. (1996). Shifting the boundaries: House of God and the politics of reading. *The Pacific Journal of Theology, 16*, 55–71.

Kamu, L. (1996). *The Samoan culture and the Christian gospel*. Apia: Methodist Printing.

Mageo, J. M. (1996). Continuity and shape-shifting: Samoan spirits in culture history. In J. M. Mageo & A. Howard (Eds.), *Spirits in culture, history, and mind*. New York: Routledge.

Maliko, T. (2000). *An analysis of the hierarchy of voice: The context of the Congregational Christian Church of Samoa in New Zealand*. Unpublished master's thesis, The University of Auckland.

Mitaera, J. (1997). Pastoral care and the real world context of Cook Islanders in Aotearoa New Zealand. In P. Culbertson (Ed.), *Counselling Issues and South Pacific Communities* (pp. 117–131). Auckland: Snedden & Cervin.

Palu, M. (2002). Pacific theology. *The Pacific Journal of Theology, 2*(28), 21–46.

Peters, L. G. (1994). Rites of passage and the borderline syndrome: Perspectives in transpersonal anthropology. *ReVision, 17*(1), 35–49.

Swain, T., & Trompf, G. (1995). *Religions of Oceania*. London: Routledge.

Taule'ale'ausumai, F. J. (1997). Pastoral care: A Samoan perspective. In P. Culbertson (Ed.), *Counselling Issues and South Pacific Communities* (pp. 215–237). Auckland: Snedden & Cervin.

Taule'ale'ausumai, F. J. (1994). *The Samoan face of God*. Unpublished master's thesis, Victoria University, Wellington.

Vaai, U. (1996). A theological reflection on God's oikos (house) in relation to the Samoan context. *Pacific Journal of Theology, II, 16*, 72–76.

Wingeier, D. (1995). Pastoral selection in Samoa. *Journal of Supervision and Training in Ministry, 16*, 217–223.

Wright, L. S., Frost, C. J., & Wisecarver, S. J. (1993). Church attendance, meaningfulness of religion, and depressive symptomatology among adolescents. *Journal of Youth and Adolescence, 22*(5), 559–569.

Psychology, Psychiatry, and Psychotherapy

Antilla, O. (1995). Some thoughts on the process of immigration. *Forum: Journal of the New Zealand Association of Psychotherapists, 1*, 77–85.

Bhugra, D., & Bhul, K. (2001). *Cross-cultural psychiatry: A practical guide*. London: Arnold.

Bowden, R. (2001). *A psychotherapist sings in Aotearoa: Psychotherapy in New Zealand*. Plimmerton: Caroy Publications.

Brickman, C. (2003). *Aboriginal populations in the mind: Race and primitivity in psychoanalysis*. New York: Columbia University Press.

Bush, A., Collings, S., Tamasese, K., & Waldegrave, C. (2005). Samoan and psychiatrists' perspectives on the self: Qualitative comparison. *Australian and New Zealand Journal of Psychiatry, 39*, 621–626.

Culbertson, P. (1999). Listening differently with Maori and Polynesian clients. *Forum: Journal of the New Zealand Association of Psychotherapists, 5*, 65–82.

Doi, T. (1976). Psychotherapy as a 'Hide and Seek.' In W. P. Lebra (Ed.), *Culture-bound syndromes, ethnopsychiatry, and alternative therapies* (pp. 22–31). Honolulu: University of Hawai'i Press.

Holmes, D. (1992). Race and transference in psychoanalysis and psychotherapy. *International Journal of Psychoanalysis, 73*, 1–11.

Hubber, T. D. (1998). *An exploration of intercultural parenting: The experience of Samoan & New Zealand-European couples*. Unpublished master's thesis, The University of Auckland.

Kitayama, S. & Markus, H. R. (1994). Culture and self: How cultures influence the ways we view ourselves. In D. Matsumoto (Ed.), *People: Psychology from a cultural perspective* (pp. 17–37). Pacific Grove: Brookes Cole.

Lui, D. (2001). Traditional healing in modern psychiatry: A Pacific perspective. In *No One is An Island: Proceedings of the 11th Annual MHS Conference 2001*. Wellington: The Mental Health Services Conference of Australia and New Zealand.

Matsumoto, D. (2000). *People: Psychology from a cultural perspective*. Long Grove, IL: Waveland Press.

Patterson, S. (2003). *Cultural matching vs. cultural collusion: How does cultural identification affect the psychotherapeutic relationship?* Unpublished master's thesis, Auckland University of Technology.

Puthenpadath, L. (2001). Culture as a variable in psychotherapy. *The Journal of the New Zealand Association of Psychotherapists, 7*, 73–80.

Rezentes, W. C. (1996). *Ka lama kukui: Hawaiian psychology: An introduction*. Honolulu: A'ali'i Books.

Saha, A. K. (1999). Individualism-collectivism revisited: Some consequences for group decision-making. In W. J. Lonner, D. L. Dinnel, D. K. Forgays, & S. A. Hayes (Eds.), *Merging past, present and future in cross-cultural psychology*. Lisse: Swets & Zeitlinger Publishers.

Seeley, K. (2000). *Cultural psychotherapy: Working with culture in the clinical encounter*. Northvale: Jason Aronson.

Tamasese, K. (2003). Honoring Samoan ways and understanding. In C. Waldegrave, K. Tamasese, F. Tuhaka, & W. Campbell (Eds.), *Just Therapy—A Journey* (pp. 183–195). Adelaide: Dulwich Centre Publications.

Tseng, W., & Streltzer, J. (Eds.). (1997). *Culture and psychotherapy: A guide to clinical assessment*. New York: Brunner/Mazel.

White, G. M., & Kirkpatrick, J. (Eds.). (1985). *Person, self, and experience: Exploring Pacific ethnopsychologies*. Berkeley: University of California Press.

Wilson, J. J., & Everts, J. F. (1995). Psychological wellbeing in New Zealand's aging population: Implications for counsellors working in a multicultural society. *New Zealand Journal of Counselling, 17*(2), 51–58.

Young, B. B. C. (1980). The Hawaiians. In J. F. McDermott, W. S. Tseng, & T. W. Maretzki (Eds.), *People and cultures of Hawaii: A psychocultural profile*. Honolulu: University of Hawai'i Press.

Research Methodology

Anae, M. (1998b). Inside out: Methodological issues on being a 'native researcher.' *Pacific Health Dialog: Journal of Community Health and Clinical Medicine for the Pacific, 5*(2), 273–279.

Baba, T., Mahina, 'O., & Williams, N. (Eds.). (2004). *Researching the Pacific and indigenous people*. Auckland: Centre for Pacific Studies, Auckland University.

Finau, S. A. (1995). Health research in the Pacific: In search of a reality. *New Zealand Medical Journal, 108*, 16–19.

Finau, S. A. (2001). Marching from the margin: A health vision for Pacificans in Aotearoa. *The New Zealand Medical Journal, 114*(1134), 296–298.

Helu-Thaman, K. (1995). Concepts of learning, knowledge, and wisdom in Tonga, and their relevance to modern education. *Prospects, 25*(4), 723.

Helu-Thaman, K. (2003). Decolonizing Pacific Studies: Indigenous perspectives, knowledge, and wisdom in higher education. *The Contemporary Pacific, 15*(1), 1–17.

Hereniko, V. (2000). Indigenous knowledge and academic imperialism. In R. Borofsky (Ed.), *Remembrance of Pacific pasts: An invitation to remake history*. Honolulu: University of Hawai'i Press.

Laing, P., & Miteara, J. (1994). Key informants and co-operative inquiry: Some reflections on a cross-cultural research team collecting health data in the South Pacific. *Sites, 28*, 64–76.

Latukefu, S. (1968). Oral traditions: An appraisal of their value in historical research in Tonga. *Journal of Pacific History, 3*, 135–143.

Latukefu, S. (1980). The definition of authentic oceanic cultures with particular reference to Tongan culture. *Pacific Studies, 4*(1), 60–81.

Mara, D. L. (1999). Why research? Why educational research for/by/with Pacific communities in Aotearoa-New Zealand? In L. Tuioti (Ed.), *Educating Pasefika Positively: Pacific Island Educators' Conference, 13–15 April 1999*. Auckland: PIERC Education.

Smith, L. T. (1999). *Decolonizing methodologies: Research and indigenous people*. Dunedin: University of Otago Press.

Spoonley, P. (1999). The challenge of cross-cultural research. In C. Davidson & M. Tolich (Eds.), *Social science research in New Zealand*. Auckland: Longman.

Tamasese Efi', T. T. (2005, July). Clutter in indigenous knowledge, research and history: A Samoan perspective. *Social Policy Journal of New Zealand, 25*, 61–69.

Teaiwa, K., & Kabutaulaka, T. (2000). Personalizing Pacific Studies: Strategies for imagining Oceania/Surfing our sea of islands: The politics of imagination. *SPAN, 50/51*, 15–42.

Tiatia, J. (2000). Listen to the silence. In M. Gilling (Ed.), *Research: The art of juggling*. Wellington: Massey University.

Trask, H-K. (1991). Natives and anthropologists: The colonial struggle. *The Contemporary Pacific, 3*, 168–171.

Tupuola, A. M. (1993). Raising research consciousness the fa'asamoa way. *New Zealand Annual Review of Education, 3*, 175–189.

Sexuality and Gender

Anae, M., Fuamatu, N., Lima, I., Mariner, K., Park, J., & Sua'ali'i-Sauni, T. (2000). *Tiute ma matafaioi a nisi tane Samoa i le faiga o aiga: The roles and responsibilities of some Samoan men in reproduction*. Auckland: Pacific Health Research Centre, The University of Auckland.

Besnier, N. (1994). Polynesian gender liminality through time and space. In G. Herdt (Ed.), *Third sex, third gender: Beyond dimorphism in culture and history*. New York: Zone Books.

Besnier, N. (1997). Sluts and superwomen: The politics of gender liminality in urban Tonga. *Ethnos, 62*(1-2), 5–31.

Besnier, N. (2002). Transgenderism, loyalty, and the Miss Galaxy beauty pageant in Tonga. *American Ethnologist, 29*(3), 534–567.

Dolgoy, R. (2000). *The search for recognition and social movement emergence: Towards an understanding of the transformation of the fa'afafine of Samoa*. Unpublished doctoral dissertation, The University of Alberta.

Douaire-Marsaudon, F. (1996). Neither black nor white: The father's sister in Tonga. *The Journal of the Polynesian Society, 105*(2), 139–164.

Farran, S. (2004). Transsexuals, fa'afafine, fakaleiti and marriage law in the Pacific: Considerations for the future. *Journal of the Polynesian Society, 113*(2), 119–142.

Faumui, A. T. (1996). *Voices of Samoan women graduates: Survival, success and contradiction*. Unpublished master's thesis, The University of Auckland.

Gailey, C. W. (1987). *Kinship to kingship: Gender hierarchy and state formation in the Tongan Islands*. Austin: University of Texas Press.

Grant, N. (1995). From Margaret Mead's fieldnotes: What counted as 'sex' in Samoa? *American Anthropologist, 97*(4), 678–682.

Griffen, V. (1982). *A healthbook for Pacific women*. Suva: Institute of Pacific Studies.

Guttmann, M. (1997). Trafficking in men: The anthropology of masculinity. *Annual Review of Anthropology, 26*, 385–409.

Hughes, C. K. (2004). Factors associated with health-seeking behaviors of Native Hawaiian men. *Pacific Health Dialog: Journal of Community Health and Clinical Medicine for the Pacific, 11*(2), 176–182.

Huntsman, J. (Ed.). (1995). *Tonga and Samoa: Images of gender and polity*. Christchurch: Macmillan Brown Centre for Pacific Studies.

James, K. (1994). Effeminate males and changes in the construction of gender in Tonga. *Pacific Studies, 17*, 39–69.

Joe, K. A., & Chesney-Lind, M. (1995). Just every mother's angel: An analysis of gender and ethnic variations in youth gang membership. *Gender and Society*, 9, 408–431.

Jones, A., Herda, P., & Sua'ali'a, T. (Eds.) (2000). *Bitter sweet: Indigenous women in the Pacific*. Dunedin: University of Otago Press.

Kanongata, K. (1995). Pacific women and theology. *Pacific Journal of Theology*, 13, 17–33.

Kanongata, K. (1997). Pacific women's theology of birthing and liberation. In W. R. Barr (Ed.), *Constructive Christian theology in the worldwide church*. Grand Rapids: Eerdmans.

Larner, W. (1989). *Migration and female labour: Samoan women in New Zealand*. Unpublished master's thesis, University of Canterbury, Christchurch, New Zealand.

Leckie, J. (2000). Gender and work in Fiji: Constraints to re-negotiation. In A. Jones, P. Herda, & T. M. Sua'ali'i (Eds.), *Bitter sweet: Indigenous women in the Pacific* (pp. 73–92). Dunedin: University of Otago Press.

Lipinski, J., & Pope, J. H. (2002). Body ideals in young Samoan men: A comparison with men in North America and Europe. *International Journal of Men's Health*, 1(2), 163–171.

Mageo, J. M. (1992). Male transvestism and cultural change in Samoa. *American Ethnologist*, 19(3), 443-459.

Mageo, J. M. (1994). Hairdos and don'ts: Hair symbolism and sexuality history in Samoa. *Man*, 29(2), 407–432.

Mageo, J. M. (1996). Samoa, on the Wilde side: Male transvestism, Oscar Wilde, and liminality in making gender. *Ethos*, 24(4), 588–627.

Mageo, J. M. (2002). Self models and sexual agency. In J. M. Mageo, *Power and the self*. Cambridge: Cambridge University Press.

Mageo, J. M. (2003). *Fa'afafine: Transvestism in Samoa*. Washington: Museum of Anthropology.

Malo, V. (2000). *Pacific people in New Zealand talk about their experiences with mental illness*. Wellington: Mental Health Recovery, Series 3.

Manderson, L., & Jolly, M. (Eds.). (1997). *Sites of desire, economies of pleasure: Sexualities in Asia and the Pacific*. Chicago: University of Chicago Press.

Matzner, A. (2001). *Transgender, queens, mahu, whatever: An oral history from Hawai'i*. Retrieved July 23, 2005, from http://wwwshe.murdoch.edu.au/intersections/issue6/matzner.html. [Intersections 6].

McIntosh, T. (1999). *Words and worlds of difference: Homosexualities in the Pacific*. Working paper 3/99, Working Papers on Sociology and Social Policy. Suva: University of the South Pacific.

Miles, P. (2003). *Fa'afafine, fakaleiti and mahu: Transgender in the Pacific*. Retrieved June 18, 2005, from http://europe/eu.int/comm/development/publicat/courier183/fr/fr_045.pdf.

Moyle, R. (1975). Sexuality in Samoan art forms. *Archives of Sexual Behavior*, 4(3), 227–247.

Murray, S. (Ed.). (1992). *Oceanic homosexualities*. New York: Garland Press.

New Zealand AIDS Foundation. (1996). *Needs assessment: Pacific Islands men who have sex with men: Report to North Health*. Auckland: NZ AIDS Foundation.

Niumeitolu, F. (2003). Kainga: Reinventing a Tongan-American feminism. In *Intersections: Critical locations of feminist rhetorical practice*, Fourth Biennial Feminism(s) & Rhetoric(s) Conference. Columbus: Ohio State University.

Ortner, S. (1981). Gender and sexuality in hierarchical societies: The case of Polynesia. In S. Ortner & H. Whitehead (Eds.), *Sexual meanings: The cultural construction of gender and sexuality*. Cambridge: Cambridge University Press.

Ortner, S. (1997). *Making gender: The politics and erotics of culture*. Boston: Beacon.

Park, J., Sua'ali'i, T., Anae, M., Lima, I., Fuamatu, N., & Mariner, K. (2002). A late-twentieth-century Auckland perspective on Samoan masculinities. In H. Worth, A. Paris, & L. Allen (Eds.), *The life of Brian: Masculinities, sexualities and health in New Zealand*. Dunedin: University of Otago Press.

Peteru, A. (1997). *The sexuality and STD/HIV risk-related sexual behaviours of single, unskilled, young adult Samoan males: A qualitative study*. Unpublished master's thesis, Mahidol University, Thailand.

Poasa, K. (1992). The Samoan fa'afafine: One case study and discussion of transexualism. *The Journal of Psychology and Human Sexuality*, *5*(3), 39–51.

Pulotu-Endemann, F. K., & Peteru, C. L. (2001). Beyond the paradise myth: Sexuality and identity. In C. Macpherson, P. Spoonley, & M. Anae (Eds.), *Tangata o te moana nui: The evolving identities of Pacific peoples in Aotearoa/New Zealand*. Palmerston North: Dunmore Press.

Ralston, C. (1992). The study of women in the Pacific. *The Contemporary Pacific*, *4*(1), 162–175.

Rogers, G. (1977). The father's sister is black: A consideration of female rank and power in Tonga. *Journal of the Polynesian Society*, *86*, 157–182.

Schmidt, J. (2001). Redefining fa'afafine: Western discourses and the construction of transgenderism in Samoa. *Intersections 6*, Retrieved August 17, 2005, from http://wwwsshe.murdoch.edu.au/intersections/issue6/schmidt.html.

Schoeffel, P. (1978). Gender, status and power in Western Samoa. *Canberra Anthropology*, *1*, 69–81.

Schoeffel, P. (1979). *Daughters of Sina: A study of gender, status and power in Western Samoa*. Unpublished doctoral dissertation, Australian National University, Canberra.

Schoeffel, P. (1979). The ladies' row of thatch: Women and rural development in Western Samoa. *Pacific Perspective*, *8*(1), 1–11.

Schoeffel, P. (1987). Rank, gender and politics in ancient Samoa. *The Journal of Pacific History*, *22*, 174–193.

Schoeffel, P. (1995). The Samoan concept of feagaiga and its transformation. In J. Huntsman (Ed.), *Tonga and Samoa: Images of Gender and Policy*. Christchurch: Macmillan Brown Centre for Pacific Studies.

Shankman, P. (1996). The history of Samoan sexuality conduct and the Mead-Freeman controversy. *American Anthropologist, 98*(3), 555–567.

Shore, B. (1976). Incest prohibitions and the logic of power in Samoa. *Journal of the Polynesian Society, 85*(2), 275–296.

Shore, B. (1981). Sexuality and gender in Samoa. In S. Ortner & H. Whitehead (Eds.), *Sexual meanings: The cultural construction of gender and sexuality.* Cambridge: Cambridge University Press.

Sua'ali'i, T. M. (2000). Deconstructing the 'exotic' female beauty of the Pacific Islands. In A. Jones, P. Herder, & T. M. Sua'ali'i (Eds.), *Bitter sweet: Indigenous women in the Pacific* (pp. 93–108). Dunedin: University of Otago Press.

Sua'ali'i, T. M. (2001). Samoans and gender: Some reflections on male, female and fa'afafine gender identities. In C. Macpherson, P. Spoonley, & M. Anae (Eds.), *Tangata o te moana nui: The evolving identities of Pacific peoples in Aotearoa/New Zealand.* Palmerston North: Dunmore Press.

Taumoefolau, M. (1999). Is the father's sister really 'black'? *Journal of the Polynesian Society, 100,* 191–198.

Tongamoa, T. (Ed.). (1988). *Pacific women: Roles and status of women in Pacific societies.* Suva: University of the South Pacific.

Tupuola, A. M. (1998). Fa'asamoa in the 1990s: Young Samoan women speak. In R. DuPlessis, & L. Alice (Eds.), *Feminist thought in Aotearoa/New Zealand: Differences and connections.* Auckland: Oxford University Press.

Tupuola, A. M. (2000). Learning sexuality: Young Samoan women. In A. Jones, P. Herda & T. Sua'ali'i-Sauni (Eds.), *Bitter sweet: Indigenous women in the Pacific* (pp. 61–72). Dunedin: University of Otago Press.

Tupuola, A. M. (2004). Talking sexuality through an insider's lens: The Samoan experience. In A. Harris (Ed.), *All about the girl: Culture, power, and identity.* New York: Routledge.

Van Trigt, J. (2000). Reflecting on the Pacific and Pacific Island women in five dominant cinematic texts. In A. Jones, P. Herder, & T. M. Sua'ali'i (Eds.), *Bitter sweet: Indigenous women in the Pacific* (pp. 109–120). Dunedin: University of Otago Press.

Wallace, L. (1999). Fa'afafine: Queens of Samoa and the elision of homosexuality. *Gay and Lesbian Quarterly, 5*(1), 25–39.

Wallace, L. (2003). *Sexual encounters: Pacific texts, modern sexualities.* Ithaca: Cornell University Press.

Worth, H. (2000). Up on K Road on a Saturday night: Sex, gender and sex work in Auckland. *Venereology: The Interdisciplinary, International Journal of Sexual Health, 13*(1), 15–24.

Worth, H. (2002). 'Tits is just an accessory': Masculinity and femininity in the lives of Maori and Pacific queens. In H. Worth, A. Paris, & L. Allen (Eds.), *The life of Brian: Masculinities, sexualities and health in New Zealand.* Dunedin: University of Otago Press.

Young, L. H. (1999). Considering the impact of gender in Tongan whaling: A framework for evaluation and suggestions for maximizing benefits to women. In M. Freeman (Ed.), *Issues in indigenous whaling: Tonga*. Qualicum Beach, BC: World Council of Whalers.

Substance Abuse and Addictions

Abrahamson, A. (2002). Yaqona, alive and signifying: Transformations and inventions of kava in Eastern Fiji. In *5th Conference of the European Society for Oceanists (ESfO): Recovering the past: Resources, representations and ethics of research in Oceania*. Vienna: ESfO.

Alcohol Advisory Council of New Zealand (ALAC). (1997). *The place of alcohol in the lives of people from Tokelau, Fiji, Niue, Tonga, Cook Islands and Samoa living in New Zealand: An overview.* Wellington: Alcohol Advisory Council of New Zealand.

Bellringer, M. E., Perese, L., Rossen, F., Tse, S., Adams, P., Brown, R., & Manaia, W. (2002). *Supporting the wellbeing of young people in relation to gambling in New Zealand: A discussion document*. Auckland: Centre for Gambling Studies and Problem Gambling Foundation.

Biersack, A. (1991). Kava'onau and the Tongan chiefs. *Journal of Pacific Studies, 100* (3), 230–267.

Bott, E. (1968). Psychoanalysis and ceremony. In J. Sutherland (Ed.), *The psychoanalytic approach*. London: Bailliere, Tindall & Caswell.

Collocott, E. E. V. (1927). Kava ceremonial in Tonga. *The Journal of the Polynesian Society, 36*, 21–47.

Feldman, H. (1980). Informal kava drinking in Tonga. *The Journal of the Polynesian Society, 89*, 101–103.

Hill, L., & Casswell, S. (1999). *Alcohol harm reduction: Research-based advice for purchasing strategy on public health issues.* Auckland: Alcohol and Public Health Research Unit, University of Auckland.

Lemert, E. (1967). Secular use of kava in Tonga. *Quarterly Journal of Studies on Alcohol, 28*, 238–241.

Lemert, E. (1972). Forms and pathology of drinking in three Polynesian societies. In E. Lemert (Ed.), *Human deviance, social problems and social control.* Englewood Cliffs: Prentice Hall.

Marshall, M. (1993). A Pacific haze: Alcohol and drugs in Oceania. In V. Lockwood (Ed.), *Contemporary Pacific societies: Studies in development and change.* Englewood Cliffs: Prentice Hall.

Newell, W. H. (1947). Kava ceremony in Tonga. *Journal of Polynesian Society, 56*, 364–417.

Pardini, D. A., Plante, T. G., Sherman, A., & Stump, J. E. (2000). Religious faith and spirituality in substance abuse recovery: Determining the mental health benefits. *Journal of Substance Abuse Treatment, 19*, 347–354.

Perese, L., & Faleafa, M. (2000). *The impact of gambling on some Samoan people's lives in Auckland*. Auckland: Compulsive Gambling Society.

Pratt, R. (1922). Kava ceremony in Tonga. *Journal of the Polynesian Society, 31*, 198–201.

Prescott, J., & McCall, G. (Eds.). (1989). *Kava: Use and abuse in Australia and the South Pacific*. Kensington: National Drug & Alcohol Research Centre.

Siataga, P. (2000). The church and alcohol related harm. In *Pacific issues workshop report: Alcohol and Pacific People*. Auckland: Target Education and Management Consultants.

Tuala, P. (1999). Alcoholism in Samoa: A disease. *Pacific Islands Report*, Retrieved June 2, 2005, from http://166.122.164.43/archive/1999/December/12-23-17.htm.

Suicidal Behaviors

Aghanwa, H. S. (2000). The characteristics of suicide attempters admitted to the main general hospital in Fiji Islands. *Journal of Psychosomatic Research*, *49*, 439–445.

Booth, H. (1999). Gender, power and social change: Youth suicide among Fiji Indians and Western Samoans. *Journal of Polynesian Society*, *108*(1), 39–68.

Booth, H. (1999). Pacific Island suicide in comparative perspective. *Journal of Biosocial Science*, *31*, 433–448.

Bourke, T. (2001). Suicide in Samoa. *Pacific Health Dialog: Journal of Community Health and Clinical Medicine for the Pacific*, *8*(1), 213–219.

Bowles, J. R. (1985). Suicide and attempted suicide in contemporary Western Samoa. In F. X. Hezel, D. H. Rubinstein & G. W. White (Eds.), *Culture, youth and suicide in the Pacific*. Honolulu: University of Hawai'i Press.

Cowling, W. (1990). Mental illness is not the only cause of suicides in Tonga. *Matangi Tonga*, *5*(6), 38–40.

Enoka, M. I. S. (2001). Letters to the editor. Weaving mental health care in Samoa: My story (O la'u tala). *Pacific Health Dialog: Journal of Community Health and Clinical Medicine for the Pacific*, *8*(1), 238–239.

Finau, S. A., & Lasalo, P. (1985). Suicide and parasuicide in paradise. *New Zealand Family Physician*, *12*, 101–104.

Hezel, F. X. (1984). Cultural patterns in Trukese suicide. *Ethnology*, *23*, 193–206.

Hezel, F. X. (1987). Truk suicide epidemic and social change. *Human Organization*, *46*(4), 283–291.

Hezel, F. X. (1989). Suicide and the Micronesian family. *The Contemporary Pacific*, *1*(1 & 2), 43–74.

Hezel, F. X. (1993). Culture in crisis: Trends in the Pacific today. *Micronesian Counselor*, Retrieved May 21, 2005, from http://www.micsem.org/pubs/counselor/frames/cultcrisfr.htm.

Hezel, F. X. (1994). What can we do to prevent suicide in the Pacific? *Pacific Health Dialog: Journal of Community Health and Clinical Medicine for the Pacific*, *1*(1), 59–62.

Macpherson, C., & Macpherson, L. (1985). Suicide in Western Samoa: A sociological perspective. In F. X. Hezel, D. H. Rubinstein, & G. W. White

(Eds.), *Culture, youth and suicide in the Pacific*. Honolulu: University of Hawai'i Press.

Macpherson, C., & Macpherson, L. (1987). Towards an explanation of recent trends in suicide in Western Samoa. *Man (N.S), 22*, 305–330.

Norton, R., Macpherson, C., & Macpherson, L. (1988). Chiefs, adolescent suicide and the transformation of chiefly authority in Western Samoa. *Man, 23*(4), 759–762.

Rose, J., Hatcher, S., & Koelmeyer, T. (1999). Suicide in Auckland 1989–1997. *New Zealand Medical Journal, 112*(1094), 324–326.

Rubinstein, D. H. (1987). Cultural patterns and contagion: Epidemic suicide among Micronesian youth. In A. Robillard & A. Marsella (Eds.), *Contemporary issues in mental health research in the Pacific Islands*. Honolulu: University of Hawai'i Press.

Rubinstein, D. H. (1992). Suicide in Micronesia and Samoa: A critique of explanations. *Pacific Studies, 15*(1), 51–75.

Rubinstein, D. H. (1994). Changes in the Micronesian family structure leading to alcoholism, suicide and child abuse and neglect. *Micronesian Counselor,* Retrieved April 14, 2005, from http://www.micsem.org/pubs/publications/microsounselor/cngmic.html.

Tatz, C. (1999). *Aboriginal suicide is different: Aboriginal youth suicide in New South Wales, the Australian Capital Territory and New Zealand: Towards a model of explanation and alleviation*. Sydney: Criminology Research Council.

Tiatia, J. (2003). *Reasons to live: NZ-born Samoan young people's responses to suicidal behaviours*. Unpublished doctoral dissertation, The University of Auckland.

Tiatia, J., & Coggan, C. (2001). Young Pacifican suicide attempters: A review of emergency department medical records. *Pacific Health Dialog: Journal of Community Health and Clinical Medicine for the Pacific*, 8(1), 124–128.

Va'a, F. (1982). Samoa's youth suicide wave. *Pacific Islands Monthly, 53*(7), 28–29.

Vivili, P. S., Finau, S. A., & Finau, E. (1999). Suicide in Tonga, 1982–1997. *Pacific Health Dialog: Journal of Community Health and Clinical Medicine for the Pacific*, 6(2), 211–212.

White, M. G. (1985). Suicide and culture: Island views. In F. X. Hezel, D. H. Rubinstein, & G. W. White (Eds.), *Culture, youth and suicide in the Pacific*. Honolulu: University of Hawai'i Press.

Yuen, N. Y. C., Nahulu, L. B., Hishinuma, E. S., & Miyamoto, R. H. (2000). Cultural identification and attempted suicide in Native Hawaiian adolescents. *Journal of the American Academy of Child and Adolescent Psychiatry, 39*(3), 360–367.

The Arts

Avia, T. (2004). *Wild dogs under my skirt*. Wellington: Victoria University Press.

Figiel, S. (1996). *The girl in the moon circle*. Suva: Mana Publications.

Figiel, S. (1996). *Where we once belonged*. Auckland: Pasifika Press.

Figiel, S. (1999). *They who do not grieve*. Auckland: Vintage.

Helu-Thaman, K. (1993). *Kakala*. Suva: Mana Publications.

Kaeppler, A. L. (1993). Poetics and politics of Tongan laments and eulogies. *American Ethnologist, 20*(3), 474–502.

Kneubuhl, V. (1987). Traditional performances in Samoan culture: Two forms. *Asian Theater Journal, 4*(2), 166–176.

Mila, K. (2005). *Dream fish floating*. Auckland: Huia.

Moore, A. C. (1995). *Arts in the religions of the Pacific: Symbols of life*. Otago: Continuum International.

Sinavaiana, C. (1992). *Traditional comic theater in Samoa: A holographic view*. Unpublished doctoral dissertation, University of Hawai'i, Honolulu.

Sinavaiana, C. (1992). Where the spirits laugh last: Comic theater in Samoa. In W. E. Mitchell (Ed.), *Clowning as critical practice*. Pittsburgh: University of Pittsburgh Press.

Taumoefolau, M. (2005). *Songs and poems of Queen Sālote*. Auckland: Auckland University Press.

Thomas, N. (1997). *In Oceania: Visions, artifacts, histories*. Durham: Duke University Press.

Wendt, A. (Ed.) (1995). *Nuanua: Pacific writing in English since 1980*. Auckland: Auckland University Press.

Wendt, A. (1999). Afterword: Tatauing the post-colonial body. In V. Hereniko & R. Wilson (Eds.), *Inside out: Literature, cultural politics and identity in the new Pacific* (pp. 399–412). Lanham: Rowman & Littlefield.

Wendt, A. (1999). *The best of Albert Wendt's short stories*. Auckland: Vintage.

Wendt, A. (2004). *The songmaker's chair*. Honolulu: University of Hawai'i Press.

Wendt, A., Whaitiri, R., & Sullivan, R. (Eds.) (2003). *Whetu Moana: Contemporary Polynesian poems in English*. Auckland: Auckland University Press.

Violence

Adinkrah, M. (2003). Men who kill their own children: Paternal filicide incidents in contemporary Fiji. *Child Abuse & Neglect, 27*, 557–568.

Asiasiga, L., Falanitule, L., Tu'itahi, S., & Guttenbeil, Y. (2004). Family violence: A Pacific perspective. In M. Burton, V. Elizabeth, L. Falanitule, J. Hind, B. Martin, & H. Rauwhero (Eds.), *Free from abuse: What women say and what can be done*. Auckland: Auckland District Health Board.

Asiasiga, L., & Gray, A. (1998). *Intervening to present family violence in Pacific communities: A literature review for Offending by Pacific Peoples Project (OOPS)*. Wellington: Ministry of Justice.

Collier, A. F., McClure, F. H., Collier, J., Otto, C., & Polloi, A. (1999). Culture-specific views of child maltreament and parenting styles in a Pacific Island community. *Child Abuse & Neglect, 23*(3), 229–244.

Counts, D. (1990). Domestic violence in Oceania: Conclusion. *Pacific Studies, 13*, 3.
Cribb, J. (1997). Being bashed is just something I have to accept: Western Samoan women's attitudes towards domestic violence in Christchurch. *Social Policy Journal of New Zealand, 9*, 164–170.
Duituturaga, E. (2998). *Pacific Islands study in attitudes to family violence: A study across cultures*. Wellington: FVPCC.
Hunt-Ioane, F. (2005). *Physical discipline in Samoan families*. Unpublished master's thesis, Massey University, New Zealand.
Mapusaga O Aiga. (1996). *A study of domestic & sexual violence against women in [Western] Samoa*. Apia: Mapusaga O Aiga.
Schultz, R. F. (1995). Child abuse in Fiji: A hidden problem. *Pacific Health Dialog: Journal of Community Health and Clinical Medicine for the Pacific, 21*(2), 31–36.
Siaosi Sumeo, K. (2005). *An exploratory study on the physical and sexual abuse of children in Samoa*. Unpublished master's thesis, Massey University, New Zealand.

Youth

Bell, Z. (2000). *Having their say: Six Pacific girls talk about their experiences in a New Zealand secondary school*. Unpublished master's thesis, Massey University, New Zealand.
Brown, T., Sheehan, R., & Hewitt, L. (2002). Child abuse in the context of parental separation and divorce. *Children Australia, 27*(2), 35–40.
Coggan, C., Patterson, P. & Tiatia, J. (1999). *Impact evaluation of the schools as first point of contact for health services*. Auckland: Injury Prevention Research Centre.
Cote, J. E. (1994). *Adolescent storm and stress: An evaluation of the Mead-Freeman controversy*. Mahwah: Lawrence Erlbaum Associates.
Fogarty, J. W. (1992). On the cutting edge of two cultures: Cultural adaption and areas of tension of Samoan adolescent girls in a New Zealand high school. *New Zealand Journal of Counselling, 14*(2), 11–18.
Freeman, D. (1984). *Margaret Mead and Samoa*. Harmondsworth: Penguin.
Herdt, G., & Leavitt, S. C. (Eds.). (1998). *Adolescence in Pacific Island societies*. Pittsburgh: University of Pittsburgh Press.
Jones, A. (1991). *At school I've got a chance: Culture/privilege: Pacific Islands and Pakeha girls at school*. Palmerston North: Dunmore Press.
Leacock, E. (1987). Postscript: The problems of youth in contemporary Samoa. In L. D. Holmes (Ed.), *Quest for the real Samoa: The Mead/Freeman controversy and beyond*. Westport: Bergin & Garvey Publishers.
McDade, T. W. (2001). Lifestyle incongruity, social integration, and immune function in Samoan adolescents. *Social Science & Medicine, 53*, 1351–1362.
McGeorge, T. (1996). *Self-esteem in New Zealand raised Pacific Islands young people*. Auckland: Health Research Council of New Zealand.

Mead, M. (1943). *Coming of age in Samoa*. London: Penguin Books.

Ministry of Pacific Island Affairs. (2003). *Ala fou, new pathways: Strategic directions for Pacific youth in New Zealand*. Wellington: Ministry of Pacific Island Affairs.

Phinney, J., Lochner, B. T., & Murphy, R. (1990). Ethnic identity development and psychological adjustment in adolescence. In A. R. Stiffman & L. E. Davis (Eds.), *Ethnic issues in adolescent mental health*. London: Sage Publications.

Ritchie, J., & Ritchie, J. (1979). *Growing up in Polynesia*. Sydney: George Allen & Unwin.

Tiatia, J. (1996). *The church: Friend or foe for our Pacific Island youth? A New Zealand born perspective*. Unpublished master's thesis, The University of Auckland.

Tupuola, A. M. (1993). *Critical analysis of adolescent development: A Samoan women's perspective*. Unpublished master's thesis, Victoria University, Wellington.

Tupuola, A. M. (1998). *Adolescence: Myth or reality for Samoan women? Beyond stage-like toward shifting boundaries and identities*. Unpublished doctoral dissertation, Victoria University, Wellington.

Tupuola, A-M. (2004). Pasifika edgewalkers: Complicating the achieved identity status in youth research. *Journal of Intercultural Studies, 25*(1), 87–100.

Vaoiva, R. (1999). *New Zealand born Pacific Island youth: Identity, place and Americanisation*. Unpublished master's thesis, University of Auckland.

Index

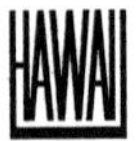

Production Notes for Culbertson / *Penina Uliuli*
Cover designed by Neli Seumanutafa
Interior design and composition by BW&A Books, Inc.
Text and display type in Monotype Dante
Printing and binding by the Maple-Vail Book Manufacturing Group
Printed on 55# Glatfelter Offset B18 cream, 360 ppi